Allan G. Farman (Ed.)

Panoramic Radiology

Allan G. Farman (Ed.)

Panoramic Radiology

Seminars on Maxillofacial Imaging and Interpretation

With 178 Figures, Mostly in Colour

Springer

Allan G. Farman, BDS, PhD (odont), DSc (odont), MBA,
Diplomate of the American Board of Oral and Maxillofacial Radiology,
Diplomate Japanese Board of Oral and Maxillofacial Radiology
Professor of Radiology and Imaging Science, Department of Surgical
and Hospital Dentistry,
Clinical Professor of Diagnostic Radiology,
Adjunct Professor of Anatomical Sciences and Neurobiology,
The University of Louisville,
Louisville, Kentucky 40292,
USA

**This book was prepared in collaboration with Panoramic Corporation,
Fort Wayne, Indiana**

Library of Congress Control Number: 2007921305

ISBN 978-3-540-46229-3 Springer Berlin Heidelberg New York

Springer-Verlag is a part of Springer Science+Business Media
springer.com

Editors: Dr. Ute Heilmann / Annette Hinze, Heidelberg, Germany
Desk Editor: Wilma McHugh, Heidelberg, Germany
Cover design: Frido Steinen-Broo, eStudio Calamar, Spain
Typesetting and Production: LE-TeX Jelonek, Schmidt & Vöckler GbR, Leipzig, Germany

Printed on acid-free paper 21/3100/YL 5 4 3 2 1 0

For my ideal wife, and fellow Oral and Maxillofacial Radiologist,

Taeko Takemori Farman

Preface

During a Chicago Midwinter Dental meeting some years ago, I was asked by representatives from Panoramic Corporation to recommend a good general textbook on panoramic radiography. I was informed there is a great deal of interest within the dental profession in obtaining clinically relevant information on how to achieve the maximum diagnostic yield from the panoramic radiograph.

On my personal library shelf, I had several texts on panoramic radiography published by such eminent sources as Manson-Hing, Langlais, and Chomenko; however, when I looked at the dates of publication inside the front covers of these books, I was disappointed to find that the latest revision was made much more than a decade ago. A thorough search of the World Wide Web, including "Bestwebbuys.com" showed that I was not mistaken in thinking that there was no available text based upon modern panoramic technology. No easy-to-access, up-to-date resource on panoramic radiography existed in the English language.

It is for this reason that I agreed to edit a newsletter on panoramic radiography that would be distributed as a service to the dental profession. My agreement was contingent upon editorial independence, strict avoidance of commercial content, and a focus on the interpretation of panoramic radiographs in general rather than radiographs made using a machine from one particular vendor. Each issue was to contain several pages of content, mostly devoted to one topic in each case. Since its inception in 2000, twenty-two episodes of *Panoramic Imaging News* have been published and, while the Newsletter is to continue, it has been decided to update and expand the subject materials published to date and present these in one convenient volume.

The editor/author-in-chief wishes to thank Panoramic Corporation for its collaboration over the past five years and for permission to reproduce prior topics from *Panoramic Imaging News* in this book format.

Allan G. Farman
Louisville, Kentucky
October 2006

Contents

1 Getting the Most Out of Panoramic Radiographic Interpretation 1
Allan G. Farman

Quality Assurance 1
Image Projection Geometry 1
Interpreting a Normal Panoramic Radiograph 3
Anatomical Comparisons 3
Test 5

2 Ghost Images: Objects Outside the Image Layer that are not Entirely Excluded from the Panoramic Radiograph 7
Allan G. Farman

Anatomic Ghosts 7
Jewelry Ghosts 7
Lead Apron 10
Prostheses 10
Test 14

3 Digital Options for Panoramic Radiology 15
Allan G. Farman
in association with William R. Jacobs

Film Disadvantages 16
Film Advantages 16
Digital X-ray Imaging Disadvantages 16
Digital X-ray Imaging Advantages 16
If I Decide To Go Digital, How Do I Get Into It? What Systems Are Available? 16
  Film Scanners and Cameras 16
  Photostimulable Phosphor Plates 17
  Solid-state Detectors 19
Radiation Dosage 19
Costs 19
Interoperability 22
References 23

4 Panoramic Radiology: Risk Within Reason 25
Allan G. Farman

National Council on Radiation Protection and Measurement: Radiation Protection in Dentistry (NCRP Report No. 145) 25
US Population Radiation Exposure 26
Principles of Radiation Protection 26
Risk within Reason 27
Risk within Reason from Panoramic Radiology 27
Patient Safety 28
Occupational Safety 28
Going Digital 29
Panoramic Dosimetry 29
Summary 31
References 31
Test 32

5 Panoramic Radiology: Role in ADA/FDA Use Guidelines 33
Allan G. Farman

The "New" Dental Patient 34
Patients Having No Signs or Symptoms of Maxillofacial Disease 34
The "Recall" Dental Patient 35
Outcomes Evidence 35
  Screening for Dental Fitness 35
  Screening General Dental Patients 35
  Screening for Periodontal Disease 35
  Screening for Periapical Disease 38
  Orthodontic Screening 38
Some Final Considerations 39
References 39
Test 40

6 Panoramic Radiologic Appraisal of Anomalies of the Dentition 41
Allan G. Farman in association with Christoffel J. Nortjé and Robert E. Wood

Anomalies in Tooth Number 42
  Hypodontia 43
  Hypodontia and Clefts 44
  Hypodontia and Down Syndrome 44
  Hypodontia and Ectodermal Dysplasias 45
  Supernumerary Teeth 46
Anomalies in Tooth Size 49
  Macrodontia 49
  Microdontia 51

Anomalies in Root Formation ... 51
  Dilaceration ... 52
  Taurodontism ... 53
  Enamel Pearl ... 53
  Connation ... 53
  Concrescence ... 53
  Supernumerary Roots ... 56
Anomalies of Tooth Crowns ... 56
  Talon Cusp ... 56
  Dens Invaginatus ... 56
  Dens Evaginatus ... 56
Panoramic Radiology: An Important Adjunct in the Assessment of Dental Morphology ... 56
Tooth Structure Anomalies ... 56
  Enamel Hypoplasia ... 56
  Amelogenesis Imperfecta ... 58
  Dentinogenesis Imperfecta ... 60
  Radicular Dentin Dysplasia ... 62
  Coronal Dentin Dysplasia ... 62
  Odontodysplasia ... 63
Concluding Remarks ... 66
References ... 66
Test ... 69

7 Tooth Eruption and Dental Impaction ... 73
Allan G. Farman

Premature Eruption ... 73
Retarded Eruption ... 73
Dental Impactions ... 74
  Impacted Third Molars ... 74
  Impacted Canines ... 76
  Other Impacted Regular Teeth ... 76
  Impacted Supernumerary Teeth ... 77
  Resorption of Impacted Teeth ... 77
  Pathoses and Impaction ... 77
Ectopic Dental Eruption ... 78
Concluding Remarks ... 78
References ... 80

8 Panoramic Radiographic Assessment in Orthodontics ... 83
Anibal M. Silveira
in association with Allan G. Farman

Pros and Cons ... 83
Root Parallelism ... 83
Quality Control ... 85
American Board of Orthodontics Panoramic Requirement ... 85
Conclusions ... 86
References ... 87
Test ... 89

9 Assessing Growth and Development with Panoramic Radiographs and Cephalometric Attachments ... 91
Allan G. Farman

Eruption Sequence and Timing ... 91
Normal Variations in Eruption Timing ... 95
  Sex ... 95
  Skeletal Pattern ... 96
  Ethnicity ... 96
Local Causes of Delayed Dental Eruption ... 96
Systemic Conditions Delaying Dental Eruption ... 96
  Low Birthweight ... 96
  Second-hand Smoke ... 97
  Syndromes ... 97
  Delayed Puberty ... 97
Factors in Premature Dental Eruption ... 97
Assessment of Biological Age Using Hand-Wrist Radiographs ... 97
Assessment of Biological Age Using Lateral Cephalograms ... 98
Biological Age and Orthodontic Intervention ... 98
Age and Identity ... 98
Concluding Remarks ... 100
References ... 103
Test ... 105

10 Panoramic Radiographic Appearance of the Mandibular Canal in Health and in Disease ... 107
Allan G. Farman
in association with Christoffel J. Nortjé

Pathological Conditions of the Mandible 109
Benign Lesions Within the Mandibular Canal ... 109
Malignant Lesions Within the Mandibular Canal ... 110
Benign Lesions Peripheral to the Mandibular Canal ... 110
Malignant Lesions Peripheral to the Mandibular Canal ... 111
Lesions Obscuring the Mandibular Canal 113
Concluding Remarks ... 114
References ... 115
Test ... 117

11 Pathological Conditions affecting the Maxillary Sinus ... 119
Allan G. Farman
in association with Christoffel J. Nortjé

Overview of alternative imaging modalities ... 119

Maxillary sinus disease frequencies 119
Inflammatory conditions 119
Mucous retention (extravasation) phenomenom 120
Adjacent dental pathoses 120
Benign cysts and neoplasms 121
Other benign radio-opacity 121
Dysplastic conditions affecting the maxillary sinuses 124
Detection of maxillary sinus malignant neoplasia 124
Summary 128
References 128
Test 130

12 Panoramic Radiology: Endodontic Considerations 133
Allan G. Farman
in association with Stephen J. Clark

Periapical Pathoses 133
Providing a Comprehensive Radiographic Overview 136
Follow Up Evaluation 138
Maxillary Sinus Disease Related to Endodontic Therapy 138
Endo-antral syndrome 138
Aspergillosis 139
Conditions that May Simulate Dental Periapical Pathoses 140
Conclusion 141
References 141
Test 142

13 Panoramic Radiology of Pericoronal Pathoses 143
Allan G. Farman in association
with Christoffel J. Nortjé
and Robert E. Wood

Follicular Cysts 143
Envelopmental Keratocystic Odontogenic Tumor 145
Ameloblastoma 146
Adenomatoid Odontogenic Tumor 146
Ameloblastic Fibroma and Fibro-odontoma 147
Odontogenic Myxoma 147
Calcifying Odontogenic Cyst 147
Calcifying Epithelial Odontogenic Tumor 148
Malignancies Associated with Envelopmental Radiolucencies 148
Regional Odontodysplasia 148
Cherubism 148
Cyst Boundaries in Radiologic Differentiation 151
Concluding Remarks 151
References 151
Test 153

14 Panoramic Radiology in Maxillofacial Trauma 155
Allan G. Farman
in association with George M. Kushner

Fractures of Teeth and Alveolar Bone 155
Fractures of the Body and Angle of the Mandible 155
Dental Impactions as Predisposing Factors to Mandibular Fracture 157
Panoramic Radiographs in Third Molar Assessment for Relationship to the Inferior Dental Canal 158
Panoramic Radiographs and Mandibular Fracture Assessment 159
Roles of Computed Tomography and Panoramic Radiology in Mandibular Fracture Detection 160
Pathological Jaw Fracture 163
Foreign Body Detection 163
Fractures of the Maxilla 163
Concluding Remarks 164
References 165
Test 166

15 Panoramic Radiographic Detection of Systemic Disease 167
Arthur H. Friedlander and Keith M. Norman in collaboration with Allan G. Farman, Christoffel J. Nortjé, and Robert E. Wood

Detection of Carotid Artery Disease and also by Inference, Coronary Artery Disease 167
Osteoporosis 171
Evidence Supporting Panoramic Radiographs to Screen for Osteoporosis 171
Evidence Against Using Panoramic Radiographs to Screen for Osteoporosis 173
Osteoporosis and Periodontal Disease 173
Diabetes Mellitus 174
Hyperparathyroidism 174
Specific Infections 176
Tuberculosis 176
Syphilis 176
Metastatic Malignancies 178
Concluding Remarks 179
References 179
Test 182

16 **Panoramic Radiology: Oncologic Dentistry Considerations** ... 183
Allan G. Farman
in association with Zafrulla Khan

What is Oncologic Dentistry? ... 183
Cancer Therapy Effects on Oral Tissues .. 186
Oral Mucositis ... 186
Xerostomia ... 186
Periodontal Disease ... 186
Osteonecrosis ... 186
Childhood Therapy ... 191
Dental Restorations Affecting Radiation Therapy Planning and Application ... 192
Dental Outcomes ... 192
References ... 193
Test ... 194

17 **Cephalometric Attachments Are Not Only of Value for Orthodontic Assessment** ... 195
Allan G. Farman

Lateral Skull Projection ... 195
Posterior-Anterior (PA) Projection ... 195
Occipitomental Projection (Waters' Technique) ... 197
Reverse Towne Projection ... 198
Submentovertex Projection ... 198
Lateral-Oblique Projection of the Jaws ... 200
Test ... 202

18 **Selected Abstracts** ... 205
Allan G. Farman

Dental Caries Assessment ... 205
Periodontal Disease Assessment ... 205
Endodontics ... 206
Selection Criteria ... 206
Safety and Risk ... 207
Digital Imaging ... 208
Dental Implants ... 209
Prosthodontics ... 210
Orthodontics ... 210
Growth and Maturity ... 212
Oncologic Dentistry ... 214
Jaw Fractures ... 214
Dental Impactions ... 215
Dental Anomalies ... 218
Jaw Pathoses ... 220
Systemic Diseases ... 221
Test ... 223

19 **Frequently Asked Questions About Panoramic Radiography** ... 225
Panoramic Radiology Corporation staff led by Steve T. Yaggy in association with Allan G. Farman

Subject Index ... 229

List of Contributors

Stephen J. Clark, DMD
Diplomate, American Board of Endodontics,
Associate Professor, Department of Periodontics,
Endodontics, Dental Hygiene,
Director, Graduate Program in Endodontics,
The University of Louisville,
Louisville Kentucky 40292, USA
E-mail: sjclar01@louisville.edu

Allan G. Farman, BDS, PhD (odont), DSc (odont), MBA
Diplomate of the American Board of Oral and Maxillofacial Radiology,
Diplomate Japanese Board of Oral and Maxillofacial Radiology
Professor of Radiology and Imaging Science,
Department of Surgical and Hospital Dentistry,
Clinical Professor of Diagnostic Radiology,
Adjunct Professor of Anatomical Sciences and Neurobiology,
The University of Louisville,
Louisville Kentucky 40292, USA
E-mail: agfarm01@louisville.edu

Arthur H. Friedlander, DMD
Diplomate, American Board of Oral and Maxillofacial Surgery,
Associate Chief of Staff and Director of Graduate Medical Education, VA
Greater Los Angeles Healthcare System,
Professor of Oral and Maxillofacial Surgery at the UCLA School of Dentistry,
The Center for the Health Sciences,
Los Angeles CA 90095-1668, USA
E-mail: arthur.friedlander@med.va.gov

William R. Jacobs
President, WRJ & Associates, Dental Marketing Consultants, Homer Glen, Illinois
E-mail: bill@thejacobsonline.com

Zafrulla Khan, DDS, MS, FACP
Professor of Prosthodontics,
School of Dentistry
Adjunct Professor, Medical and Radiation Oncology
School of Medicine
Director, Maxillofacial/Oncologic Dentistry
James Graham Brown Cancer Center
University of Louisville,
Louisville Kentucky 40292, USA
E-mail: zafkhan@louisville.edu

George M. Kushner, MD, DMD
Diplomate, American Board of Oral and Maxillofacial Surgery,
Director, Graduate Program in Oral and Maxillofacial Surgery,
The University of Louisville,
Louisville Kentucky 40292, USA
E-mail: gmkush01@gwise.louisville.edu

Keith M. Norman, BA
Research Associate, VA Greater Los Angeles Healthcare System, Los Angeles, CA 90073, USA
E-mail: keithmasao@aol.com

Christoffel J. Nortjé, BChD, PhD (odont), DSc (odont)
Diplomate American Board of Oral and Maxillofacial Radiology,
Professor of Oral and Maxillofacial Radiology,
University of the Western Cape, Belleville 7535,
Republic of South Africa
E-mail: cnortje@uwc.ac.za

Anibal Silveira, DDS
Diplomate American Board of Orthodontics
Associate Professor, Department of Orthodontics and Pediatric Dentistry,
Associate Director, Graduate Orthodontic Program,
The University of Louisville,
Louisville Kentucky 40292, USA
E-mail: amsilv01@gwise.louisville.edu

Robert E. Wood, DDS, Dip Oral Radiol, MSc, PhD, FRCD (C)
Oral and Maxillofacial Radiologist,
Associate Professor, University Health Network/
Princess Margaret Hospital,
Toronto, ON Canada
E-mail: Bob.Wood@uhn.on.ca

Stephen T. Yaggy
President, Panoramic Corporation
Fort Wayne, Indiana, 46818, USA

Getting the Most Out of Panoramic Radiographic Interpretation

1

Allan G. Farman

Learning Objectives

After reading this chapter, the following knowledge should be gained:

- Appreciation of the formation of the panoramic image
- The ability to identify normal hard tissue and soft tissue anatomic structures depicted in the dental panoramic radiograph

Quality Assurance

As with any other radiographic method, optimum interpretable diagnostic images can only be achieved with careful quality assurance in patient positioning, in selecting appropriate exposure parameters and during processing. While panoramic radiography is easy to perform well if all the manufacturer's instructions are followed, it is equally easy to perform badly. Most errors are due to incorrect patient positioning, leading to excessive and sometimes disproportionate distortion. A correctly positioned patient's panoramic radiograph generally shows symmetry of the size of the mandibular rami and condyles, and the dental segments are "in focus" with a gentle downward convexity of the maxillary arch. Provided the patient bites correctly on the bite-block, the anterior structures are portrayed in the midline and the apices of the mandibular incisor teeth should be in full "focus." Provided that the tongue is kept up in the roof of the mouth during exposure, the roots of the maxillary teeth are clearly demonstrated. It is less expensive in time and materials—and in radiation to the patient—to perfect your panoramic technique, than to make unnecessary repeat exposures. And the diagnostic yield from an excellent panoramic radiograph is far superior to one made under less rigorous quality control.

Image Projection Geometry

To gain the maximum amount of diagnostic information from a dental panoramic radiograph (pantomograph), it is necessary to understand that panoramic radiographs are "flattened out" schemes of a curved image layer. Think of the plan view of the head (Fig. 1.1). The panoramic radiograph provides a plan of one side, then the midline, then the other side of the face and jaws. Imagine the panoramic detector (e.g., X-ray film) wrapped around the outside of the face. The actual panoramic film seems large in comparison with a 3M human phantom (Fig. 1.2). This is because the actual image from most panoramic systems is enlarged by about 20%. Figures 1.3 and 1.4 show a printed panoramic image reduced to life size superimposed on the phantom. These graphically explain the association between the panoramic radiograph and the represented structures. In reality the image is formed section by section behind the secondary slit. Figure 1.5 illustrates this process by putting the same printed panoramic image in place of the film cassette. The relative movement of the X-ray source and the "camera" during exposure creates the effect of "wrapping the film about the patient's face" (Fig. 1.6). This analogy to "film" wrapped around the face is equally applicable to the distribution of anatomic

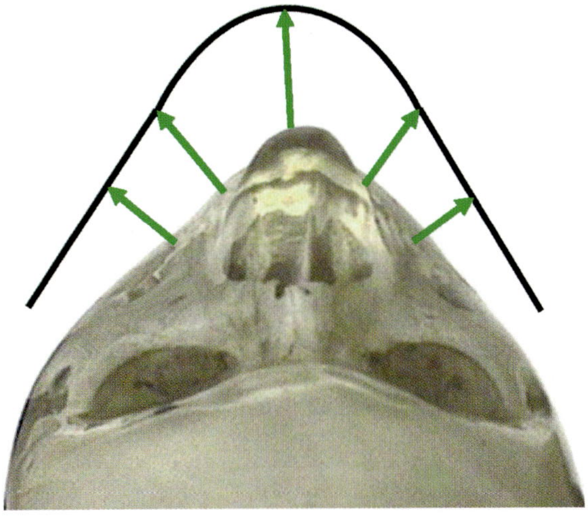

Fig. 1.1 A panoramic radiograph simultaneously presents views from both sides of the patients face as well as providing a frontal perspective

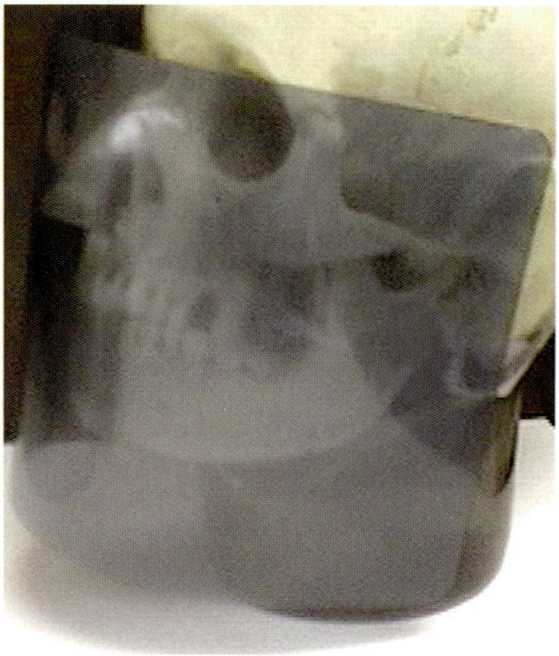

Fig. 1.2 You can best understand the relative position of structures shown in a panoramic radiograph if you imagine the image layer to be bent around the patient's face

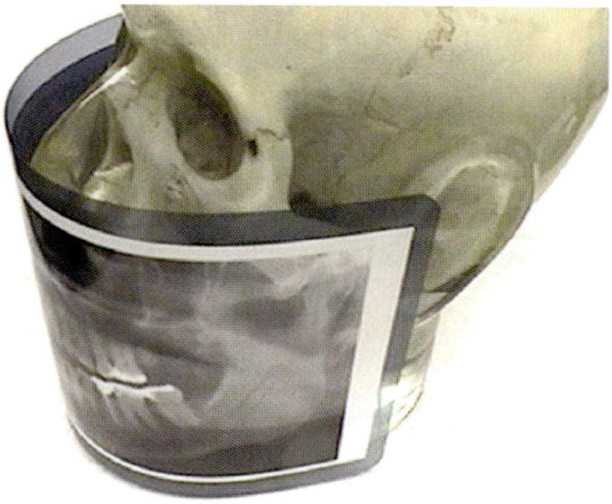

Fig. 1.3 The lateral and more posterior structures are projected to each side of the panoramic radiograph

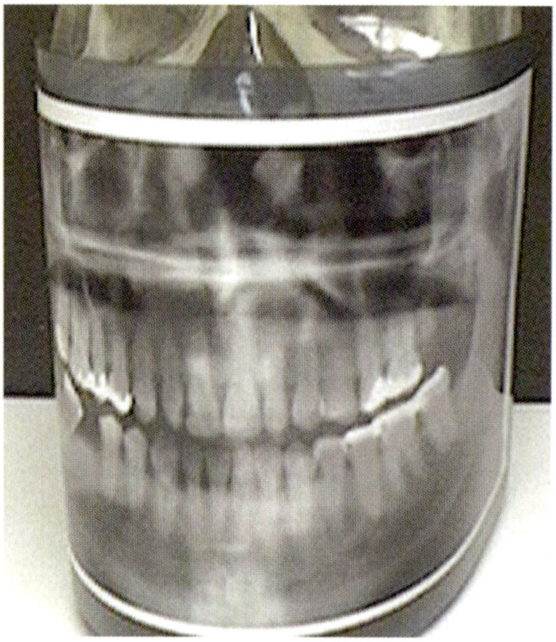

Fig. 1.4 The anterior structures are shown in the midline of the standard panoramic projection

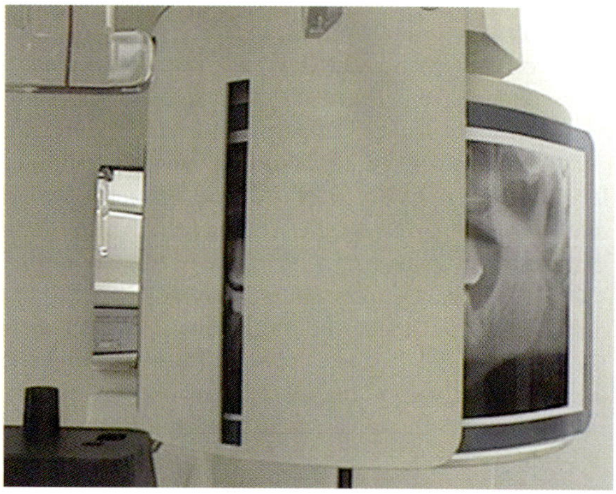

Fig. 1.5 The panoramic image is formed sequentially from information passing through the machine's secondary slit collimator. The film or photostimulable phosphor detector moves past the secondary slit at the appropriate rate necessary to minimize mechanical distortion. For solid-state systems the movement is virtual rather than actual

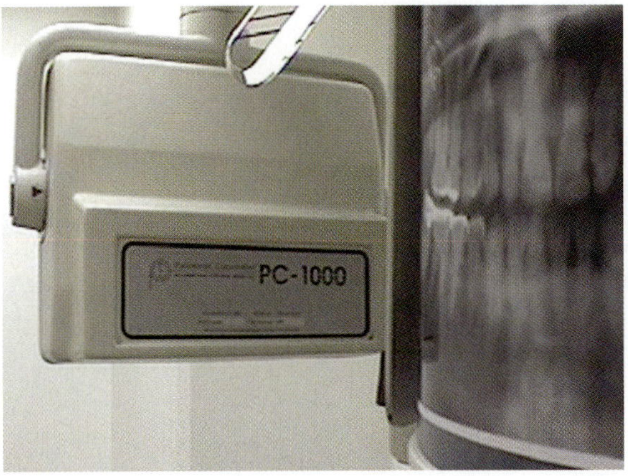

Fig. 1.6 The panoramic latent image is created as the film cassette moves past the secondary slit. The production of the latent image is simulated using the print of a panoramic radiograph

structures displayed in the image created by digital panoramic systems as it is their analog predecessors.

Interpreting a Normal Panoramic Radiograph

A normal panoramic radiograph contains a substantial amount of information. Figure 1.7 is the PC-1000 (Panoramic Corporation, Fort Wayne, Indiana) panoramic radiograph of a 12-year-old male patient. Fifty distinct soft tissues, bony and dental landmarks have been labeled on this radiograph. This is merely a selection from vast amount of information that is actually present. When was the last time that you consciously and thoroughly inspected all of the structures that are demonstrated? As you probably are making the radiograph with the intent of dental diagnosis at the forefront, the dental arches should be left to last in your systematic evaluation of the image. You can sequence your evaluation in many ways; however, it is very important to develop a consistent approach that ensures that all diagnostic information in the radiograph is indeed read. To see all of the subtle variations in contrast, it is imperative that with film imaging: (1) a view box be used (preferably having a variable light intensity), (2) any extraneous light from the view box be blocked out, and (3) the diagnostic evaluation is performed under subdued ambient lighting away from distractions. Similar rules apply for digital panoramic radiography, but of course the computer monitor replaces the view box. It is suggested that you review all panoramic radiographs made in a given day when all patients have left the practice. It will be surprising how much can be gained from such a second look when the atmosphere is likely to be more relaxed!

You can sequence your evaluation in many ways; however, it is very important to develop a consistent approach that ensures that all diagnostic information in the radiograph is indeed read.

Anatomical Comparisons

I approach reading the radiograph roughly in the numerical sequence shown in Fig. 1.7; namely starting with the bony landmarks from the midline of the upper jaw and nasal cavity, then working back in the maxilla and zygomatic complex on each side. The soft tissue shadows of the tongue and soft palate are incorporated at this stage. This is followed by evaluation of the cervical spine and associated structures. I then evaluate the contents of the mandible starting from the midline and then progressing posteriorly on each side. Any examination would be incomplete without a thorough evaluation of the soft tissues anterior to the spine and inferior to the mandible. The last part of the evaluation should be the area of chief complaint and the dental arches. These regions automatically draw your attention whereas the other features within the radiograph can be missed without careful sequencing.

Using the same numerical key as that for the annotated radiograph (Fig. 1.7), Figs. 1.8 and 1.9 shows the normal anatomical structures viewed from the lateral and frontal facial aspects of a 3M phantom. It should be remembered that the radiograph shows all features within the panoramic image layer whether facial or lingual. It should also be remembered that only the structures that are within the selected image layer will be in "focus." This image layer is generally narrower for the anterior regions than for the posterior segments.

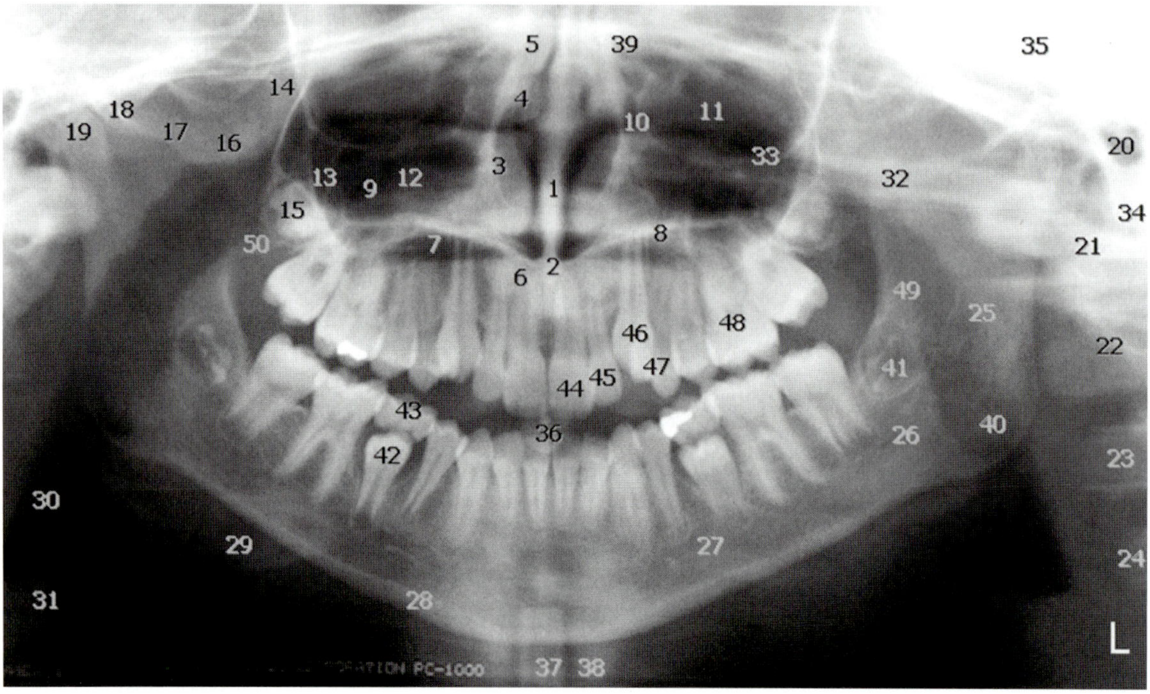

Fig. 1.7 Annotated panoramic radiograph. *1* Nasal septum, *2* anterior nasal spine, *3* inferior turbinate, *4* middle turbinate, *5* superior turbinate, *6* soft tissue shadow of the nose, *7* airspace between soft tissue shadow of upper border of tongue and hard palate, *8* lateral wall of nasal passage, *9* maxillary sinus (antrum), *10* nasolacrimal canal orifice, *11* orbit, *12* infraorbital canal, *13* zygomatic process of the maxilla, *14* pterygomaxillary fissure, *15* maxillary tuberosity with developing third permanent molar tooth, *16* zygoma, *17* zygomatico-temporal structure, *18* articular eminence of temporal bone, *19* mandibular condyle, *20* external auditory meatus, *21* first cervical vertebra (atlas), *22* second cervical vertebra (axis), *23* third cervical vertebra, *24* fourth cervical vertebra, *25* mandibular foramen and lingula, *26* mandibular canal, *27* mental foramen, *28* inferior border of mandible, *29* hyoid, *30* pharyngeal airspace, *31* epiglottis, *32* coronoid process of mandible, *33* inferior orbital rim, *34* mastoid process, *35* middle cranial fossa, *36* bite-block for patient positioning during panoramic radiography, *37* chin holder (cephalostat), *38* shadow of cervical spine, *39* ethmoid sinus, *40* angle of mandible, *41* crypt of developing mandibular third permanent molar tooth, *42* developing mandibular second premolar tooth, *43* primary second molar tooth showing physiological root resorption, *44* maxillary permanent central incisor tooth, *45* maxillary permanent lateral incisor tooth, *46* maxillary permanent canine tooth, *47* maxillary first premolar tooth, *48* maxillary permanent first molar tooth, *49* ramus of mandible, *50* pterygoid plates

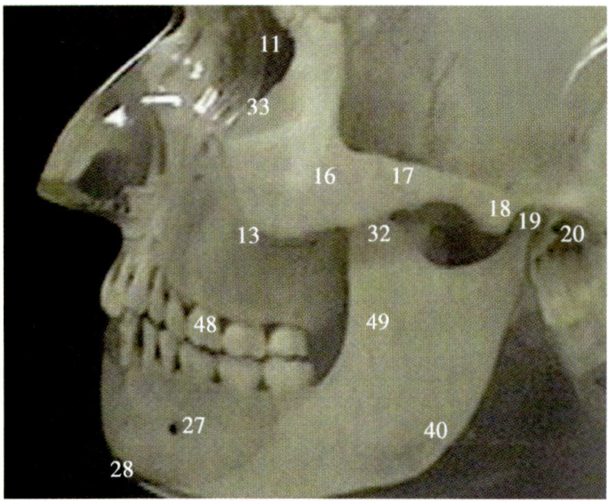

Fig. 1.8 Annotated lateral view of a 3M head phantom. (*Numbers* as in Fig. 1.7)

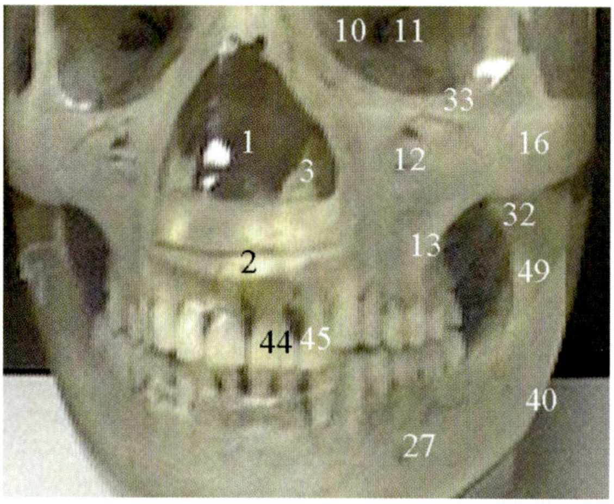

Fig. 1.9 Annotated anterior view of a 3M head phantom. (*Numbers* as in Fig. 1.7)

TEST: Getting the most out of panoramic interpretation

1. In panoramic radiology, the image layer is generally narrower for the anterior regions than for the posterior segments.

   True ☐ **False** ☐

2. Bright ambient lighting is to be preferred when reading panoramic radiographs.

   True ☐ **False** ☐

3. Only the structures that are within the selected image layer will be in "focus."

   True ☐ **False** ☐

4. The sequence for evaluation of a panoramic radiograph should be consistent to ensure that all diagnostic information in the radiograph is read.

   True ☐ **False** ☐

5. The panoramic image is formed sequentially from information passing through the machine's secondary slit.

   True ☐ **False** ☐

6. The lateral and more posterior structures of the maxillofacial region are projected to each side of the panoramic radiograph.

   True ☐ **False** ☐

7. Since panoramic radiographs are primarily to evaluate the teeth and jaws evaluation of the soft tissues anterior to the spine and inferior to the mandible is superfluous.

   True ☐ **False** ☐

Ghost Images: Objects Outside the Image Layer that are not Entirely Excluded from the Panoramic Radiograph

2

Allan G. Farman

Learning Objectives

After reading this chapter, the following knowledge should be gained:

- Appreciation of the causes of "ghost" image artifacts in panoramic images
- Cognizance of the causes of specific projection artifacts
- Ability to reduce the chances of projecting "ghost images" during panoramic radiographic procedures

Panoramic radiographs consist of a series of narrow tomograms sequentially scanned onto the detector (film or storage phosphor in a cassette, or a solid-state digital detector) beneath a secondary slit. Panoramic radiology aims to produce a complete view of both dental arches and their adjacent structures with minimal geometric distortion and with minimal overlap of anatomic details from the contralateral side. To achieve this, the patient's head is maintained stationary in a cephalostat about which the radiation source and X-ray detector rotate. A curved image layer is generally achieved using a continuously changing center of rotation. Objects that are within the selected image layer are clearly visible in the image, while objects outside the image layer are deliberately blurred out of recognition. The degree to which the blurring of extraneous details is successful is dependent upon a number of factors. These factors include: (1) the atomic density of the contents of the object; (2) the bulk of the content of the object; (3) the proximity of the object to the image layer; and (4) the bulk and density of the patient's soft tissues.

Anatomic Ghosts

All panoramic radiographs include ghost images even though these have been minimized following more than 50 years of trial and error by the various manufacturers of panoramic dental radiographic systems. Many ghost images are actually from normal anatomic structures. For example, in the edentulous patient having relatively thin soft tissues, it is not uncommon for the ghost image of the mandibular ramus to be clearly demonstrated in magnified form over the contralateral mandibular body (Fig. 2.1). The presence of such a ghost shadow of normal anatomic structures is not an error in technique, but rather a normal finding when using panoramic radiology on some patients.

While ghost images of some anatomic structures cannot be avoided, most ghost images can be excluded or reduced.

While ghost images of some anatomic structures cannot be avoided, most ghost images can be excluded or reduced. A very common unwanted image is that of the cervical spine reflected over the mandibular incisor teeth (Fig. 2.2). This is best prevented by having the patient stand, or sit, upright with their neck straight and extended, rather than slouched during panoramic exposures. If the patient's neck is slouched, the X-ray beam traverses several cervical vertebrae on the way to exposing the incisor view causing an opaque shadow of the spine to obscure details of the incisor teeth.

Jewelry Ghosts

Jewelry, such as earrings, is usually constructed of materials with high atomic density, and is generally outside the image layer. It can frequently lead to ghost image formation. All patients (male and female) should be asked to remove the jewelry around the head and neck before panoramic radiography is performed. Ghost images of earrings are generally magnified and displayed over the maxillary sinus and body of the mandible on the opposite side of the radiographic image (Fig. 2.3). Their actual appearance will be dictated by their orientation (Fig. 2.4).

Particular care needs to be taken if the earring is unilateral and solid as the ghost image might be mistaken for an odontoma or other radio-opaque disease entity. Bullets and shrapnel in the soft tissues may also cause ghost images to appear magnified and contralaterally in the panoramic radiographic image (Fig. 2.5).

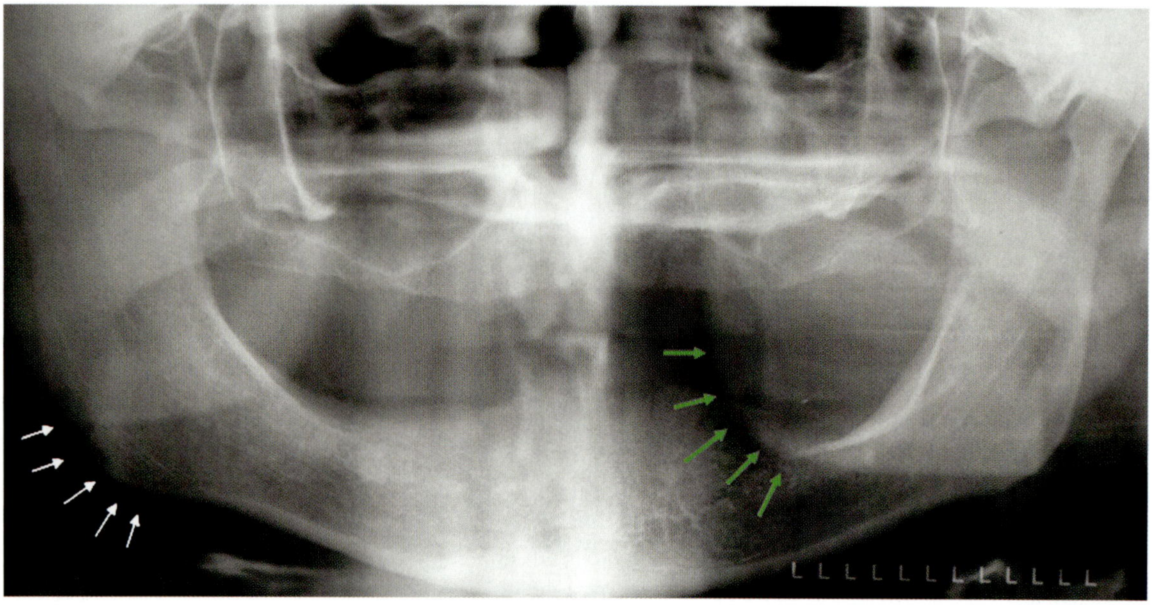

Fig. 2.1 Panoramic radiograph of an edentulous patient. The true image of the right mandibular angle is outlined by *white arrows*. The ghost image of the same structure is outlined using *green arrows*

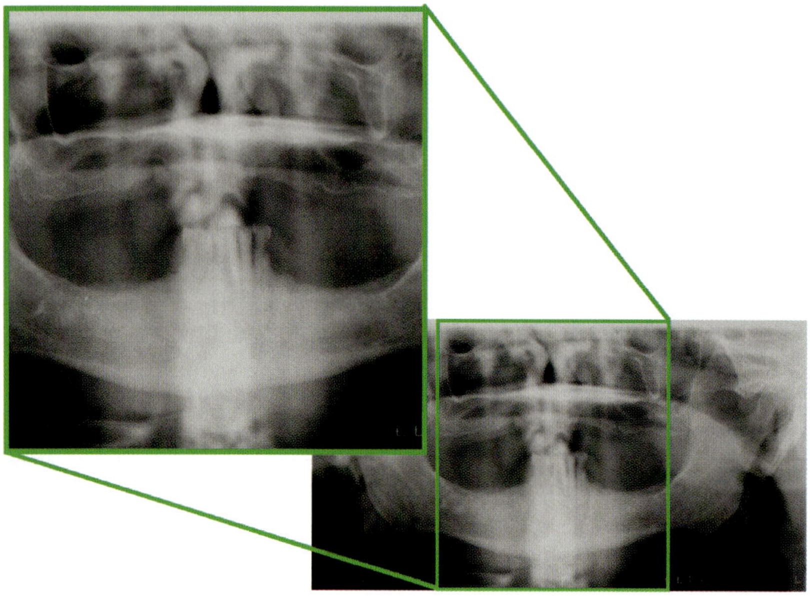

Fig. 2.2 Detail of panoramic radiograph showing how the shadow of the spine can obscure detail of the mandibular anterior teeth if the patient's neck is not kept erect during panoramic radiography

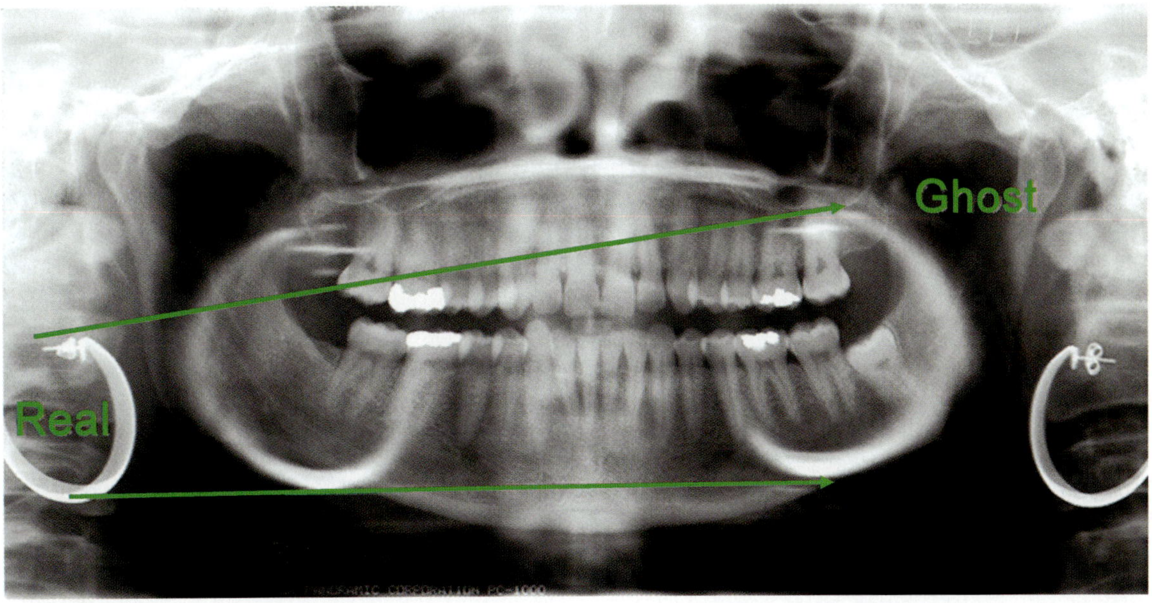

Fig. 2.3 Bilateral earrings casting ghost images

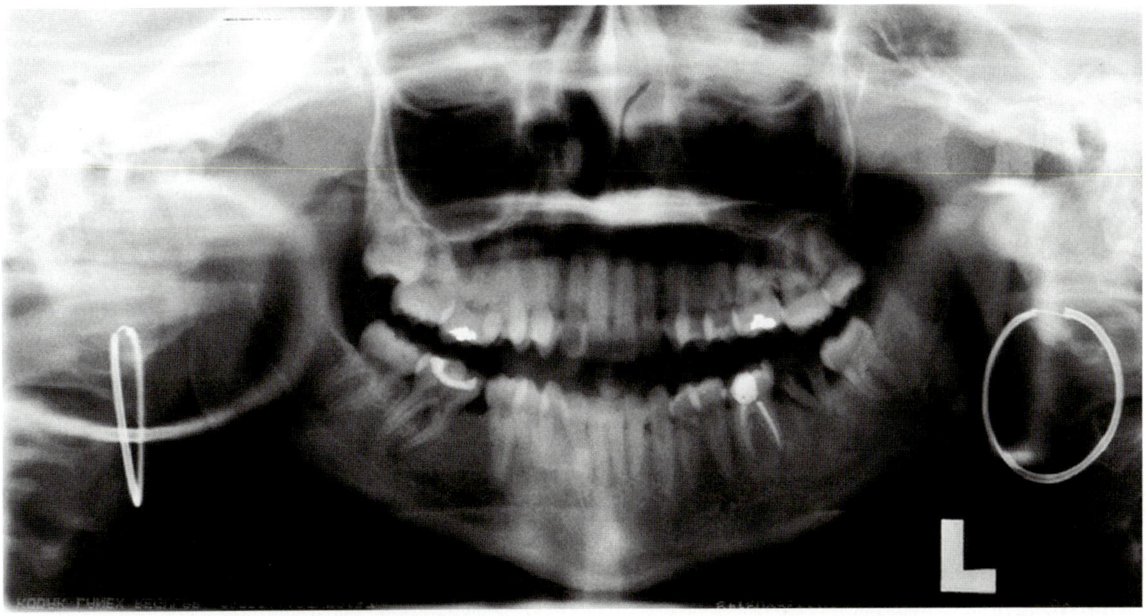

Fig. 2.4 Appearance of the earrings is dependent upon their relative position with respect to the incoming X-ray beam. In this case, the right earrings are rotated so both the real and ghost images differ in appearance from the earring on the other side

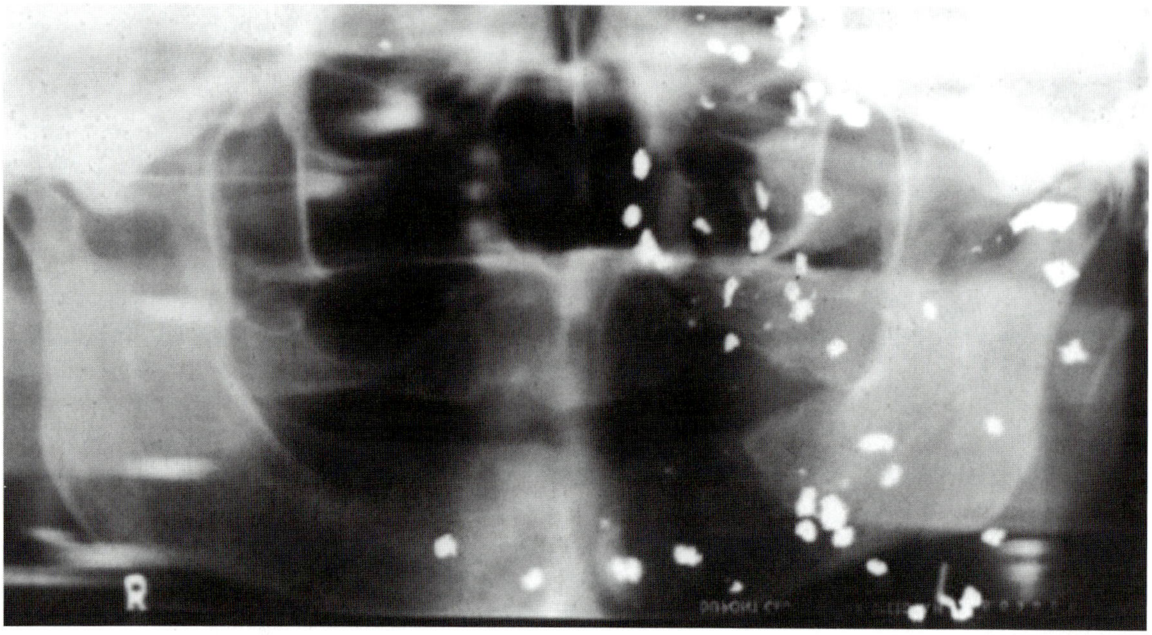

Fig. 2.5 Sharp opaque images on the left side of the image are buckshot. The indistinct opaque images on the right side are ghost images

Tongue rings are centrally positioned and can cast a radio-opaque shadow upward over the nasal passageway (Fig. 2.6). The actual shadow depends on where the tongue is positioned during the making of the panoramic image.

Lead Apron

As the X-ray beam is well collimated for panoramic dental radiography, a lead apron is now not required for patient safety in many parts of the world; however, regulatory requirements do remain in some places. The use of a leaded garment is to protect the patient against radiation; hence, if worn it should face the incoming beam. In panoramic radiography the beam comes from the rear of the patient. The apron should be draped around the patients back rather than over their chest. In any event, it is necessary to make sure that the lead apron is placed smoothly over the patient's shoulders. A lead apron rising up at the patient's shoulder will produce an artifact in the same manner as occurs with earrings; namely, contralaterally (Fig. 2.7) over the body of the mandible, possibly extending over the maxillary sinus.

Prostheses

Dental prostheses are generally within the image layer, and cast primary rather than ghost images. When the denture base is entirely radiolucent, the denture can be left in place to aid patient positioning during panoramic radiography, without loss of needed image details (Fig. 2.8). However, if the denture base is radio-opaque (e.g., chrome-cobalt or stainless steel) the denture should always be removed prior to panoramic radiographs being made (Fig. 2.9). Finally, eyeglasses should also be removed before panoramic radiology as these can also obscure important image details (Fig. 2.10).

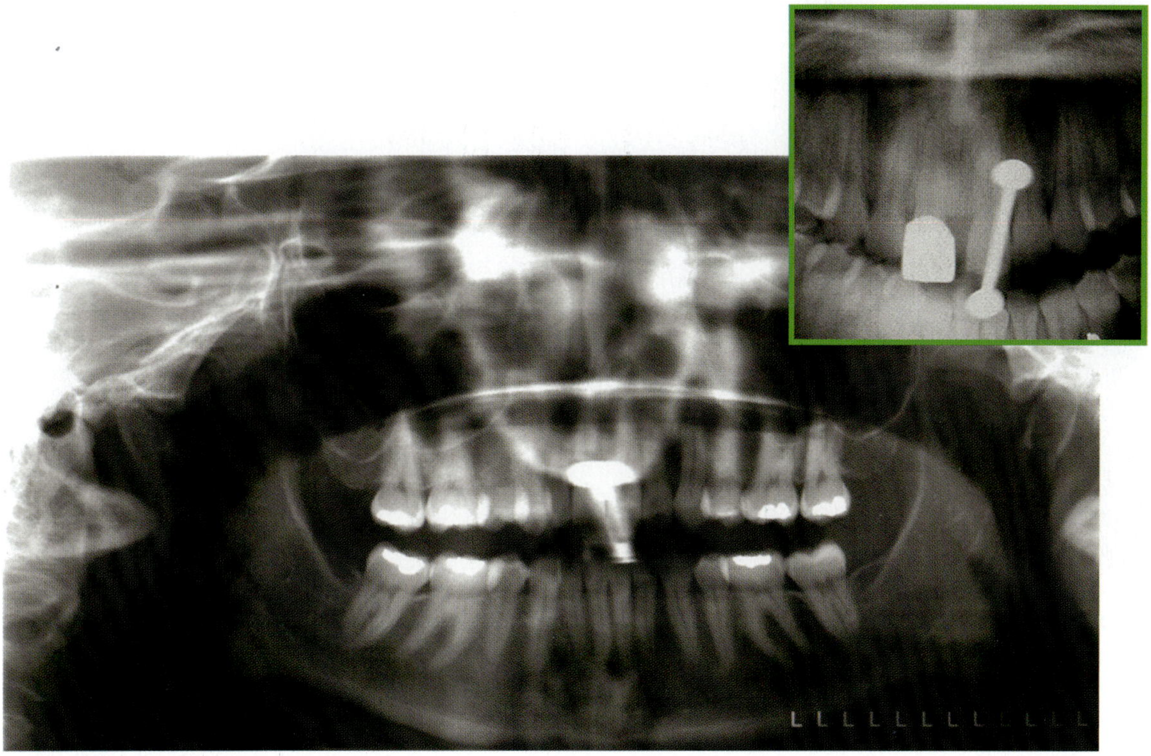

Fig. 2.6 Tongue rings have become evermore frequent. The patient is often reluctant to remove this device. It can cast a radio-opaque shadow upward superimposed in the midline over the nasal passageway. The insert (upper right) shows that holding the tongue ring close to the teeth eliminates the scatter effect

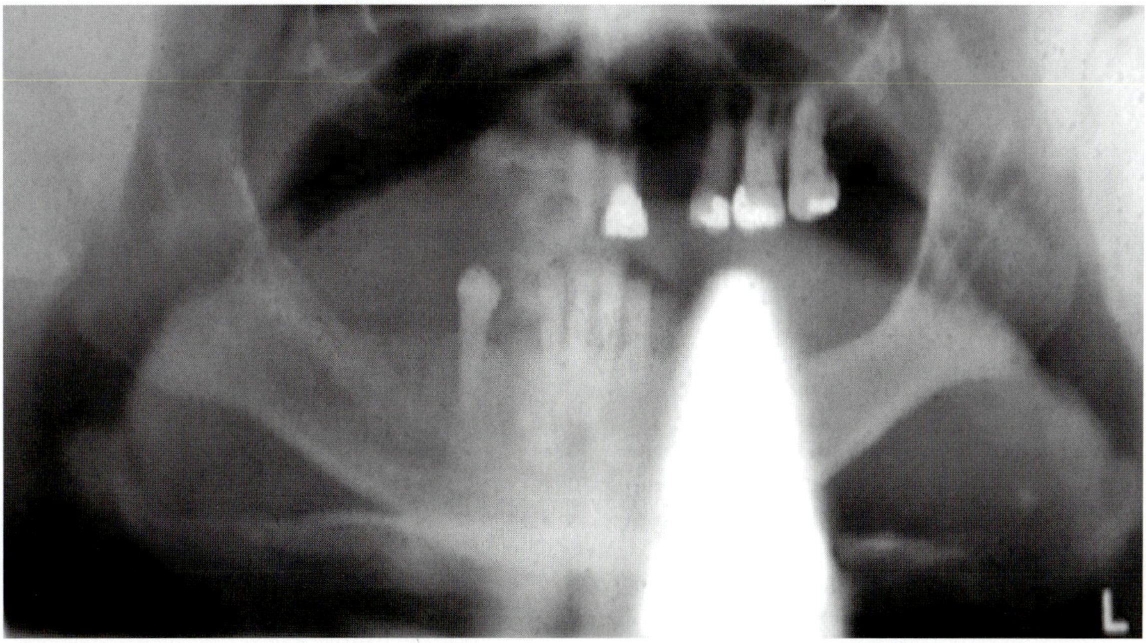

Fig. 2.7 A lead apron raised up on the right shoulder has cast a radio-opaque image on the left side of the image in the premolar region

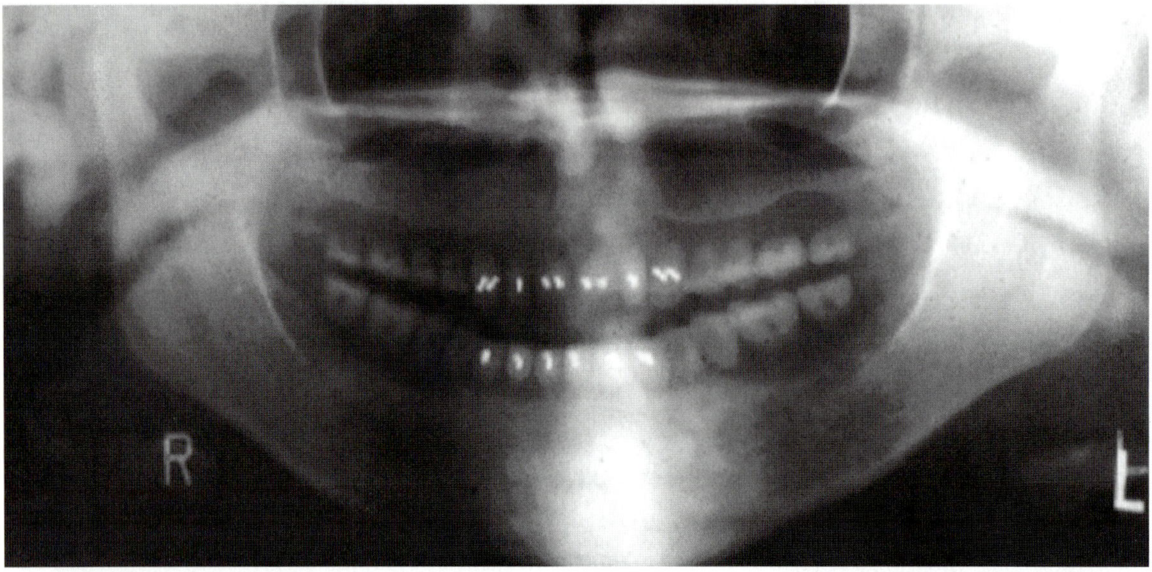

Fig. 2.8 Sometimes it is not a bad idea to leave dentures with entirely radiolucent bases in place to facilitate patient positioning for panoramic radiography. In such cases the artificial teeth are usually radio-opaque but rarely hide important details so long as the patient is properly positioned

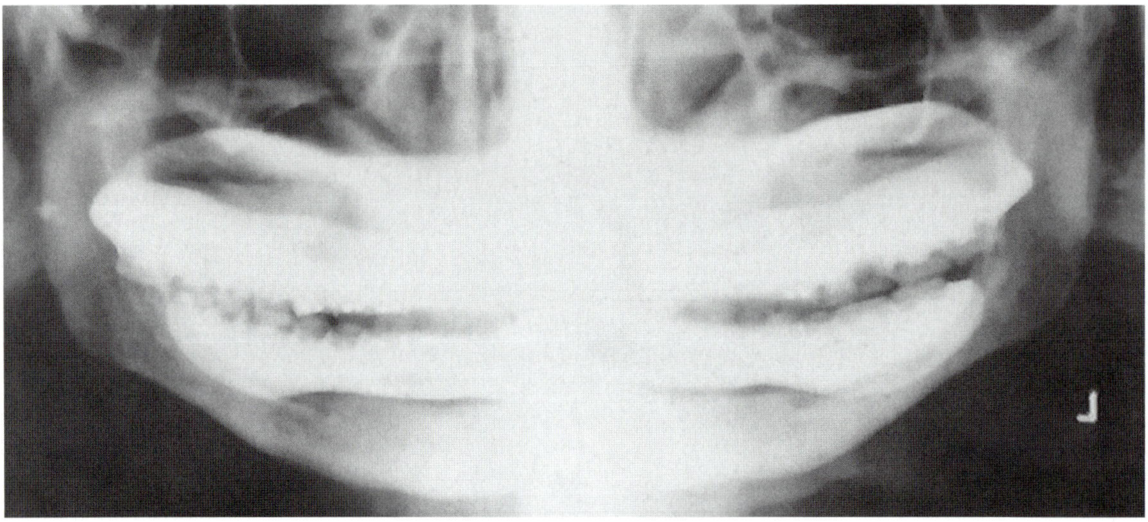

Fig. 2.9 Where denture bases are radio-opaque the denture should always be removed prior to panoramic radiology being performed. Otherwise the primary image of the denture base will exclude necessary details from the interpretation

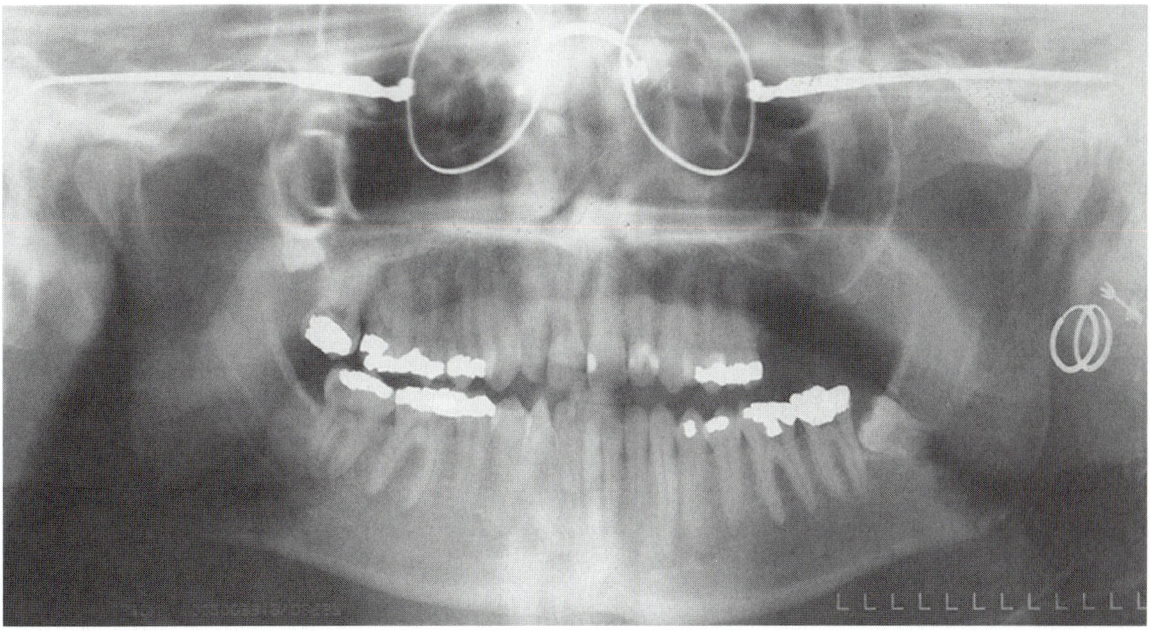

Fig. 2.10 This patient has not removed the eyeglasses and also has a unilateral earring on the left side. The primary image of the eyeglasses, while not desired, probably does not obscure relevant information. The left earring has cast a ghost image over the maxillary right tuberosity region and obscures important information concerning an unerupted third molar tooth

TEST: Ghost images

1. In panoramic radiology, the patient's head is maintained stationary in a cephalostat about which the radiation source and X-ray detector rotate.

   True ☐ **False** ☐

2. Dental prostheses must always be removed from the patient's mouth prior to panoramic radiographs being made.

   True ☐ **False** ☐

3. Lead apron artifacts are invariably caused by the apron being placed too high behind the patient's neck.

   True ☐ **False** ☐

4. Ghost images of earrings are generally magnified and displayed over the maxillary sinus and body of the mandible on the opposite side of the radiographic image.

   True ☐ **False** ☐

5. Ghost images of some anatomic structures cannot be avoided entirely during panoramic radiology.

   True ☐ **False** ☐

Digital Options for Panoramic Radiology

Allan G. Farman
in association with William R. Jacobs

3

Learning Objectives

- Gain understanding of digital system options available for panoramic radiography
- Learn the basic concept behind each approach along with the advantages and disadvantages of each option
- Review points to consider in analyzing options for your practice

Digital X-ray imaging is making substantial inroads into the dental practice. The purpose of this chapter is to provide a succinct overview of the various digital options for panoramic dental radiography.

The move to panoramic digital radiography in dentistry has been slower than the move toward intraoral digital radiography but is now accelerating. Every dental practice is different and has unique needs and wants. Before making a decision on digital panoramic radiography, you must weigh carefully your unique operation, the type of practice and patient mix, your staffing, your goals and objectives, the systems available, the overall economics and costs involved, the timing, the state of the technology, and anticipated changes in technology. If you already have a digital intraoral system the move might make sense. If you do not, then maybe going to digital intraoral first is best. Perhaps it is something you want to delay to see how things develop and what new technologies are introduced in the next year or so. Perhaps you wish to take small steps, first incorporating secondary capture using a scanner to help you determine the best long-term approach for your practice. The decision is not an easy one and takes much thought and investigation. This chapter will address the basics of digital radiography and show the alternative approaches available today.

Digital radiography encompasses all the techniques that produce digital (or computerized) images, as opposed to conventional radiography, which uses analog X-ray film. The first commercial dental intraoral detector was approved by the FDA/CDRH in late 1990 and became available in the US market in 1991. Since that year, a number of different systems have become available, and picking the right system for the job is not an easy task. Systems are different in nature, and comparison is made difficult because physical specifications do not easily translate into day-to-day dental operations.

An image is said to be digital when it is composed of separate (distinct) elements [1, 2]. Each element is called a "picture element" or pixel. If an image is displayed on the computer monitor, and the pixel is smaller than the smallest detail the viewer's eye can see, it is hard to determine that the image is indeed a digital one. If this is not the case, that is the individual pixels can be spotted, the eye views the image as a mosaic of pixels.

Each pixel can only take on a limited number of gray shades. The number of possible gray shades depends on the number of bits (binary digits) that are used to store a pixel. A 1-bit pixel can only take two values (0 or 1—that is black or white). An 8-bit pixel can take any one of 256 (2^8) values. A 16-bit pixel can take more than sixty-five thousand grayscale values (2^{16}). It is generally accepted that the human eye can only distinguish about 20 magnitudes of light intensity, and is probably unable to discern all 256 gray levels that a standard computer monitor can display. The total number of bits that are used to store an image is the number of pixels times the number of bits per pixel.

There are three methods available to produce digital images. First, it is possible to digitize conventional analog film radiographs through secondary capture using transparency scanners or specialized digital cameras.

Film scanners and digital cameras can be used to produce a digital image from an analog film radiograph.

Alternatively, digital images can be produced using storage phosphor plates or with solid-state systems, usually involving use of a charge-coupled device (CCD) or complementary metal oxide semiconductor (CMOS) comparable to the computer chip found in a digital photographic camera.

Properties essential for digital panoramic radiography include:

- Images of diagnostic quality

- Radiation dose similar or reduced compared to film radiography
- Compatibility with existing panoramic X-ray generators
- Lossless archiving (storage of the full original radiographic image)
- Interoperability of image format so that the patient's information can be conveniently shared when professionally necessary

Film Disadvantages

The following are some of the key disadvantages to using analog film radiography:

- Cost of consumables such as film and processing solutions
- Cost of processing equipment and darkroom space
- Time consumption in film processing and processor maintenance
- Processed film images are rarely optimal
- Used processing chemicals are toxic to the environment
- Film radiograph storage and retrieval can be problematic
- Duplicates made from film radiographs are invariably inferior to the original radiograph

Film Advantages

The following are some of the key advantages to using film radiography:

- Low initial cost, especially for manual processing
- Often already in place
- No changes or additional training required
- Known entity—proven output
- Relatively low cost of operation
- Excellent diagnostic clarity possible if exposed and processed optimally
- Widely accepted

Digital X-ray Imaging Disadvantages

The following are some of the key disadvantages of digital radiography:

- Added initial cost for equipment given you are presently using film imaging
- Need for additional computers, monitors, networking and backup storage
- Detectors (both solid-state and phosphor systems) can add $15,000 to $25,000 to the cost of the panoramic system
- Changes in operations, systems and procedures require an investment in time and involve a learning curve
- Not all digital image formats are identical at this moment so interoperability can be problematic both in the same office and when making outside referrals
- Eventual hardware obsolescence

Digital X-ray Imaging Advantages

The following are some of the key advantages of digital radiography:

- Digital X-ray imaging saves time as there is no chemical processing
- Digital images are more consistent in quality for the same reason
- Digital images ease communication with patients
- Digital images are readily stored and retrieved
- Digital radiology opens the way to electronic interchange
- Consultation can be expedited
- Digital images allow perfect "clone" duplication and backup
- Post-processing can help optimize the diagnostic yield
- Digital radiology eliminates environmental silver contamination from spent fixer

If I Decide To Go Digital, How Do I Get Into It? What Systems Are Available?

There are two ways to get into digital panoramic radiography:

1. Buy a totally new integrated digital system; or
2. Use your current panoramic system [3–5].

If you wish to use your current panoramic system, there are three alternatives to look at:

1. Secondary capture of analog film images using scanners—undoubtedly the most economical method;
2. Photostimulable phosphor plates; and
3. Retrofit ("add on") solid-state digital detector systems [6].

Film Scanners and Cameras

Film scanners and digital cameras can be used to produce a digital image from an analog film radiograph. In general, secondary capture is best achieved with a good quality scanner having a radiograph adaptor (i.e., scanning light in the lid to pass light through the radiograph (Fig. 3.1). Nikon and Epson produce excellent scanners for this purpose with the costs varying from around $600 to $1,500 for a sufficiently high quality system. A sharp black and white photograph setting is preferred. Scanners are preferred to digital cameras as they practically eliminate optical distortion and the reflection

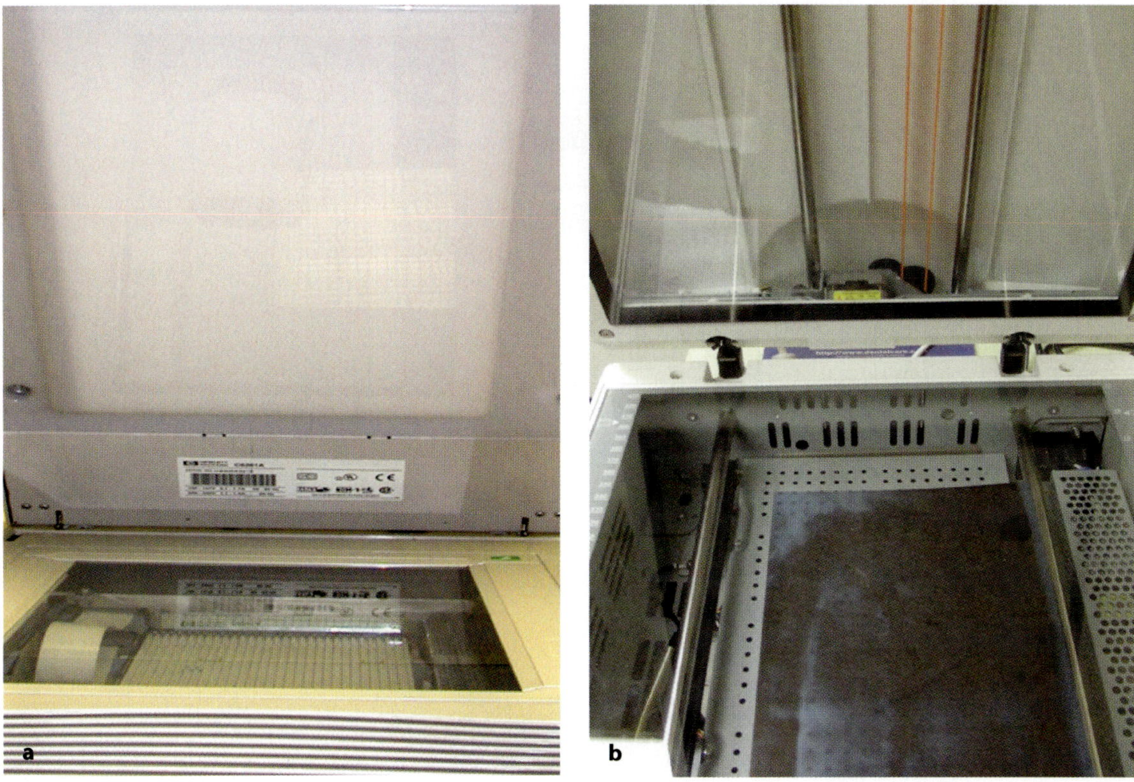

Fig. 3.1 **a** Nikon CoolPix scanner with transparency adaptor in lid sufficient for extraoral radiograph duplication. **b** Panoramic radiograph placed for digitization in an alternative flat bed scanner, the Epson FinePix Z2 with transparency adaptor

from the surface of the radiograph that would otherwise reduce image quality. Film scanners do not change the need to continue making radiographs with X-ray film. They introduce additional time-consuming activity to scan the images, but that is the price you pay to continue to use analog film radiographs while digitally storing images. No matter how good your film scanner is, scanned images can only be as good as the original film radiographs. The advantage here is that you can scan and archive your existing film files over time and you can also determine if digital panoramic imaging is for you without spending a lot of money in purchasing sophisticated equipment While Schultz et al. (2002) found the sensitivity for detection of low contrast simulated bone lesions was greater with film than after digitization, the absolute differences were small [7].

Photostimulable Phosphor Plates

A phosphor plate reader works very much like a film scanner, except that an imaging plate is used instead of analog X-ray film (Figs. 3.2, 3.3). Such reusable plates can have the same sizes as dental panoramic X-ray films. They contain a phosphor layer that "remembers" the image; hence, the name "storage phosphor." To read the image, phosphor plates need to be illuminated by a solid-state laser beam. When a portion of the plate is illuminated, it emits light that is photomultiplied and collected by a digital imaging chip.

Photostimulable phosphor systems dedicated to dentistry are available from a number of manufacturers. Each system is comprised of the phosphor plates and a laser scanner that interfaces with a computer. The plates can be quite expensive, costing $500 to $1,000 each for extraoral purposes. While extraoral plates are not as sensitive to scratching as are the intraoral plates, care must still be taken not to scratch or contaminate them. The plates are very sensitive to ambient light, which can erase much of the latent image. Furthermore, they need extensive exposure to light in order to completely erase the image before reuse. On the other hand, storage phosphor systems are versatile in that they can be used with a wide range of different X-ray systems.

Storage phosphor systems (photostimulable phosphors) specific to dentistry are available from a number of different manufacturers.

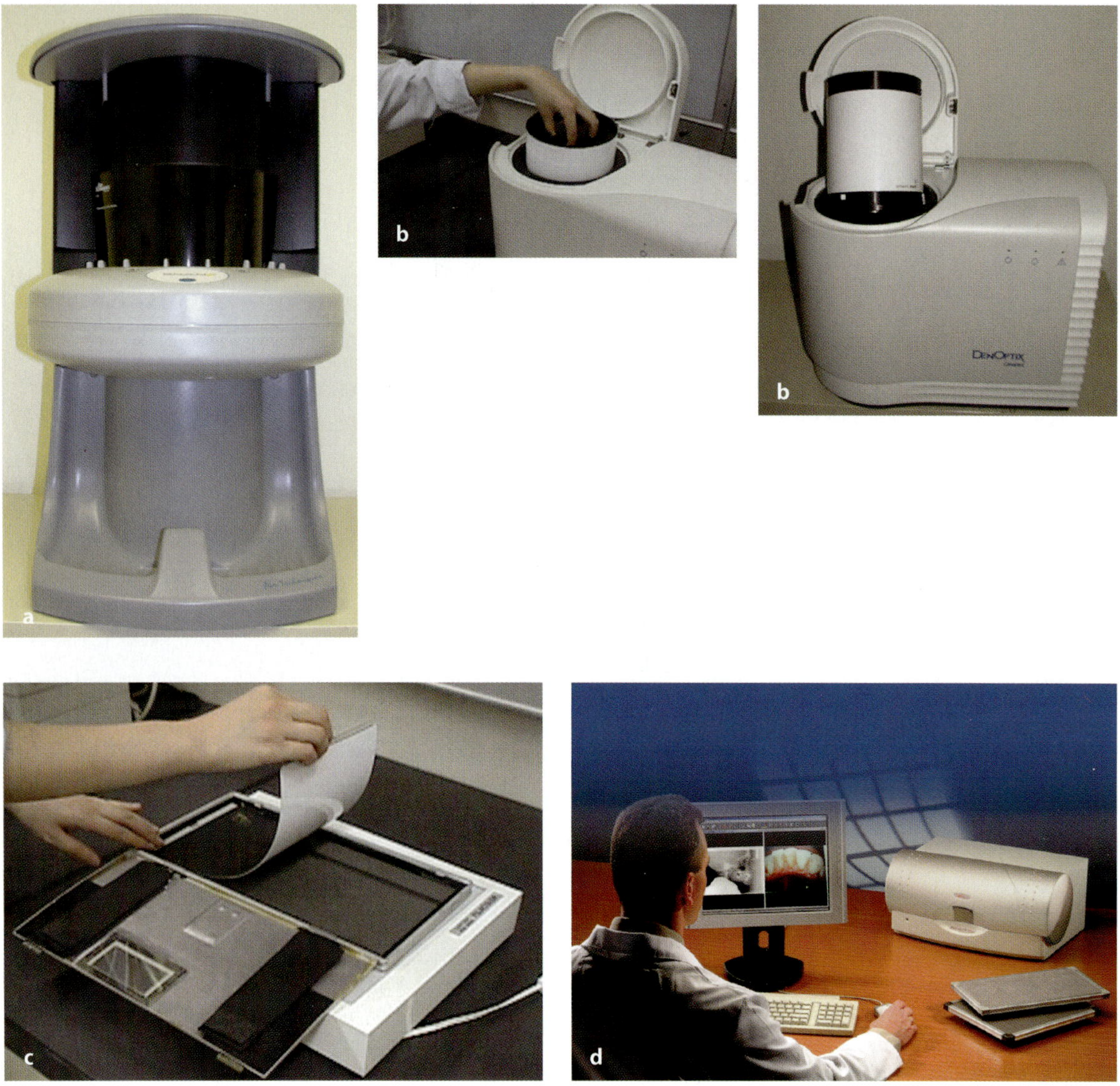

Fig. 3.2 **a** Air Techniques (NY) ScanX photostimulable phosphor plate laser scanner. **b** DenOptix (Danaher/Gendex, Des Plaines, IL) laser scanner with a photostimulable phosphor plate attached to drum ready for processing together during the scan. **c** Loading a photostimulable phosphor plate into a soft cassette. **d** Kodak/Orex Paxorama works with existing X-ray generator and photostimulable phosphor plate

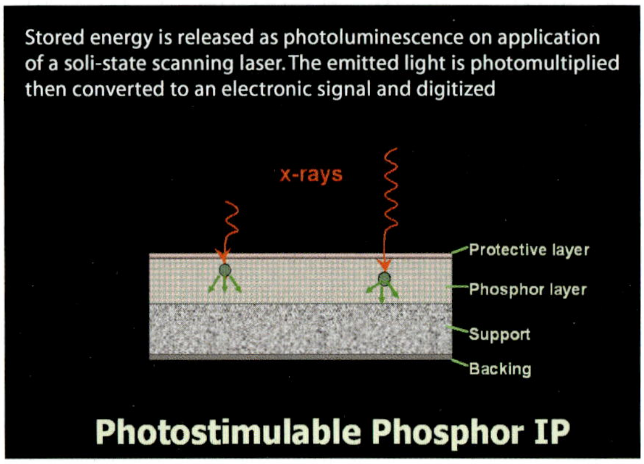

Fig. 3.3 Imaging using storage phosphor plate

Solid-state Detectors

Solid-state digital X-ray detectors are based on a silicon chip that permits the acquisition of an image. Such a chip consists of a myriad of pixels; each pixel captures a small quantity of energy (usually light from a scintillator) and converts this radiant energy into electricity. For panoramic radiography, this generally involves a charge-coupled device (CCD) or complementary metal oxide semiconductor (CMOS) of sufficient dimensions to cover the secondary slit of the panoramic machine (i.e., tall and narrow). The solid-state chip (CCD or CMOS) converts radiant light photons into electrons when a scintillator is used. The ability of detectors to capture radiant energy is no longer limited to visible photon as cadmium telluride can produce electrons directly on impact of X-ray photons. Most systems, however, still use a scintillator layer, similar to the Scintillators that are used as intensifying screens in analog film panoramic radiography (Fig. 3.4). An example of one of the earliest commercialized digital panoramic systems was that of the Trophy Digipan adaptor for the Instrumentarium OP 100 (Fig. 3.5a). Trophy is now part of the Kodak Dental Imaging Division. Instrumentarium and Kodak now manufacture competing dedicated digital panoramic systems, the Kodak RVG 8000 and the Instrumentarium OP 200D.

As with analog film, the panoramic image is pieced together during the scan. Unlike analog film radiography, the receptor is stationary and the image for each segment is read-out in appropriate sequence. Solid-state systems are available both to retrofit an existing panoramic system and as integrated units dedicated to a specific panoramic X-ray generator (Fig. 3.6). A potential concern with retrofitting a unit is that if something does go wrong you may find yourself working with the manufacturer of the panoramic system, the manufacturer of the retrofit system, and the installer.

There are several excellent dedicated digital panoramic systems on the market, however, the costs of such systems range from around $30,000 to $70,000 depending on the degree of sophistication desired.

Radiation Dosage

Unlike intraoral radiology, the switch to digital panoramic imaging does not generally result in a substantial dose reduction to the patient. In fact it is sometimes necessary to actually increase dosage to optimize image quality when using digital systems [6].

With intraoral X-ray film radiography, the emulsion is directly sensitive to X-rays, so adding a scintillating screen can improve the efficiency with which X-rays are detected. However, for extraoral radiography, an intensifying screen is generally employed—and this is not so very different from the scintillating layer used with solid-state detectors. Gijbels et al. (2001) found no difference in exposure settings or organ doses between analog X-ray film and digital panoramic radiography using photostimulable phosphor plates [9].

Costs

Determining the true cost of system ownership is not an easy matter. Certainly the basic expenditure on the system is easily measured. However, one also needs to factor in possible savings in terms of consumables such as film and processing solutions, the possible value of time-savings, or of the increased time used. Even more difficult to determine is the diagnostic gain or loss.

A good quality scanner will cost between $600 and $1,500 and can be used for general scanning purposes beyond radiographs. The system can be attached to the practice management computer, and many practice management software packages include modules for the capturing and can be used for general scanning purposes beyond radiographs. The system can be attached to the practice management computer, and many practice management software packages include modules

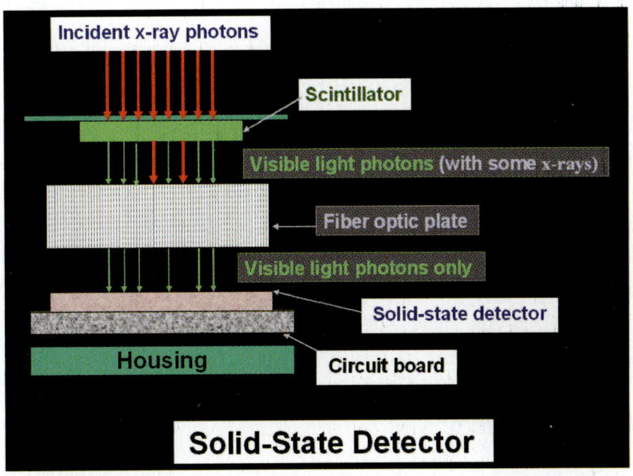

Fig. 3.4 Schematic representation of a solid-state detector. Unlike analog X-ray film radiography, the receptor is stationary and the image for each segment is read-out in appropriate sequence

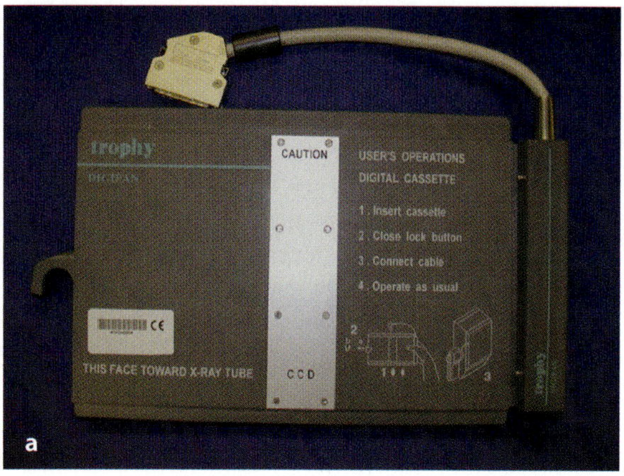

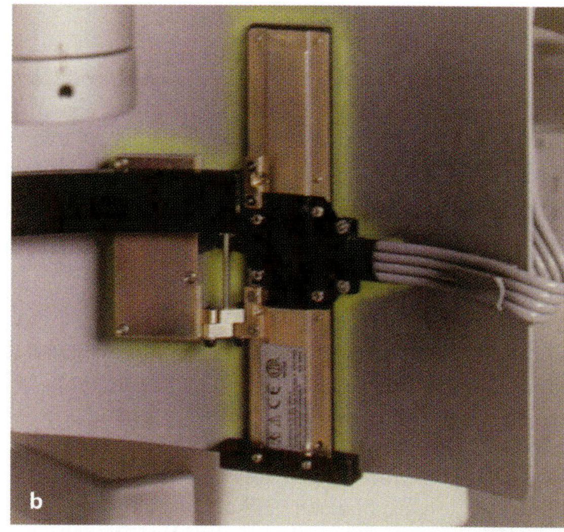

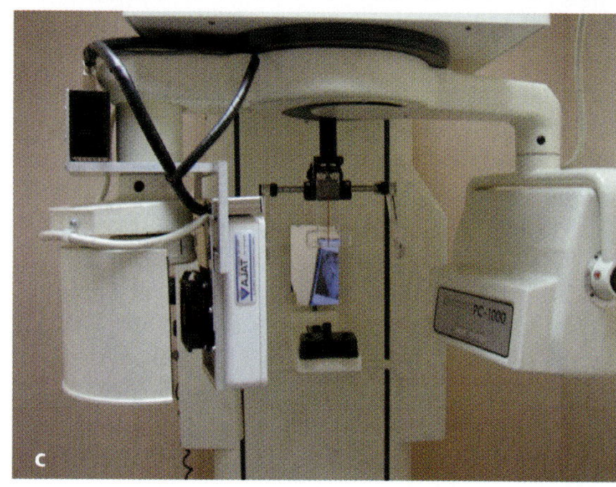

Fig. 3.5 **a** One of the earliest commercialized digital panoramics was the Trophy Digipan used with the Instrumentarium OP 100 panoramic system in place of the film cassette. A variety of "add-on" systems from several different vendor sources are now available for most panoramic systems. **b** Schick CDRPan (Long Island City, NY) digital retrofits are available for a number of panoramic systems including the Panoramic Corporation PC-1000. **c** Video Dental Concept's AJAT retrofit digital attachment to a Panoramic Corporation PC 1000. This system collects 500 Mbyte of information and the software automatically makes adjustments to the focal trough to customize to the individual patient before saving a file size approximately one hundredth the size of the original raw data following operator approval. It is also possible to make separate optimal images for the maxilla and mandible if there is a skeletal discrepancy. If one is not worried about storage space, the whole of the raw data can be saved. The unit displayed is the basic system prior to esthetic plastic covers

for the capturing and storage of secondary images. This is certainly an inexpensive way to become familiar with digital images—and it also replaces the need to use duplicating film and a duplicator to create duplicates. Such a system could be worthwhile in any dental office regardless of whether or not other digital methods are also to be incorporated. Furthermore, a scanner allows you to incorporate prior radiographic images into the electronic patient record. Problems with relying on scanning are: (1) this does not remove the darkroom issues that often lead to suboptimal analog radiographs and (2) scanning is an added task for your assistants to perform; time for which you are not being additionally reimbursed.

Storage phosphor systems (photostimulable phosphors) specific to dentistry are available from a number of different manufacturers. In most cases the cost of the basic package is roughly $15,000 to $20,000—but that price can escalate if you purchase multiple extraoral phosphor plates at as much as $1,000 each. In most instances, the plate cassette has been loaded and unloaded manually. Without using caution, this can lead to wear of the expensive plates—and also can lead to suboptimal images through the effects of ambient lighting on exposed plates being loaded into the scanner. Further, processing of extraoral plates in medium to high resolution can be quite time consuming—no big time savings, if any, over film processing. The advantage of such a system is that the images are stored digitally in computer memory and can be easily duplicated for safe archiving/storage and retrieval. Moreover, a single storage phosphor processor can be used with multiple X-ray generators.

Retrofit solid-state digital panoramic imagers have the advantage of providing a virtually instant image on the screen—so if you are in a high volume practice or have other reasons for needing immediate images, these are an excellent alternative (Figs. 3.5, 3.6). They can provide most, if not all, of the digital capabilities of the integrated digital units without the cost of buying a new machine. Retrofit systems generally cost around $20,000. If you have a relatively inexpensive panoramic system and do not utilize it to a substantial degree, then this added cost might not be warranted given your business situation.

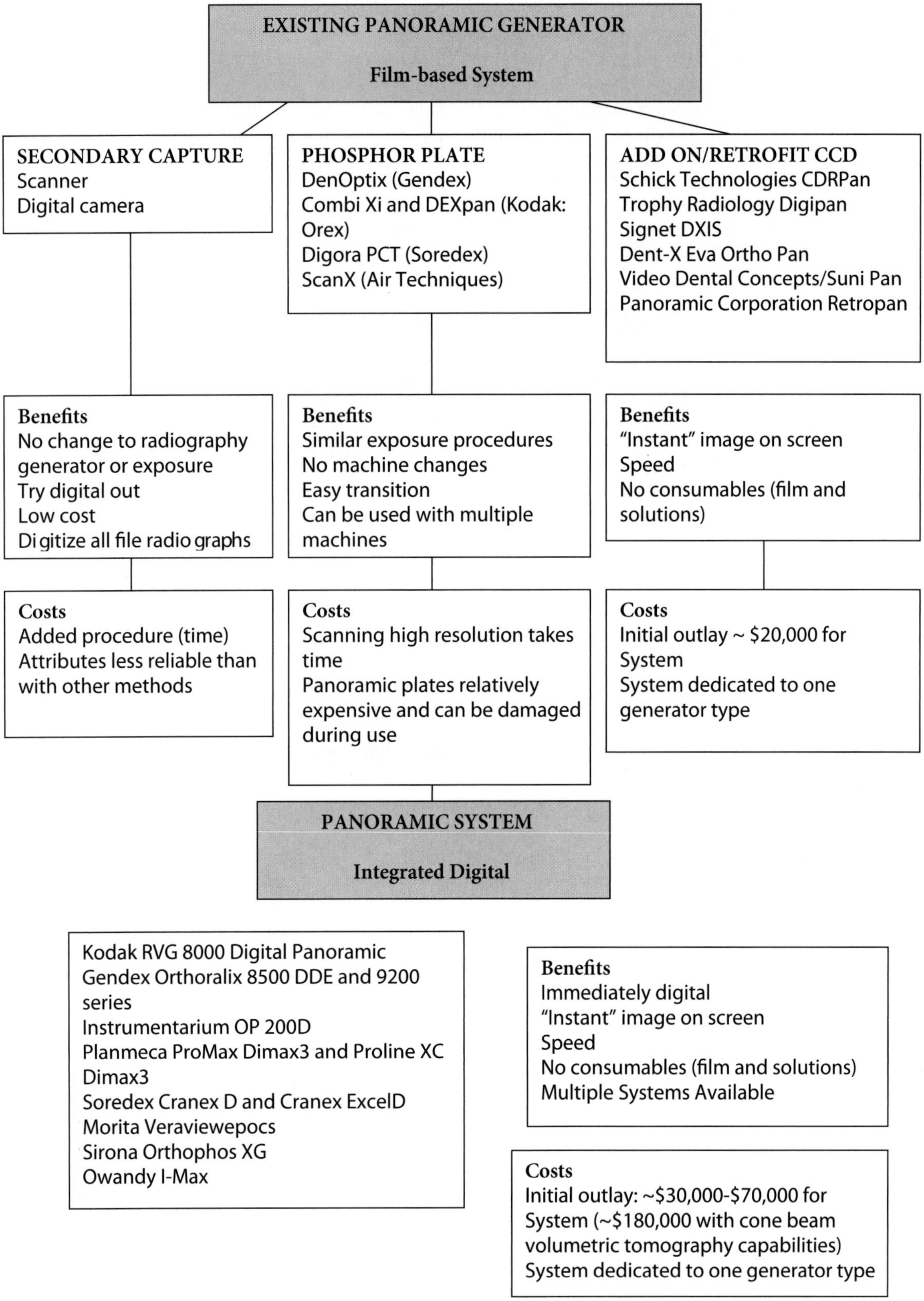

Fig. 3.6 Alternative digital approaches

There are several excellent dedicated digital panoramic systems in the market (e.g., Figs. 3.6, 3.7), however, the costs of such systems range from $30,000 to $70,000 depending on the degree of sophistication desired. To select such a unit requires a careful assessment of your practice and an individualized cost-benefit analysis. It should be remembered that reimbursements per panoramic procedure are not generally proportional to your investment. Whatever device you select should fit with the type of practice and patients you serve.

Interoperability

It is not unusual to review film radiographs that are decades old—especially when demonstrating "classical" radiographic features of disease entities at a continuing education forum [10]. Archived film images that are decades old are usually still of high quality and can be viewed by anyone who happens to have a view box to transmit light through the radiographs. One might question whether the digitized or digital versions will be

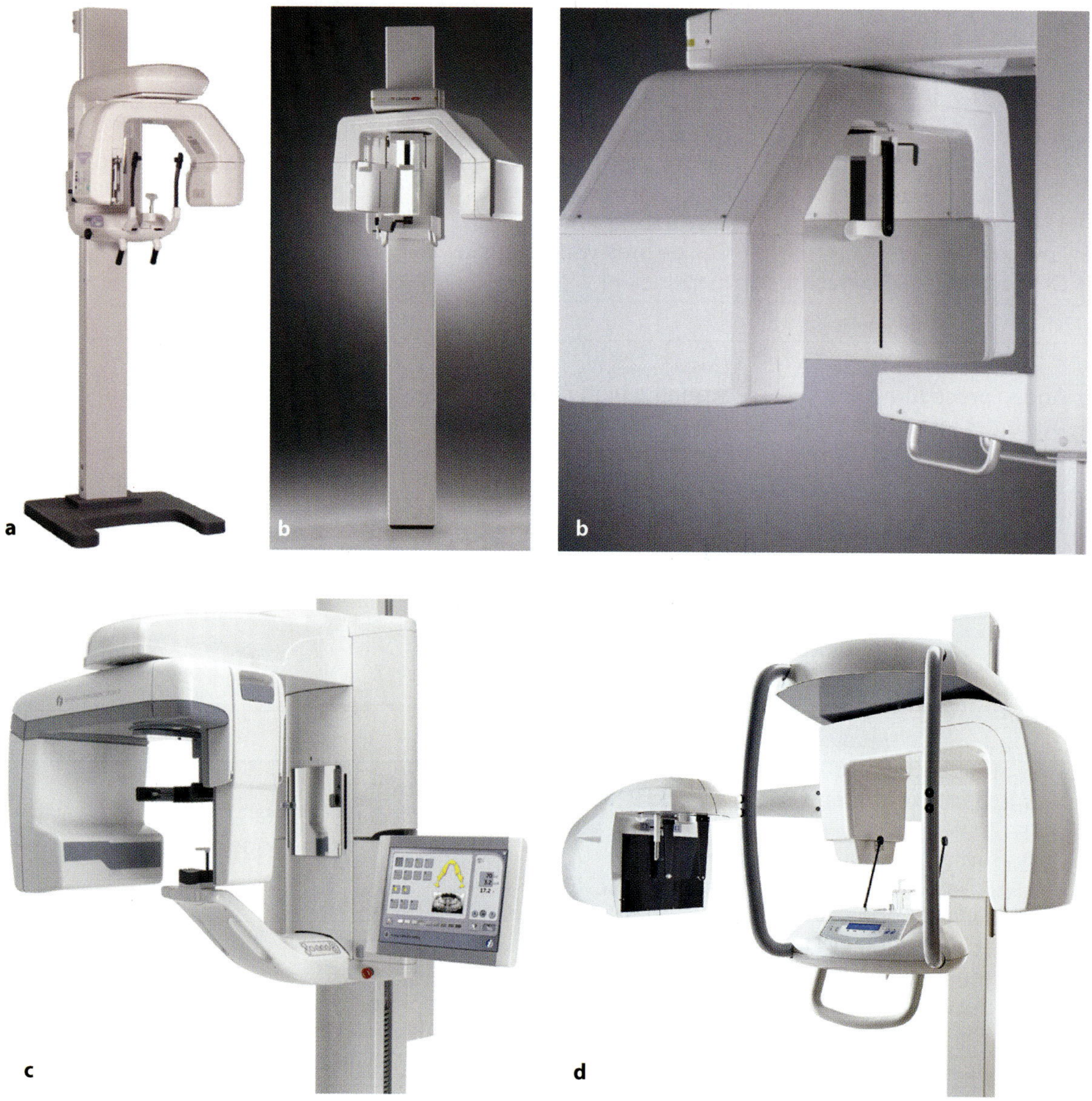

Fig. 3.7 **a** Veraviewepocs dedicated digital panoramic system (J. Morita, Kyoto, Japan). **b** Soredex Excel (PaloDEx, Helsinki, Finland). Example of a dedicated digital panoramic system. **c** Another example of a dedicated solid-state digital panoramic system is the Instrumentarium OP 200D (PaloDEx, Tuusula, Finland). **d** Another dedicated solid-state panoramic system is the Kodak RVG 8000C (Kodak Dental Imaging, Atlanta, GA). The system illustrated here includes a single-shot digital cephalometric system

as readily accessible as the analog film versions decades into the future. The likelihood of being able to retrieve digital images is dependent upon both hardware and software/file format considerations. Regarding hardware issues, one simply needs to back up all files on new media as they become accepted. For example, you cannot play music from an old record directly using a tape player or 8-track—and you cannot play a music tape on a CD or MP3 player. Similarly, it is now difficult to find a computer with a 5.25 inch floppy disk drive and standard "A" drives are rapidly disappearing to be replaced by CD-RW, DVD-RW, Flash Memory, and USB-Mass Storage Devices. If you intend to use digital images then you should expect to make periodic storage hardware upgrades.

Regarding the matter of software/file format interoperability, the digital X-ray industry and practice management system vendors are presently working together to facilitate digital image interoperability using specifications from the DICOM (Digital Image Communication) standards that were developed initially for medical radiology. This specification includes image format rules and associated information for transmission of radiographs used in dentistry including intraoral surveys and panoramic images. Working Group 12.1 of the American Dental Association's Standards Committee on Dental Informatics has been tasked with developing appropriate specifications. It must be cautioned, however, that no guidelines or specifications will guarantee interoperability. Interoperability needs to be demonstrated practically. Such practical demonstrations were initiated at the ADA Annual Congress in New Orleans in 2002 where ten companies demonstrated that interoperability of their image files could be achieved satisfactorily. Similar interoperability demonstrations have been made with DICOM validation at all ADA Annual Sessions, through at least until the time of publication of this book. Each time there are more vendors involved. Interoperability within the DICOM Standard is important so that the dentist can integrate data from different digital sources and read diagnostic images referred from outside sources where different systems may have been used. Otherwise there could be inconvenience both for the patient and for the practitioner.

References

1. Farman AG, Scarfe WC. Pixel perception and voxel vision: constructs for a new paradigm in maxillofacial imaging. Dentomaxillofac Radiol 1994;23:5–9
2. Farman AG, Farman TT. Extraoral and panoramic systems. Dent Clin North Am 2000;44:257–272
3. Farman TT, Kelly MS, Farman AG. The OP 100 Digipan: evaluation of the image layer, magnification factors, and dosimetry. Oral Surg Oral Med Oral Pathol Oral Radiol Endod 1997;83:281–287
4. Farman AG, Farman TT. Panoramic dental radiography using a charge-coupled device receptor. J Digit Imaging 1998;11(3Suppl.1):166–168
5. Farman TT, Farman AG. Clinical trial of panoramic dental radiography using a CCD receptor. J Digit Imaging 1998;11(3Suppl.1):169–171
6. Farman AG, Farman TT. A comparison of image characteristics and convenience in panoramic radiography using charge-coupled device, storage phosphor and film receptors. J Digit Imaging 2001;14(2Suppl.1):48–51
7. Schulze RK, Rosing ST, D'Hoedt B. Contrast perception in digitized panoramic radiographs compared with their film-based originals. Oral Surg Oral Med Oral Pathol Oral Radiol Endod 2002;94:388–394
8. Benediktsdottir IS, Hintze H, Petersen JK, Wenzel A. Image quality of two solid state and three photostimulable phosphor plate digital panoramic systems, and treatment planning of mandibular third molar removal. Dentomaxillofac Radiol 2003;32:39–44
9. Gijbels F, Sanderink G, Serhal CB, Pauwels H, Jacobs R. Organ doses and subjective image quality of indirect digital panoramic radiography. Dentomaxillofac Radiol 2001;30:308–313
10. Farman AG. Use and implication of the DICOM standard in dentistry. Dent Clin North Am 2002;46:565–573

TEST: Digital options for panoramic radiology

1. Duplicate images of digital radiographs made with charge-coupled devices or photostimulable phosphors are inferior to the original image.

   True ☐ **False** ☐

2. Digital imaging systems not utilizing analog X-ray film are environmentally friendly.

   True ☐ **False** ☐

3. Solid-state digital technologies include photostimulable phosphor plates.

   True ☐ **False** ☐

4. Digital panoramic radiographs generally require a reduced dosage in comparison with traditional film/screen radiography.

   True ☐ **False** ☐

5. Strict adherence to DICOM file formats is a guarantee of interoperability between different digital systems used in dentistry.

   True ☐ **False** ☐

6. Hardware upgrades in storage devices are likely to be needed periodically to preserve the availability of digital images.

   True ☐ **False** ☐

7. Scanning generally using a laser is necessary to process the latent image when using photostimulable phosphors for panoramic radiography.

   True ☐ **False** ☐

8. Achievement of digital imaging using an existing panoramic unit is possible using secondary capture, phosphor plate or retrofit (add-on) solid-state systems.

   True ☐ **False** ☐

9. For digital panoramic radiography using a solid-state system, the solid-state detector moves in a similar manner to analog film during the exposure.

   True ☐ **False** ☐

10. Gijbels et al. (2001) found a substantial difference in exposure settings and organ doses between analog X-ray film and digital panoramic radiography using photostimulable phosphor plates.

    True ☐ **False** ☐

Panoramic Radiology: Risk Within Reason

4

Allan G. Farman

Learning Objectives

After studying this chapter, the reader should be able to:

- Explain the ALARA principle as it applies to panoramic dental radiography
- Understand the concepts of background dose equivalence
- Promote the safe and effective use of ionizing radiation for maxillofacial diagnosis, treatment planning and treatment guidance
- Differentiate between administrative radiographs and the administrative use of diagnostic radiographs

The absolute risk from low levels of radiation used in dental radiography is estimated to be less than one in a million; certainly much lower than many normal pursuits that go unquestioned, including automobile transportation. Nonetheless, unless there is a balancing gain in terms of clinical diagnosis or treatment guidance, radiographs should not be made. The underlying principle should be to keep exposure to ionizing radiation 'As Low As Reasonably Achievable.'

National Council on Radiation Protection and Measurement: Radiation Protection in Dentistry (NCRP Report No. 145)

Brand and Gibbs ably co-chaired the NCRP Report on *Radiation Protection in Dentistry* [1]. In the introduction to their report, it is stated that while available data clearly shows ionizing radiation can result in biological damage if delivered in sufficiently high dose, it is not clear that radiation doses required for dental radiography present any risk. However, neither is it clear that such small doses are entirely free from risk. Benefits from a dental radiographic examination are considered to outweigh the radiation exposure incurred provided that:

- The radiographic examination is clinically indicated and justified (see Chapter 5 for a review of ADA/FDA dental radiograph selection criteria)
- The technique is optimized to ensure high-quality diagnostic images
- Appropriate safety measures are adopted to minimize unnecessary exposure to the patient, staff, and public

Exposure levels for the operators of X-ray equipment and the public must be within regulated limits established by regulatory bodies, but the 'As Low As Reasonably Achievable' principle (ALARA) also applies [2]. This principle was originally coined to promote minimizing operator dose rather than accepting any dose so long as it falls below regulatory limits. It has been extended to encompass the patient. Reasonable efforts should be made to reduce or eliminate all avoidable radiation exposure.

The three principles that are incorporated in ALARA are that:

1. Exposures are clinically justified
2. Optimization of technique is applied to minimize exposure to the patient
3. Dose limitations are applied to ensure than nobody is exposed to an unacceptably high risk

Patient exposures are only warranted if they will supply beneficial clinical information. No radiograph should be made simply as a routine and none should be prescribed without study of the patient history and a thorough clinical examination. While radiographs may be used for administrative uses subsequent to their use for clinical diagnosis or treatment guidance, no radiograph should be made simply for administrative purposes when not needed clinically. It is unethical to irradiate a patient without there being a clinical reason for the exposure. The administrative use of clinically needed radiographs is acceptable. Making administrative radiographs *per se*, in the absence of clinical need, is not an acceptable practice.

Recommended limitations set by the NCRP are higher for occupational exposures than for exposure of the general public [3]. The recommendation for maximum occupational exposure is an equivalence of 50 milliSievert (mSv) per annum for individuals aged 18 years or older but only 10 mSv × age in years for the cumulative effective dose. For the public, the maximum recommended equivalent effective dose is 1 mSv per annum for continuous or frequent exposure, or 5 mSv effective dose for infrequent exposure. Equivalent dose is the mean absorbed dose in an organ or tissue modified by the radiation weighting factor for the types of radiation. For X-radiation the modifying weighting factor is unity (one).

US Population Radiation Exposure

The average per capita exposure to radiation for US citizens is around 3.6 mSv with the largest source being radon gas (~2 mSv = 56% of total) (Fig. 4.1; Table 4.1) [4]. The next highest contributors to the US population exposure are ingested radioisotopes (internal) and diagnostic X-ray exposure, both at around 11% of the total. To get dental X-ray in perspective, the percentage of all diagnostic X-ray exposure attributable to dentistry is very small.

Principles of Radiation Protection

There are three primary concerns in radiation protection. These are:

1. Minimizing length of exposure
2. Maximizing distance from radiation source
3. Using shielding

The best means to minimize the total length of exposure is to reduce the number of radiographic procedures performed by dint of appropriate selection. Only radiographs that are professionally judged necessary for diagnosis or treatment guidance purposes should be made. Following the judicial use of selection criteria, the next step to reducing unnecessary patient and occupational exposure is to assure that the procedures are carried out by trained personnel capable of achieving technical perfection with a minimum number of remakes. Finally, each individual exposure should be made at the lowest dose commensurate with obtaining an image of excellent diagnostic quality.

Image quality should not be sacrificed in an attempt to reduce dose. If this were to happen, the correct treatment may be delayed, or alternatively there may be a subsequent increased dose due to the necessity of remaking the diagnostic radiograph.

For the patient, distance is not really an issue of radiation safety as this is largely a factor of the chosen technique; however, for the operator (and also for the public), the inverse square law applies where complete shielding from radiation is not feasible. According to the inverse square law, the intensity of radiation decreases proportionately to the square of the distance from the source. Hence, if one moves from 2 to 4 m from the source, the radiation intensity is reduced to one fourth, and at 6 m to one ninth of that at 2 m. This is a consideration when choosing where to position an X-ray unit. By the way, scattered radiation from a panoramic unit is usually minimal due to tight collimation of the beam and the bulk of the detector. While radiation use rules and statutes do vary between jurisdictions, it is generally recommended that the operator be at least two meters from the source in the absence of protective shielding.

Of course, the operator should never stand in front of the useful X-ray beam. Preferably, stand behind a radiation barrier when operating X-ray equipment. The safest position for the operator—and for the general public—is to be protected behind a radiation barrier. The necessary barrier construction should be determined following analysis by an appropriately certified

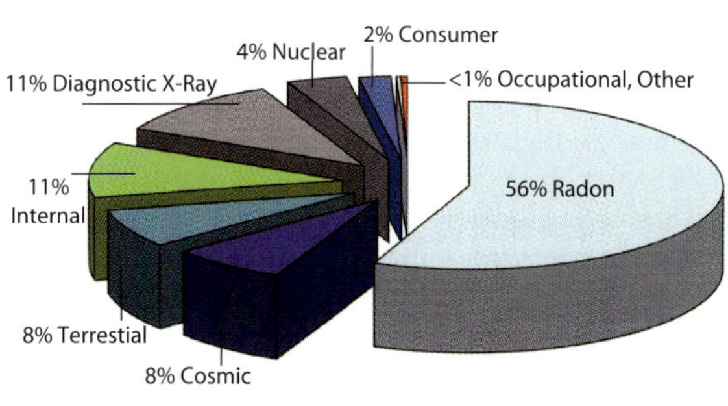

Fig. 4.1 US average dose equivalence and sources per capita based on NCRP data [4]

Table 4.1 Radiation exposure for US citizens

Source	Percentage
Radon	56
Diagnostic X-ray	11
Internal	11
Terrestrial	8
Cosmic	8
Nuclear	4
Consumer products	2
Occupational and other	<1

health physicist. Often for dentistry such a barrier can be fabricated very simply using various thicknesses of regular dry wall combined with a leaded-acrylic panel to permit observation of the patient during the exposure. Panoramic radiographic systems require only very minimal shielding in comparison with other systems such as intraoral X-ray generators. Concerning the draping of patients in lead aprons and thyroid shields, you will need to follow local regulations; however, scientific study questions the need for a lead apron when panoramic radiography is employed [5].

With panoramic radiography, beam collimation is precise. If a lead apron is to be used, remember that the beam is directed largely from behind the patient, so the apron should be placed to protect the patient's back.

Risk within Reason

The risk of a dental radiographic procedure has been estimated at approximately one-in-a-million for causing a fatal malignancy. This estimate is based upon multiple assumptions, and also needs to be viewed against a lifetime probability of more than one-in-five of developing a fatal malignancy that would be indistinguishable from one caused by diagnostic X-rays. Other one-in-a-million risks of fatal outcome in everyday life include 20 minutes of simply living and dying from natural causes for a 60-year-old male, 1 hour of working in a coal mine and dying from black lung—or 3 hours in the same mine and dying from an accident, or 10 days in a typical factory and succumbing to accidental death [6]. This risk has also been compared to fatal accidents during various types of transportation. There is a one-in-a million risk of fatality from 300 miles traveling in an automobile, 1,000 miles in an airplane from a regular airline, 10 miles cycling, or 6 miles paddling in a canoe. And there is also a one-in-a-million risk from smoking 1.4 cigarettes or drinking 500 cc of wine [6]. Risk is weighted differently in the perception of individuals, but the real relative risk of dental radiography in general, and panoramic radiography in particular, is extremely low (Fig. 4.2) [7].

Risk within Reason from Panoramic Radiology

When individual tissue dosages (Fig. 4.3) and overall dose is considered for both panoramic and intraoral radiographic procedures, differences in total values could be considered "half of nothing" rather than "continued cause for concern." This in no way belittles the need to follow the ALARA principle, but perhaps puts into perspective claims and counter-claims that will perhaps never be subject to real outcomes measures based upon morbidity or mortality measures.

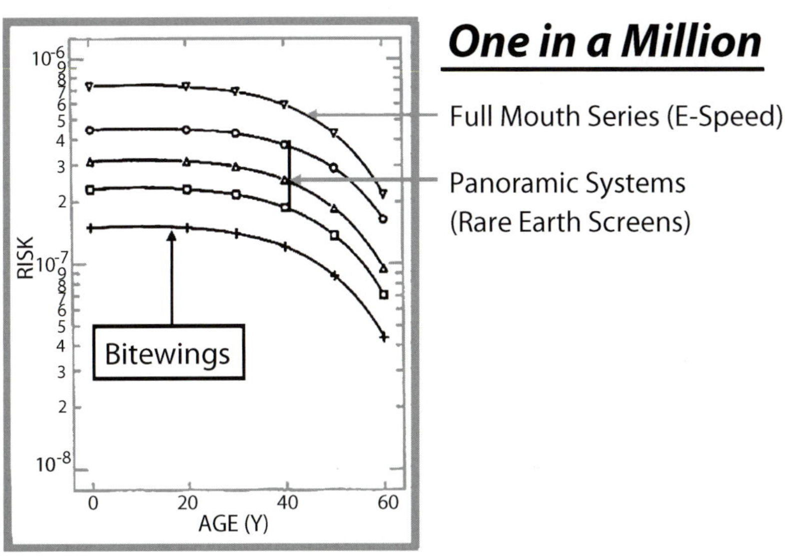

Fig. 4.2 The relative risks of panoramic and intraoral radiography vary between different studies depending on assumptions that are applied concerning the tissues irradiated, and also depending upon the detector speeds and collimation applied. The calculated relative risks made by Gibbs et al. [7] compare standard panoramic radiology imaging using rare earth screens (*middle three curves*) with relatively fast (ANSI Speed Group E; *top curve*) full mouth intraoral radiography. *Bottom curve* Bitewings. It should be noted that the risk is provided on a logarithmic scale; hence, differences depicted are actually greater than they seem

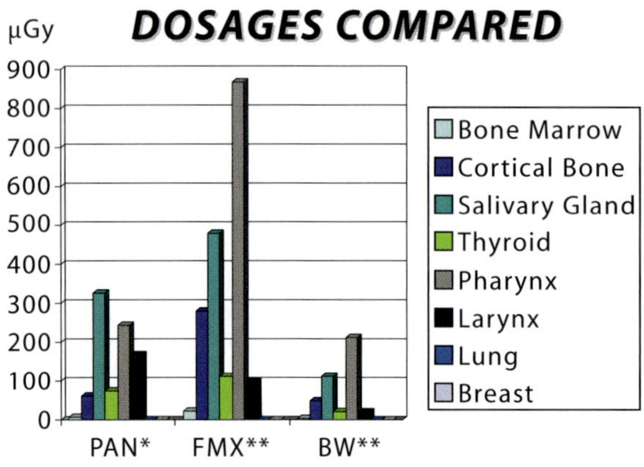

Fig. 4.3 Comparative organ dosages from selected panoramic (*PAN*) and intraoral X-ray procedures (*FMX, BW*). *Asterisk* rare earth screen, *double asterisk* ANSI Speed Group E. (Based on the work of Julian Gibbs)

Patient Safety

Gijbels et al. measured patient radiation dose during panoramic exposure with various panoramic units for five digital panoramic imaging systems [8]. An anthropomorphic phantom was filled with thermoluminescent dosimeters (TLD 100) and exposed using the different panoramic generators for ten consecutive exposures. Four machines were equipped with a charge-coupled device (CCD) detector, whereas one of the units used storage phosphor plates. The exposure settings recommended by the different manufacturers for the particular patient size were used: tube potential settings ranged between 64 and 74 kV, current between 4 and 7 mA, and exposure times between 8.2 and 19.0 seconds. The effective radiation dose was calculated with inclusion of the salivary glands. Effective radiation doses ranged between 4.7 and 14.9 μSv for one exposure. Salivary glands absorbed the most radiation for all panoramic units. When phosphor and CCD digital panoramic systems were compared, the effective dose of the digital unit using the storage phosphor (8.1 μSv) was within the range of the effective doses for the CCD units (4.7–14.9 μSv). It was concluded that a rather wide range of patient radiation doses can be found for digital panoramic units. There is a tendency for lower effective doses for modern digital panoramic systems compared with analog panoramic imaging reported in earlier studies. However, the measured dosages were all comparatively low. The current risks from dental radiography are much lower than they may have been in the past. There has been a two-order of magnitude decline in the radiation dose needed for an intraoral radiograph since the second decade of the twentieth century [9].

Longstreth et al. (2004) investigated whether the risk of intracranial meningioma was associated with past dental radiography—specifically, posterior bitewings, full-mouth series, and lateral cephalometric and panoramic radiographs [10]. The authors conducted a population-based case-control study of residents of certain counties in western Washington State. Case subjects ($n = 200$) had an intracranial meningioma that was confirmed histologically between January 1995 and June 1998.The authors used random-digit dialing and Medicare eligibility lists to identify two control subjects to be matched to each case patient based on age and sex. Prior dental radiographic exposures were determined during an in-person interview. The authors compared self-report and dental records in a subset of study participants. Of the four dental X-ray procedures evaluated, only the full-mouth series (specifically six or more exposures) over a lifetime was associated with a significantly increased risk of meningioma (odds ratio, 2.06; 95% confidence limits, 1.03–4.17); however, evidence for a dose response relation was lacking (p for trend = 0.33). The risk was elevated with the aggregate number of full-mouth series in 10-year periods from approximately 15–40 years before intracranial meningioma diagnosis, with significant elevations in the 10-year periods beginning 22–30 years before diagnosis. The risks were even greater when only women were considered. It was concluded that dental X-rays involving full-mouth series performed 15–40 years ago, when radiation exposure from full-mouth series was much greater than it is now, were associated with an increased risk of meningioma. The authors did not find increased risk with bitewings, lateral cephalometric, and panoramic radiographs [10].

Occupational Safety

Gijbels et al. (2005) measured occupational radiation dose during panoramic exposure from five digital panoramic radiographic systems four of which were equipped with a charge-coupled device (CCD) detector, and one used storage phosphor plates [11]. An anthropomorphic phantom served as the patient. An ionization chamber recorded the scattered radiation at one meter from the phantom at five different locations around the panoramic generators both at the level of the thyroid gland and the level of the gonads and effective organ doses were calculated. Exposure parameters were set as recommended by the manufacturers for the particular patient size: tube potential settings were in the range of 64–74 kV, exposure cycles ranged between 8.2 and 19.0 seconds, and tube and current values ranged between 4 and 7 mA. The maximum organ equivalent dose at one meter from the panoramic unit was merely 0.60 μGy, and the maximum organ effective dose was only 0.10 μSv. Organ equivalent doses varied between 0.18 and 0.30 μGy and organ effective doses between 0.01 and 0.05 μSv for the different positions around the units (average for the different panoramic units).The variations in organ doses for the various machines were 0.04–0.53 μGy organ equivalent dose and 0.01–0.08 μSv organ effective dose. Assuming that 500 panoramic radiographs per year are made by a practitioner at 1 m distance from the panoramic unit, he or she would receive an annual additional organ effective dose of 5–15 μSv for the thyroid gland 5–40 μSv for the gonads, depending on the type of digital panoramic system employed.

Going Digital

When converting to digital radiography, it should be remembered that traditional panoramic radiography used a screen-film combination, whereas analog intraoral radiography uses direct-exposure film. Hence, when going digital there is usually little gain in terms of dose reduction for panoramic systems. This is not the case for intraoral radiography where the addition of a scintillator, or the use of a storage phosphor imaging plate, can result in dose savings of around 50% in comparison with use of fast intraoral X-ray films. The traditional differences found in the Gibbs et al. study [7] where panoramics were preferred on a simple dose comparison does not always apply when going digital [12]. The decision to use digital panoramic versus digital intraoral radiographic imaging should be made on such issues of desired area of coverage rather than being based upon radiation dose.

Kiefer et al. (2004) investigated the dose to the head and neck region comparing analog and digital radiographic dental systems [12]. Four radiographic devices were tested: panoramic radiography (analog and digital) and 14-image full-mouth-survey (FMS; analog and digital). Organ doses were measured on a Rando-phantom by use of CaF_2 dosimeters. The effective dose was lowest in digital FMS (41 μSv) and highest in analog FMS (78 μSv), i.e., dose was reduced by 47% by using a digital device for intraoral radiography. In panoramic radiography, doses were 17% lower using digital technique (digital 45 μSv versus analog 54 μSv). Thus, FMS using 14 films is no longer associated with higher doses than panoramic radiography when conventional films are replaced by digital techniques. Caution is needed in interpretation of these findings; however, as the FMS in the USA commonly comprises 20 images meaning that the results for the FMS would need to be increased by more than 40% to provide results that can be compared with the classic findings of Gibbs et al. [7].

Panoramic Dosimetry

Tierris et al. (2004) used a dose-area product (DAP) meter to compare DAP between panoramic and intraoral radiology [13]. DAP was measured for 62 panoramic X-ray units using three types of exposure (male, female, and child) and in 20 intraoral X-ray units of 50, 60, and 70 kVp. DAP reference levels for panoramic radiography were 117, 97, and 77 mGy cm^2 for exposure of a male, female, and child, respectively. Results showed that DAP from a panoramic dental examination approximated only twice that from a single intraoral examination.

A pencil ionization chamber is commonly used to measure the CT dose index for CT scanners. In 2004, Perisinakis et al. investigated using such a pencil ionization chamber for the determination of dose-width product (DWP) and DAP in panoramic radiography [14]. A Rando anthropomorphic phantom appropriately loaded with thermoluminescent dosimeters (TLDs) was used to obtain organ dose and effective dose values from panoramic radiography. Reproducibility of DWP determination using the pencil ionizing chamber was better than 1.5%. DWP measured using the pencil chamber was found to be up to 11% higher than the corresponding values determined using TLD array. The panoramic exposure obtained with settings appropriate for the typical adult patient was found to result in 0.008 mSv patient effective dose, 0.0002 mGy gonadal dose, and 11.3 cGy cm^2 DAP. This confirms that the gonadal dose due to scatter during panoramic radiology is minimal.

Buch and Fensham (2003) used traditional lithium fluoride TLDs to determine dosages from dental radiography to the head and neck region [15]. Selected TLDs were placed in a Rando female phantom in a position corresponding to the lens of the eye-three in the left and three in the right eye. A standard panoramic radiograph was made of the phantom. The TLDs were then replaced by another two groups of three in the same positions in the phantom and a lateral cephalogram made with the same machine.. Six of the 12 TLDs were then randomly selected for re-use. Three were placed in the phantom in the region of the thyroid and a panoramic radiograph again made. The procedure was repeated for a cephalogram and the TLDs again read. In all cases the readings of each group of three TLDs did not vary by more than 10% on either side of the mean readings. The TLD readings were then converted to actual dose measurements. The doses to left and right eyes and to the thyroid were found to be 0.015, 0.022, and 0.090 mSv, respectively, for the panoramic radiographs and 0.035, 0.018, and 0.018 mSv for the cephalogram—all insignificant doses in terms of the "background equivalent" concept (Fig. 4.4).

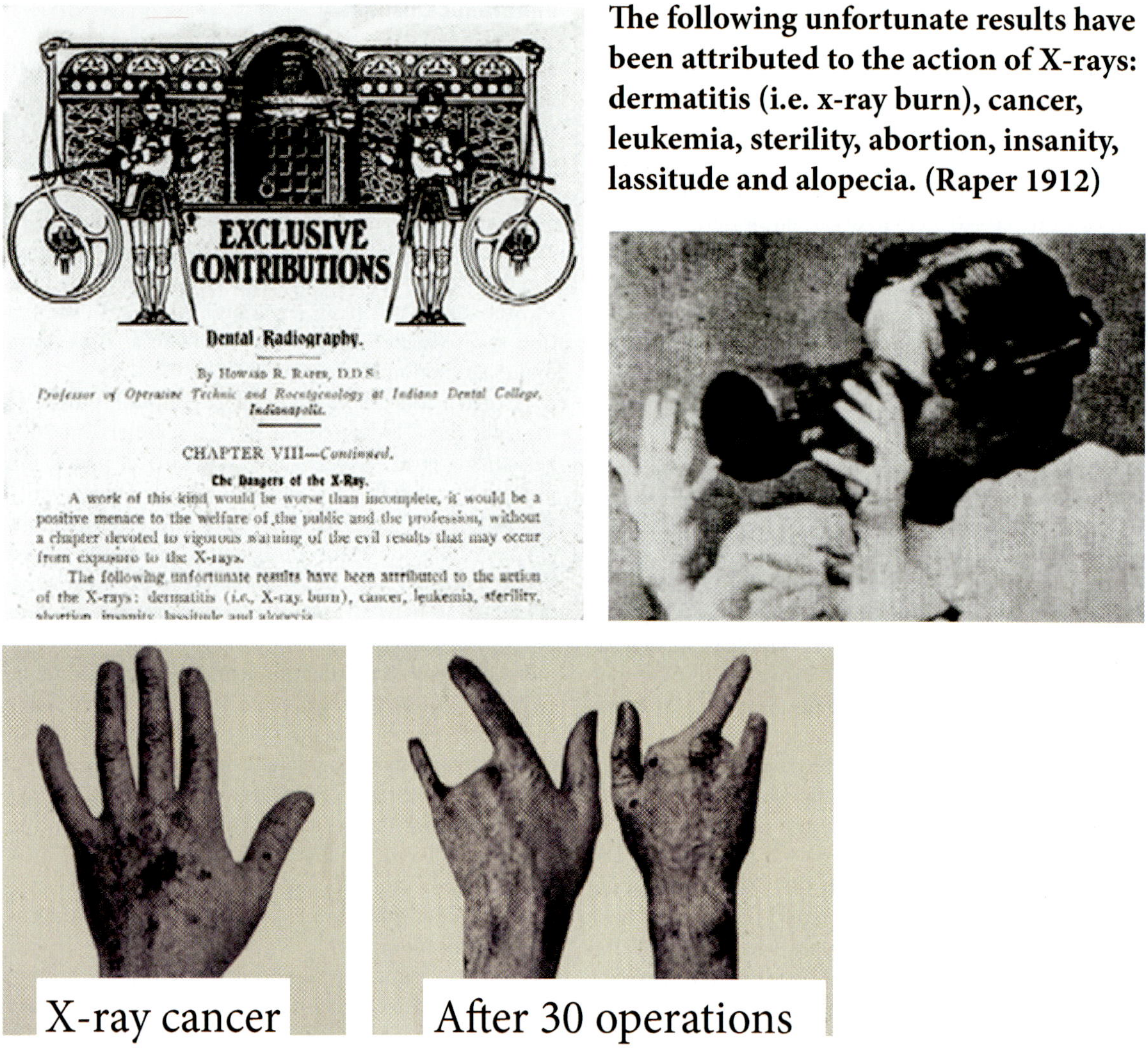

Fig. 4.4 There is no doubt that high dosages of radiation can be harmful to the operator. This was proven more than 100 years ago with radiation-induced cancer affecting the hands of such dental radiology pioneers as Dr. C. Edmund Kells. Dental radiology pioneers tested the quality of X-ray production using a fluoroscopic view of their own hands. Dr. Howard Riley Raper, father of dental radiology instruction in the USA, covered the issue of radiation safety concerns in Chapter VIII of his series of papers on dental radiography published in *Dental Items of Interest*. This was several decades before the development of panoramic dental radiography by Paatero in the middle of the twentieth century

Summary

No activity is entirely free from risk. There might be more risk in the journey to the dentist than in the radiographs that are made for justifiable diagnostic purposes in consequence of professional prescription.

Despite modern dental radiography being designated as of low risk potential, professionalism demands adherence to the ALARA principle. Unnecessary radiographic procedures should be avoided. Radiographs should only be made when there is a diagnostic purpose determined by history taking and clinical evaluation of the patient. Whatever radiographs are selected, it is the duty of the dental team to ensure radiation exposure is kept to the lowest level consistent with production of a high quality diagnostic image. Compromising image quality merely to reduce an already low dose is not a good service to the patient. If a radiograph is needed it should be performed optimally. Further dose savings are probably "half of nothing" rather than "continued cause for concern" [16].

References

1. NCRP. Radiation Protection in Dentistry. NCRP Report No. 145. 2003. Bethesda, MD: National Council on Radiation Protection and Measurement
2. NCRP. Implementation of the Principle of As Low As Reasonably Achievable. NCRP Report No. 107. 1990. Bethesda, MD: National Council on Radiation Protection and Measurement
3. NCRP. Limitation of exposure to ionizing radiation. NCRP Report No. 116. 1993. Bethesda, MD: National Council on Radiation Protection and Measurement
4. NCRP. Ionizing Radiation Exposure of the Population of the United States. NCRP Report No. 93. 1987. Bethesda, MD: National Council on Radiation Protection and Measurement
5. Nortjé CJ, Harris AM, Lackovic KP, Wood RE. Does the lead apron and collar always reduce radiation dose? S Afr Dent 2001;56:502–504
6. Wilson R. Risk caused by low levels of pollution. Yale J Biol Med 1978;51:37–51
7. Gibbs, SJ, Pujol A, McDavid WR, Welander U, Tronje G. Patient risk from rotational panoramic radiography. Dentomaxillofac Radiol 1988;17:25–32
8. Gijbels F, Jacobs R, Bogaerts R, Debaveye D, Verlinden S, Sanderink G. Dosimetry of digital panoramic imaging. Part I: Patient exposure. Dentomaxillofac Radiol 2005;34:145–149
9. Farman AG. ALARA still applies. Oral Surg Oral Med Oral Pathol Oral Radiol Endod 2005;100:395–397
10. Longstreth WT Jr, Phillips LE, Drangsholt M, Koepsell TD, Custer BS, Gehrels JA, van Belle G. Dental X-rays and the risk of intracranial meningioma: a population-based case-control study. Cancer 2004;100:1026–1034
11. Gijbels F, Jacobs R, Debaveye D, Bogaerts R, Verlinden S, Sanderink G. Dosimetry of digital panoramic imaging. Part II: Occupational exposure. Dentomaxillofac Radiol 2005;34:150–153
12. Kiefer H, Lambrecht JT, Roth J. Dose exposure from analog and digital full mouth radiography and panoramic radiography. Schweiz Monatsschr Zahnmed 2004;114:687–693
13. Tierris CE, Yakoumakis EN, Bramis GN, Georgiou E. Dose area product reference levels in dental panoramic radiology. Radiat Prot Dosimetry 2004;111:283–287
14. Perisinakis K, Damilakis J, Neratzoulakis J, Gourtsoyiannis N. Determination of dose-area product from panoramic radiography using a pencil ionization chamber: normalized data for the estimation of patient effective and organ doses. Med Phys 2004;31:708–714
15. Buch B, Fensham R. Orthodontic radiographic procedures: how safe are they? S Afr Dent J 2003;58:6–10
16. Bonkowski JH, Farman AG, Scheible L. A matter of professional conscience: maximizing patient radiation safety. J Mich Dent Assoc 1988;70:525–531

TEST: Panoramic radiology: risk within reason

1. ALARA is the acronym for As Low As Reasonably Achievable.

   True ☐ **False** ☐

2. Panoramic radiography has been linked to an increased incidence of intracranial meningioma.

   True ☐ **False** ☐

3. According to the work of Gibbs et al. panoramic radiography using rare earth screens is somewhat less risky than standard full mouth series, though both are low risk.

   True ☐ **False** ☐

4. When converting to digital imaging, the dose savings from the change is likely to be similar for both panoramic and intraoral radiography

   True ☐ **False** ☐

5. When comparing results for full mouth series, one important factor to consider is the number of individual exposures that comprises the full mouth series in each study.

   True ☐ **False** ☐

6. When comparing results for full mouth series, one important factor to consider is the number of individual exposures that comprises the full mouth series in each study.

   True ☐ **False** ☐

7. Dose-area product can be determined for panoramic radiography using a pencil ionization chamber.

   True ☐ **False** ☐

8. The risk of a panoramic radiograph is approximately equivalent to smoking 1.4 cigarettes or drinking 500 cc of wine.

   True ☐ **False** ☐

9. There is no proof that X-radiation causes cancer.

   True ☐ **False** ☐

10. Three important factors in occupational radiation dose minimization are time, distance, and shielding.

    True ☐ **False** ☐

Panoramic Radiology: Role in ADA/FDA Use Guidelines

5

Allan G. Farman

Learning Objectives

After studying this chapter, the reader should be able to:

- Define criteria for patient high and low risk for dental caries
- Describe appropriate radiograph selection for the asymptomatic child, adolescent, and adult patient
- Differentiate between radiograph selection for the asymptomatic new versus recall dental patient

The proper selection of a radiographic examination requires professional judgment based upon the individual patient's clinical history and examination. The ADA/FDA Selection Criteria are meant as a Guideline to supplement professional judgment in radiograph selection for the asymptomatic dental patient. The latest version of the Guidelines include greater emphasis on the use of panoramic radiography than hithertofore.

A comprehensive oral and dental screening is part of the baseline pretreatment workup for all first time appointments of "new" dental patients. This workup generally includes selected radiographic examinations based both upon the oral history of signs and symptoms of dental disease and clinical inspection of the patient by the dentist. Selected radiographs are also needed in asymptomatic patients to examine areas at high risk of insidious disease that cannot be readily inspected directly. Moreover, selected radiographic examinations are also needed at periodic follow up of patients, again dependent primarily on signs and symptoms of disease, but also based upon clinical evaluation of disease risk in patients free of symptoms of oral disease. The first FDA Guidelines for the dental patient radiograph selection were developed in the early 1980s under the leadership of Dr. Stephen R. Matteson with representation and feedback from numerous professional organizations and public review announced in the Federal Register.

Matteson et al. (1983) reported the results of a 1980 survey of a 27% random sample of all practicing dentists in North Carolina [1]. The objective of the survey was to establish then current practice standards regarding panoramic, full-mouth series, and bitewing radiographs. A total of 414 dentists (76% of those surveyed) responded.

A questionnaire was used to record demographic data on the dentists, age-specific prevalence data on the type of radiograph most often made at a patient's initial visit, and the prevalence of radiographs based on need as perceived by the dentist and assessed separately for a variety of patient characteristics (age, oral hygiene, caries activity, fluoride treatment, and systemic medical problems). Results of the survey of a subset of 338 dentists in general practice showed their median age to be 40 years with a median length of experience of 13 years. At an initial visit, for patients younger than 12 years, bitewing radiographs only were most commonly made; for patients older than 12 years, bitewings plus a panoramic radiograph were made. Full-mouth series plus bitewings were rarely made on patients younger than 6 years (~2% of the time), but were more commonly performed as patients aged (29% for patients aged 40 years and older).

A variety of patient characteristics were considered for their impact on the need for bitewing radiographs at recall. Caries activity was ranked most important for selecting the frequency of bitewing radiographs at follow up visits, followed by oral hygiene status and periodontal activity. The first FDA guidelines had specifically refrained from making many statements on the selection of panoramic radiographs for asymptomatic dental patients in view of a lack of systematically obtained scientific knowledge.

Shortly after development of the first FDA guidelines, White et al. investigated patient-selection criteria for panoramic radiography [2]. A total of 1,424 patients were included in this 10-month study. Clinicians were asked to indicate what signs or symptoms caused them to order a panoramic radiograph. After the radiograph was made, the referring clinician was asked to indicate the extent that the panoramic radiograph influenced the patient's care. The panoramic examination was found to be most productive in dentulous patients when no other radiographs were ordered and least productive in dentulous patients who had already had a full-mouth set of radiographs. It can be inferred that the intraoral radiographic series was most productive when a panoramic radiograph was not first ordered. Considering all patients, it would have been possible to reduce the number of panoramic examinations by 73% while missing 6% of the findings that influence patient treatment. Alternatively, it is possible that the intraoral series added little to the knowledge attained from the panoramic radiograph alone. The most important selection criteria for the panoramic examination were determined to be whether the radiograph was ordered for a "general screening examination" (a negative predictor if an intraoral full mouth series were also performed) and whether the radiograph was ordered for any specific examination (a positive predictor).

Panoramic technology has certainly improved over the past two decades. Today there is now better system movement based on scientific evaluation of anatomic variability, improved X-ray tubes, and customized detectors. For these reasons the new ADA/FDA Guidelines specify the use of panoramic radiographs plus bitewings as an acceptable alternative to the multi-film full mouth intraoral survey, especially when examining the "new" dental patient [3].

The "New" Dental Patient

When there are obvious signs or symptoms of disease, radiographic examinations usually assist in making the diagnosis. For example, if there is an obvious expansion of the mandible beyond the scope of coverage of an intraoral periapical radiograph, the choice of a panoramic image is easy to make (Fig. 5.1). Further, when a patient happens to be unable to open their mouth (i.e., lock jaw situations) a panoramic radiograph might well be the first diagnostic image made to investigate the circumstances. The ADA/FDA Guidelines for radiograph selection are not applicable in these circumstances, and are never meant to over-rule professional judgment. They are specifically directed toward the timely use of radiographs for periodic review of asymptomatic dental patients, moving the process of selection in such instances away from routine and toward criteria-based selection.

Patients Having No Signs or Symptoms of Maxillofacial Disease

This is the situation where the ADA/FDA selection criteria are valuable as guidelines. Panoramic radiography as a baseline study can be advocated as an alternate to the full mouth intraoral series for the child with transitional dentition, the adolescent with permanent dentition or the adult dentate and partially edentulous patient. It may also be used for the adult edentulous patient if signs and symptoms indicate a need. For the child with a primary dentition (prior to eruption of the first permanent tooth), radiographs on the asymp-

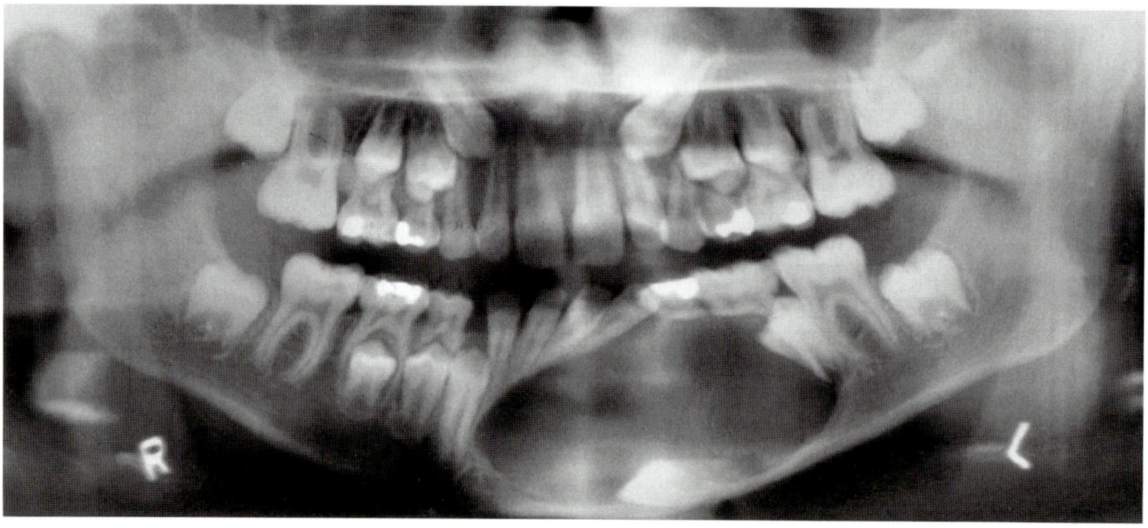

Fig. 5.1 Panoramic radiography is needed to demonstrate the extent of this large dentigerous cyst. Clinical judgment indicates that intraoral periapical radiographs would not provide sufficient coverage. The selection decision is a matter simple of professional judgment and does not require additional selection criteria

tomatic patient without signs of disease might not be needed. Intraoral radiographs of specific areas are advocated based upon professional judgment.

The "Recall" Dental Patient

For detecting dental caries progression, bitewing intraoral radiographs are usually the diagnostic images of choice, with the frequency depending upon clinical assessment of risk (see Tables 5.1, 5.2). For periodontal disease progression, clinical assessment is paramount in assessment and radiograph selection. Radiographs are secondary to clinical assessment for monitoring growth and development. The panoramic radiograph is a useful adjunct for this purpose, particularly for adolescents during the mixed dentition. In all circumstances, the guidelines are to support rather than to replace sound professional clinical judgment.

Outcomes Evidence

Screening for Dental Fitness

Chaffin et al. (2004) at the US Army Dental Command, Fort Sam Houston, Texas examined the validity of classifying initial entry training (IET) soldiers into dental fitness groups based solely on examining panoramic radiographs [4]. The dental readiness classification, derived from clinical screening, was compared to that made from panoramic radiology alone for 1,050 basic training recruits during a 1-month period at Fort Sill. The dentist who determined dental classifications by reviewing the panoramic radiograph was blinded to the earlier dental grouping made by clinical examination. Spearman's rank order correlation test was used to determine if a statistically significant correlation existed between the classifications based on the clinical examination and that from review of the panoramic radiograph alone. The project identified that 18% ($n = 186$) and 24% ($n = 249$) of the sample population had at least one high dental need condition identified respectively from the clinical screening examination and the panoramic radiograph review. Of the 186 high need dental fitness category conditions identified from the clinical inspection, 82% (152) were also identified from the blinded review of the panoramic radiograph. Spearman's rank order correlation test statistic was 0.633 for a $p < 0.001$, indicating a statistically significant correlation in the identification of IET soldiers with high dental needs conditions using a screening examination versus review of a panoramic radiograph. These findings suggest that panoramic radiograph review alone can identify IET soldiers with high treatment need and implies that a policy change may be prudent to allow this type of initial classification based on panoramic radiology alone [4].

Screening General Dental Patients

Rushton et al. (2002) attempted to measure the radiological diagnostic yield of panoramic radiographs made on new adult dental patients in 1998–99 [5]. Findings from 1,817 consecutive panoramic radiographs made to screen new dental patients were compared with clinical inspection results. The radiographs were obtained from 41 general dental practitioners, who also provided the clinical information about the patient obtained by history and examination. Two oral and maxillofacial radiologists recorded the radiological findings on each of the panoramic radiographs by consensus. Indices of diagnostic yield were devised and calculated for each radiograph from the data on radiological findings. Clinical indicators of a high-modified diagnostic yield were identified using stepwise multiple regression analysis. The clinical variables for which the significance was high ($p < 0.001$) were: increased number of teeth with clinical suspicion of periapical pathoses, presence of partially erupted teeth, increasing number of clinically evident carious lesions, partially dentate status, and presence of fixed restorations. Using clinical factors derived from the history and examination as radiographic selection criteria undoubtedly improves the odds of achieving a high diagnostic yield from panoramic radiography [5].

Screening for Periodontal Disease

Tugnait et al. (2000) surveyed radiographic practices for periodontal disease in UK and Irish dental teaching hospitals to assess current radiographic practices in the management of patients with periodontal diseases [6]. All 17 dental teaching hospitals in UK and Ireland were sent a questionnaire on radiographic equipment and radiograph selection currently used for assessment of patients with destructive periodontal diseases. Opinions were recorded for advantages and disadvantages of the most frequently used radiographic views. A 100% response rate was achieved. A protocol for selection of radiographs for periodontal patients was operated at 24% of dental hospitals. All dental hospitals used panoramic and specific periapical radiographs as one of their radiographic regimes for patients with periodontal disease: 53% of respondents most frequently took panoramic and selected periapical radiographs, 24% took full mouth periapical radiographs most frequently, and 18% took a panoramic radiograph alone.

Table 5.1 ADA/FDA guidelines for prescribing dental radiographs

Type of encounter	Patient age and dental developmental stage[a]				
	Child with primary dentition (prior to eruption of first permanent tooth)	Child with transitional dentition (after eruption of first permanent tooth)	Adolescent with permanent dentition (prior to eruption of third molar)	Adult dentate or partially edentulous	Adult edentulous
New patient being evaluated for dental disease and dental development	Individualized radiographic exam consisting of selected periapical/occlusal views and/or posterior bitewings if proximal surfaces cannot be visualized or probed. Patients without evidence of disease and with open proximal contacts may not require a radiographic exam at this time	Individualized radiographic exam consisting of posterior bitewings with **panoramic** exam or posterior bitewings and selected periapical images	Individualized radiographic exam consisting of posterior bitewings with **panoramic** exam or posterior bitewings and selected periapical images. A full mouth intraoral radiographic exam is preferred when the patient has clinical evidence of generalized dental disease or a history of extensive dental treatment		Individualized radiographic exam consisting of posterior based on clinical signs and symptoms
Recall patient with clinical caries or at increased risk for caries[b]	Posterior bitewing exam at 6- to 12-month intervals if proximal surfaces cannot be examined visually or with a probe			Posterior bitewing exam at 6- to 18-month intervals	Not applicable
Recall patient with no clinical caries and not at increased risk for caries	Posterior bitewing exam at 12- to 24-month intervals if proximal surfaces cannot be examined visually or with a probe		Posterior bitewing exam at 18- to 36-month intervals	Posterior bitewing exam at 24- to 36-month intervals	Not applicable
Recall patient with periodontal disease	Clinical judgment as to the need for and type of radiographic images for evaluation of periodontal disease. Imaging may consist of, but is not limited to, selected bitewing and/or periapical images of areas where periodontal disease (other than nonspecific gingivitis) can be identified clinically				Not applicable

Table 5.1 *(continued)* ADA/FDA guidelines for prescribing dental radiographs

Type of encounter	Patient age and dental developmental stage[a]				
	Child with primary dentition (prior to eruption of first permanent tooth)	Child with transitional dentition (after eruption of first permanent tooth)	Adolescent with permanent dentition (prior to eruption of third molar)	Adult dentate or partially edentulous	Adult edentulous
Patient for monitoring growth and development	Clinical judgment as to the need for and type of radiographic images for evaluation and/or monitoring of dentofacial growth and development		Clinical judgment as to the need for and type of radiographic images for evaluation and/or monitoring of dentofacial growth and development. **Panoramic** or periapical exam to assess developing third molars	Usually not indicated	
Patient with other circumstances including, but not limited to, proposed or existing implants, pathology, restorative/endodontic needs, treated periodontal disease and caries remineralization	Clinical judgment as to the need for and type of radiographic images for evaluation and/or monitoring in these circumstances				

[a]The recommendations in this chart are subject to clinical judgment and may not apply to every patient. They are to be used by the dentist only after reviewing the patient's health history and completing a clinical examination. Because every precaution should be taken to minimize radiation exposure, protective thyroid collars and aprons should be used wherever possible. This practice is strongly recommended for children, women of childbearing age and pregnant women

[b]Factors increasing the risk for caries may include but are not limited to: (1) high levels of caries experience; (2) history of recurrent caries; (3) high titers of cariogenic bacteria; (4) existing restoration(s) of poor quality; (5) poor oral hygiene; (6) inadequate fluoride exposure; (7) prolonged nursing (bottle or breast); (8) frequent high sucrose content in diet; (9) poor family dental history; (10) developmental or acquired enamel defects; (11) developmental or acquired disability; (12) xerostomia; (13) genetic abnormality of teeth; (14) many multisurface restorations; (15) chemo/radiation therapy; (16) eating disorders; (17) drug/alcohol abuse; and (18) irregular dental care

Table 5.2 Clinical situations possibly requiring radiographs

Type of encounter	ADA/FDA provided examples
A. Positive historical findings	1. Previous periodontal or endodontic treatment 2. History of pain or trauma 3. Familial history of dental anomalies 4. Postoperative evaluation of healing 5. Remineralization monitoring 6. Presence of implants or evaluation for implant placement
B. Positive clinical signs/symptoms	1. Clinical evidence of periodontal disease 2. Large or deep restorations 3. Deep carious lesions 4. Malposed or clinically impacted teeth 5. Swelling 6. Evidence of dental/facial trauma 7. Mobility of teeth 8. Sinus tract ("fistula") 9. Clinically suspected sinus pathology 10. Growth abnormalities 11. Oral involvement in known or suspected systemic disease 12. Positive neurological findings in the head and neck 13. Evidence of foreign objects 14. Pain and/or dysfunction of the temporomandibular joint 15. Facial asymmetry 16. Abutment teeth for fixed or removable partial dentures 17. Unexplained bleeding 18. Unexplained sensitivity of teeth 19. Unusual eruption, spacing or migration of teeth 20. Unusual tooth morphology, calcification or color 21. Unexplained absence of teeth 22. Clinical erosion

The most commonly used projections made in UK and Irish dental hospitals to assess periodontal status were panoramic radiographs with selected periapicals.

Screening for Periapical Disease

Patients are referred to the endodontist to have root canal therapy performed to treat pulpal and periradicular diseases [7]. Frequently the only radiograph to accompany the patient is a periapical radiograph of the region of concern. This radiograph is inadequate in the detection of asymptomatic pathoses that can be present in other areas of the maxilla and mandible. According to Bodey et al. (2003), the military's readiness mission requires that a panoramic radiograph be part of the dental recruit's dental record. In addition to its use for personal identification purposes, the panoramic radiograph is an excellent diagnostic tool that can give the clinician an overall view of the dentoalveolar structures [7]. They retrospectively evaluated randomly selected panoramic radiographs and recorded the presence of radiolucent and radio-opaque areas not evident on a referral periapical radiograph and determined a 4.2% prevalence of pathoses that would have otherwise gone undiagnosed.

Orthodontic Screening

... panoramic radiographs were as reliable as the intraoral radiographs for the detection of abnormalities.

An investigation was undertaken at Selly Oak Hospital, Birmingham, UK to assess the reliability of radiographic diagnosis of abnormalities of orthodontic significance in the anterior region of the maxilla from intraoral and panoramic radiographs [8]. Panoramic radiographs of 200 patients were scrutinized by two observers on two separate occasions, who also examined intraoral radiographs of the same patients. Sixty-three of these patients were selected because they had previously been diagnosed as presenting with a defined abnormality of orthodontic relevance. The remaining cases had been assessed as depicting normal radiographic appearances. Each radiograph was allocated a unique, randomly selected code number as the only means of identification. It was not possible for the observers to match the panoramic to the corresponding intraoral radiographs, and this information was only available to the principal investigator. Both observers were asked to record the presence or otherwise of any abnormalities at each observation of each radiograph, and to record their findings. The overall level of diagnostic accuracy and reproducibility was high, and the panoramic radiographs were as reliable as the intraoral radiographs for the detection of abnormalities. It was concluded that in most instances supplementary intraoral radiographs would not contribute additional information to use of the panoramic radiograph alone.

Bruks et al. (1999) examined 70 consecutive adolescents to evaluate radiographic examinations as an aid to orthodontic diagnosis and treatment planning in combination with clinical examination [9]. The clinical examination included dental impressions and extra- and intraoral photographs. The radiographic examination comprised a panoramic radiograph, a lateral cephalogram, and six intraoral anterior periapical radiographs. Initially, only records from the clinical examination were used for diagnosis and treatment planning. If required, the practitioner could choose any of the radiographs to accomplish the task. The number of radiographs ordered, the sequence of ordering, and any change in diagnosis and treatment plan caused by the radiographs were registered. In 29% of the cases the initial diagnosis, based on the clinical examination, study models and photographs, coincided with the final diagnosis. In 93% of all cases the initial treatment plan coincided with the final one. Although the panoramic examination was the most common choice, it had only a minor effect on diagnostic and treatment decisions, while the cephalometric examination had a major impact on the diagnosis. In most cases the clinical examination, supplemented with study models and photographs, provided adequate information for orthodontic treatment planning in this limited presenting sample of Scandinavian adolescents. Individually based selection criteria for radiographic examination could prevent unnecessary radiographs being obtained routinely.

Some Final Considerations

The radiation dosage used during the dental examinations is relatively small, but as dental radiographic diagnostics represents almost 25% of the entire radiological examinations, particular attention needs to be paid to this kind of examination in terms of radiation protection. Article 2 of the European Union's "patients' directive" stipulates that dentists are to show skills in radiation protection [10].

The appropriate selection of radiographic examinations for dental patients constitutes a balance between minimizing the use of ionizing radiation exposure and not loosing critical diagnostic information. Panoramic radiographic systems have advanced in terms of the quality of radiographic images they can produce when used correctly. For this reason, the use of panoramic radiography as a choice in baseline imaging of most new dental patients is provided for in the latest ADA/FDA Radiographic Selection Criteria [3].

References

1. Matteson SR, Morrison WS, Stanek EJ 3rd, Phillips C. A survey of radiographs obtained at the initial dental examination and patient selection criteria for bitewings at recall. J Am Dent Assoc 1983;107:586–590
2. White SC, Forsythe AB, Joseph LP. Patient-selection criteria for panoramic radiography. Oral Surg Oral Med Oral Pathol 1984;57:681–690
3. American Dental Association/United States Department of Health and Human Services. The Selection of Patients for Dental Radiographic Examinations. Revised 2004, pp 1–23
4. Chaffin JG, Hennessy BJ, Cripps KA. Validity of using a panoramic radiograph for initial dental classification of Army recruits. Mil Med 2004;169:368–372
5. Rushton VE, Horner K, Worthington HV. Screening panoramic radiography of new adult patients: diagnostic yield when combined with bitewing radiography and identification of selection criteria. Br Dent J 2002;192:275–279
6. Tugnait A, Clerehugh DV, Hirschmann PN. Survey of radiographic practices for periodontal disease in UK and Irish dental teaching hospitals. Dentomaxillofac Radiol 2000;29:376–381
7. Bodey TE, Loushine RJ, West LA. A retrospective study evaluating the use of the panoramic radiograph in endodontics. Mil Med 2003;168:528–529
8. Ferguson JW, Evans RI, Cheng LH. Diagnostic accuracy and observer performance in the diagnosis of abnormalities in the anterior maxilla: a comparison of panoramic with intraoral radiography. Br Dent J 1992;173:265–271
9. Bruks A, Enberg K, Nordqvist I, Hansson AS, Jansson L, Svenson B. Radiographic examinations as an aid to orthodontic diagnosis and treatment planning. Swed Dent J 1999;23:77–85
10. van der Stelt PF. Radiation protection and quality assurance in dental radiography. A treatise from the European Community. Rev Belge Med Dent 1996;51:111–122

TEST: Panoramic radiology: role in ADA/FDA use guidelines

1. ALARA is the acronym for As Low As Reasonably Achievable.

   True ☐ **False** ☐

2. Panoramic radiography has been linked to an increased incidence of intracranial meningioma.

   True ☐ **False** ☐

3. According to the work of Gibbs et al. panoramic radiography using rare earth screens is somewhat less risky than standard full mouth series, though both are low risk.

   True ☐ **False** ☐

4. When converting to digital imaging, the dose savings from the change is likely to be similar for both panoramic and intraoral radiography.

   True ☐ **False** ☐

5. When comparing results for full mouth series, one important factor to consider is the number of individual exposures that comprises the full mouth series in each study.

   True ☐ **False** ☐

6. Compromising image quality for continued savings in dose is not a good idea when making dental radiographs.

   True ☐ **False** ☐

7. Dose-area product can be determined for panoramic radiography using a pencil ionization chamber.

   True ☐ **False** ☐

8. The risk of a panoramic radiograph is approximately equivalent to smoking 1.4 cigarettes or drinking 500 cc of wine.

   True ☐ **False** ☐

9. There is no proof that X-radiation causes cancer.

   True ☐ **False** ☐

10. Three important factors in occupational radiation dose minimization are time, distance and shielding.

    True ☐ **False** ☐

Chapter

Panoramic Radiologic Appraisal of Anomalies of the Dentition

6

Allan G. Farman in association
with Christoffel J. Nortjé and Robert E. Wood

Learning Objectives

- Gain understanding of detection of developmental anomalies of the dentition
- Be able to identify radiographically the following anomalies: hypodontia, supernumerary teeth, macrodontia, microdontia, dilaceration, taurodontism, enamel pearl, connation, concrescence, talon cusp, dens invaginatus, dens evaginatus, supernumerary roots, enamel hypoplasia, amelogenesis imperfecta, dentinogenesis imperfecta, radicular dentin dysplasia, coronal dentin dysplasia, and odontodysplasia

Following FDA guidelines for radiographic examinations, the American Academy of Pediatric Dentistry in 1997 reaffirmed its recommendation for radiographic assessments of the dentition, growth and development during the transitional dentition and in adolescence [1]. This recommendation can be followed by making panoramic radiographs of your patients when they are approximately 5–7 years, 9–12 years, and 16–18 years old.

Whittington and Durward (1996) used panoramic radiographs to survey anomalies in primary teeth and their correlation with the permanent dentition of 1,680 5-year-old children. Anomalies of the primary teeth were detected in 23 children (1.4%) [2]. Six children (three boys and three girls) had hypodontia, three children (two boys and one girl) had a supernumerary tooth, and 14 children (nine boys and five girls) had connate teeth. Six of the affected teeth (in four boys and two girls) were diagnosed as fusion, and eight (five boys and three girls) as gemination. The panoramic radiographs of the 23 children with anomalies of the primary teeth revealed that 14 (61%) also had anomalies of the succedaneous permanent teeth.

Children with hypodontia in the primary dentition all had corresponding permanent teeth missing. The results of the study confirm that, when there is hypodontia, hyperdontia, gemination, or fusion of teeth in the primary dentition, there is an increased likelihood of anomalies of the succedaneous permanent teeth. Because of this close relationship between the dentitions, early identification of anomalies of the primary teeth can allow the dentist to investigate further and plan for treatment at the appropriate time.

Early detection of dental anomalies allows for timely intervention. Failure to achieve timely detection often results in more extensive treatment combined with a poorer outcome prognosis.

Locht (1980) evaluated panoramic radiographs of 704 Danish children aged 9–10 years and found 631 malpositioned teeth, caries in 224 primary and 32 permanent teeth, 60 malformed permanent teeth, 53 periapical inflammatory radiolucencies, and 42 dentigerous cysts. Hypodontia was present in 7.7% and supernumerary teeth in 1.7% of the studied population. These radiographic findings were certainly important for dental treatment planning [3]. Neal and Bowden (1988) also examined the diagnostic value obtained from panoramic radiographs made on individuals at 9–10 years of age [4]. Radiographs from 982 patients were examined and 261 (26.5%) showed findings of significance for orthodontic diagnosis and treatment planning.

Cholitgul and Drummond (2000) examined panoramic radiographs of 1,608 children and adolescents aged 10–15 years (797 males and 811 females) to determine the prevalence of tooth and jaw abnormalities. Abnormalities were detected in 21% of the radiographs (23% of females and 17% of males); 879 teeth were diagnosed with abnormalities from 331 radiographs [5]. The most common abnormalities were malpositioned teeth, missing teeth, misshaped teeth, and teeth appearing hypoplastic. Bony abnormalities and growth problems were also detected. This study demonstrated the value of panoramic radiography in detecting or confirming dental abnormalities, and supports the use of panoramic radiography to aid in the assessment of dental development.

Early detection of dental anomalies allows for timely intervention. Failure to achieve timely detection often results in more extensive treatment combined with a poorer outcome. Making a panoramic radiograph at the appropriate time is a matter of professionalism. Failure to do so might well constitute professional negligence.

Teeth develop *in utero* and during the first two decades after birth, with maturation and regressive changes occurring throughout life. It is important to understand the biological sequence and range in tooth development if one is to adequately assess anomalous dental developments and their clinical consequences. The reader's knowledge of normal developmental stages will be assumed for the purpose of this chapter. Development anomalies of the dentition can be divided according to the stage of tooth formation when the abnormality initiated. Stages of tooth development (Fig. 6.1) start with initiation of tooth formation by ectomesenchymal stimulation and subsequent proliferation of the overlying epithelium to form first the dental lamina and subsequently the tooth bud.

Abnormalities in the number of teeth can be caused by a failure in tooth bud formation (too few teeth) or formation of an excess number of tooth buds (too many teeth). This is followed by stages of histodifferentiation and morphodifferentiation. Anomalies in tooth shape likely occur during one or both of these stages. The developing tooth next moves to the stage of mineralization. Anomalies in structure of the mineralized tissues can occur at this stage. Mineralization of the crown is followed by tooth eruption that can also be aberrant causing dental impaction, malocclusion, transposition or ectopia. Maturation includes the completion of the tooth root(s) normally 3 years following eruption for permanent teeth, and subsequent increasing thickness of the dentin surrounding the pulp. Mild attrition such as the wearing down of enamel mamelons on the incisive edges of incisors can also be considered a process of maturation. More severe attrition, abrasion, erosion, dental caries, and exodontias can be considered regressive changes beyond the scope of this chapter.

Anomalies in Tooth Number

The full human dentition is composed of 20 primary teeth (eight incisors; four canines; eight molars) followed by transition to 32 adult teeth (eight incisors; four canines; eight premolars; 12 molars) with equal numbers of teeth in each jaw. If less than the normal complement of teeth develops, the patient is said to have hypodontia. If a patient develops an excessive number of teeth, the extra teeth are termed supernumeraries. Panoramic radiographs are of particular importance for

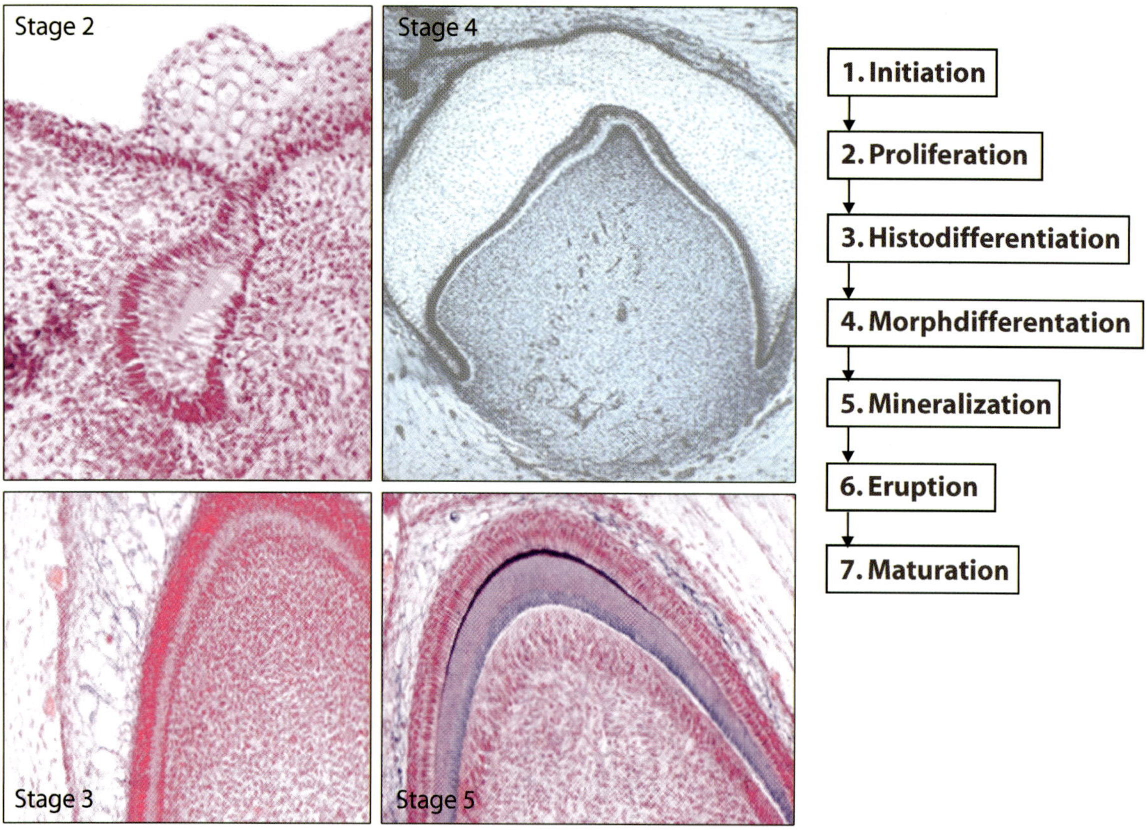

Fig. 6.1 Stages of tooth development. The type of developmental anomaly is probably dictated by the stage at which it is initiated

evaluating the number of teeth present as they provide "the whole picture" rather than just small segments of coverage. Furthermore, both regular and supernumerary teeth can be displaced to positions still within the panoramic view but beyond the bounds of a periapical radiograph.

Hypodontia

For hypodontia to be diagnosed, the missing tooth, or teeth, must not be accounted for by extraction. Dental extractions result in "pseudohypodontia." Pseudonyms for hypodontia are oligodontia and "partial anodontia." The latter term, while still used in several texts, is a misuse of the English language as it conditions an absolute. Anodontia, the complete absence of teeth, can rarely occur in consequence of the several ectodermal dysplasia syndromes, but is extremely rare. Large numbers of missing teeth, and teeth with stunted root formation, can also be a complication of chemotherapy and radiation therapy applied to treat childhood cancers.

The most frequently missing permanent teeth are the third molars and maxillary lateral incisors, followed by the premolars in either jaw. While missing third molars rarely if ever cause clinical problems, missing maxillary lateral incisors have cosmetic consequences that require working with the child's parents or legal guardians to establish a treatment strategy of space maintenance plus prosthetic replacement versus canine substitution. Similarly, missing premolars require consideration of orthodontic consequences, planning space maintenance, or closure (Fig. 6.2). Where permanent teeth are absent there is often an associated reduction in alveolar bone height and width, and drifting of adjacent teeth. If the primary tooth is retained, there are several possible outcomes. In the case of the maxillary lateral incisor, the crown size is small and short and its retention rarely provides a good cosmetic result. Crowning the primary tooth is not usually an option as the neck of the tooth is too narrow, and the root has frequently been resorbed to a greater or lesser extent. In the case of the missing premolar, the retained primary molar has a crown height that is much shorter than that of the adjacent permanent molar. The resulting malocclusion can predispose the patient to localized periodontal disease and compromise the survival of the adjacent tooth or teeth. Alternatively, the primary molar can be ankylosed (fused) to the underlying bone. In such cases, normal growth and development can cause resubmergence of the retained primary tooth. One can only surmise the difficulty that an orthodontist would have if an attempt were made to move a permanent tooth through such a submerged primary.

Ith-Hansen and Kjaer investigated persistent primary second molars in a group of young people in their late twenties with agenesis of one or two second premolars [6]. In 1982–83 it had been decided, in connection with the orthodontic evaluation of 25 patients, to allow 35 primary molars (one or two in each patient) to remain *in situ*. All patients had mixed dentitions and agenesis of one or two premolars. The primary teeth were generally in good condition, although root resorption and infraocclusion (compensated by occlusal composite onlays) occurred. In 1997, 18 of the 25 adjacent regular teeth patients with a total of 26 retained primary molars were re-examined, comprising a clinical examination for exfoliation, extraction, loosening, and ankylosis, and a radiographic examination for root resorption, tooth morphology (crown and root), and alveolar bone contour. The examination showed that the degree of root resorption was unaltered in 20 of the 26 primary molars. Three of the six remaining primary molars had been extracted and three showed extensive resorption. In three of the 26 primary molars the infraocclusion had worsened. Hence, it was concluded that persistence of primary second molars in subjects with agenesis of one or two premolars can be an acceptable, semipermanent solution. It was emphasized that further studies would be needed to establish whether this could also be an acceptable long-term solution. Obviously, if it is decided to retain a primary molar when there is premolar agenesis, the patient should be followed carefully. Periodic radiographs would be needed.

Yanagida and Mori (1990) researched congenital hypodontia using 4,009 panoramic radiographs of pedodontic patients (1,036 boys aged 2–5 years, 905 boys aged 6–11 years, and 22 boys aged 12 years or older; 1,032 girls aged 2–5 years, 985 girls aged 6–11 years 985, and 29 girls aged 12 years or older) [7].

Congenital hypodontia of primary teeth was found in 62 children (78 teeth). Congenital hypodontia of permanent teeth was found in 314 patients (566 teeth). Obviously, the majority of cases were unilateral, further complicating the treatment interventions by lack of symmetry. No significant differences were found between the right and left sides of the jaw or in relation to the patient's sex. Further, in view of the age of the patients studied, it was not possible to assess the agenesis of third permanent molars; hence, the numbers are lower than would otherwise be the case.

Peltrola et al. (1997) examined panoramic radiographs of 392 Estonian schoolchildren aged 14–17 years and found that, excluding third molars, 14% had missing teeth; 17% had missing third molars [8]. Comprehensive dental examinations and panoramic radiographs were used to determine the prevalence of hypodontia in 662 Australian military recruits [9]. Of the sampled population, 6.3% exhibited some degree of hypodontia (third molar agenesis excluded). Third molar agenesis occurred in 22.7% of the sample. There was no statistical difference between the sexes in terms of third molar agenesis; however, women exhibited an extremely low incidence of absence of maxillary lateral incisors.

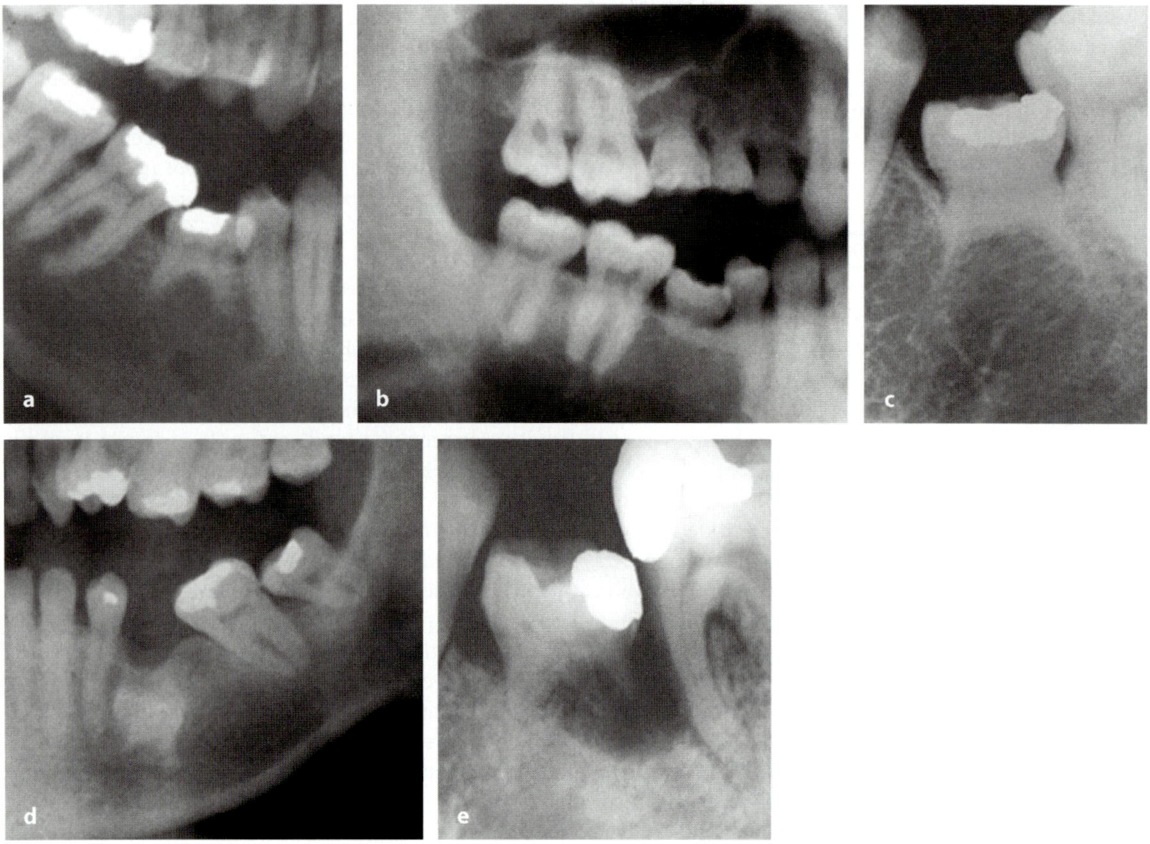

Fig. 6.2 Hypodontia with missing second mandibular premolar teeth and retained primary second molars. Each example shows a different clinical outcome. From *upper left* to *lower right* the cases show: **a** slight root resorption of retained primary and some tilting of adjacent permanent teeth; **b** marked root resorption of primary molar; **c** root resorption with bony ankylosis of retained primary molar; **d** re-submergence of retained primary tooth; **e** severe periodontal disease affecting the adjacent first permanent molar tooth

Hypodontia and Clefts

Shapira et al. (1999) studied panoramic and periapical radiographs of 278 patients with cleft lip, cleft palate, or both (158 males and 120 females), age 5–18 years, to determine the frequency of missing second premolars and the possible association between the cleft side and the side from which the premolar was absent [10]. The prevalence (18%) of missing premolars found in this study was thought to be significantly higher than that found in the general population. A considerably higher incidence of missing second premolars was found in the maxilla compared with the mandible both for unilateral and bilateral missing teeth. The second premolar was absent more frequently on the left than on the right side, both in males and females and in both jaws, corresponding to the side where clefts occurred more often.

Hypodontia and Down Syndrome

Study findings suggest a higher than normal risk of hypodontia in subjects with Down syndrome.

Kumasaka et al. (1997) used panoramic radiographs and clinical records to investigate developmentally absent permanent teeth in 98 subjects with Down syndrome (trisomy-21) [11]. This retrospective study was made using the records and panoramic radiographs of subjects from approximately five years of age through to their most recent records. The time period covered by records ranged from six to 28 years. The majority of subjects with Down syndrome (63%) exhibited hypodontia, and many subjects were missing two or more teeth (53%). Unlike in the general population, the most frequently absent teeth were the lower lateral incisors

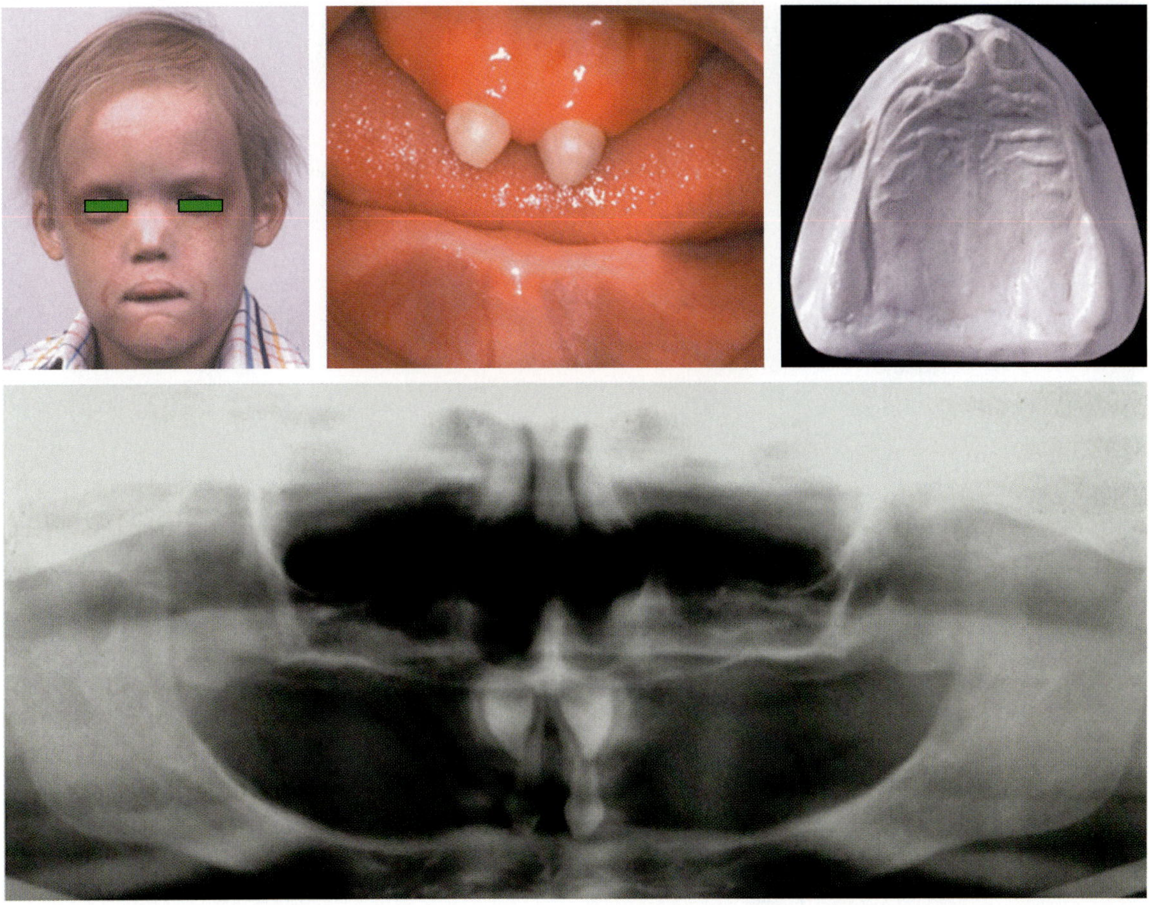

Fig. 6.3 Case of sex-linked hypohidrotic ectodermal dysplasia with severe hypodontia. The only teeth present are the primary and adult central incisors, and these are conical in shape. The child also demonstrates dry skin and sparse hair, including absence of eyebrows and eyelashes

(23.3%). The next most frequent agenesis was the upper second premolars (18.2%), the upper lateral incisors (16.5%), and the lower second premolars (15.3%). This study's findings suggest a higher than normal risk of hypodontia in subjects with Down syndrome. Shapira et al. (2000) showed a notably high prevalence of third molar agenesis in Down syndrome patients (74% of individuals older than 14 years) [12].

Hypodontia and Ectodermal Dysplasias

Teeth are essentially ectodermal appendages so dysplasia of ectoderm can affect tooth development. There is a variety of syndromes associated with severe hypodontia—or even anodontia—in view of ectodermal abnormalities (Fig. 6.3). Guckes et al. (1998) assessed the pattern of permanent teeth present in a self-selected sample of 17 female and 35 male patients with ectodermal dysplasia presenting for treatment placing dental implants [13]. The mean age of the sample was 18.7 years (age range: 5.9–60.9 years). Panoramic radiographs were examined independently by two investigators to determine the permanent teeth present. None of the sample reported extractions of permanent teeth prior to presenting for implants. The permanent teeth most likely to be present, reported as a percentage of the patient sample with that tooth, were: maxillary central incisors (42%), maxillary first molars (41%), mandibular first molars (39%), maxillary canines (22%) mandibular second molars (17%), maxillary second premolars (15%), and mandibular premolars (12%). Comparing dentition by quadrants, mandibular anterior teeth (canines and incisors) were the teeth least likely to be present.

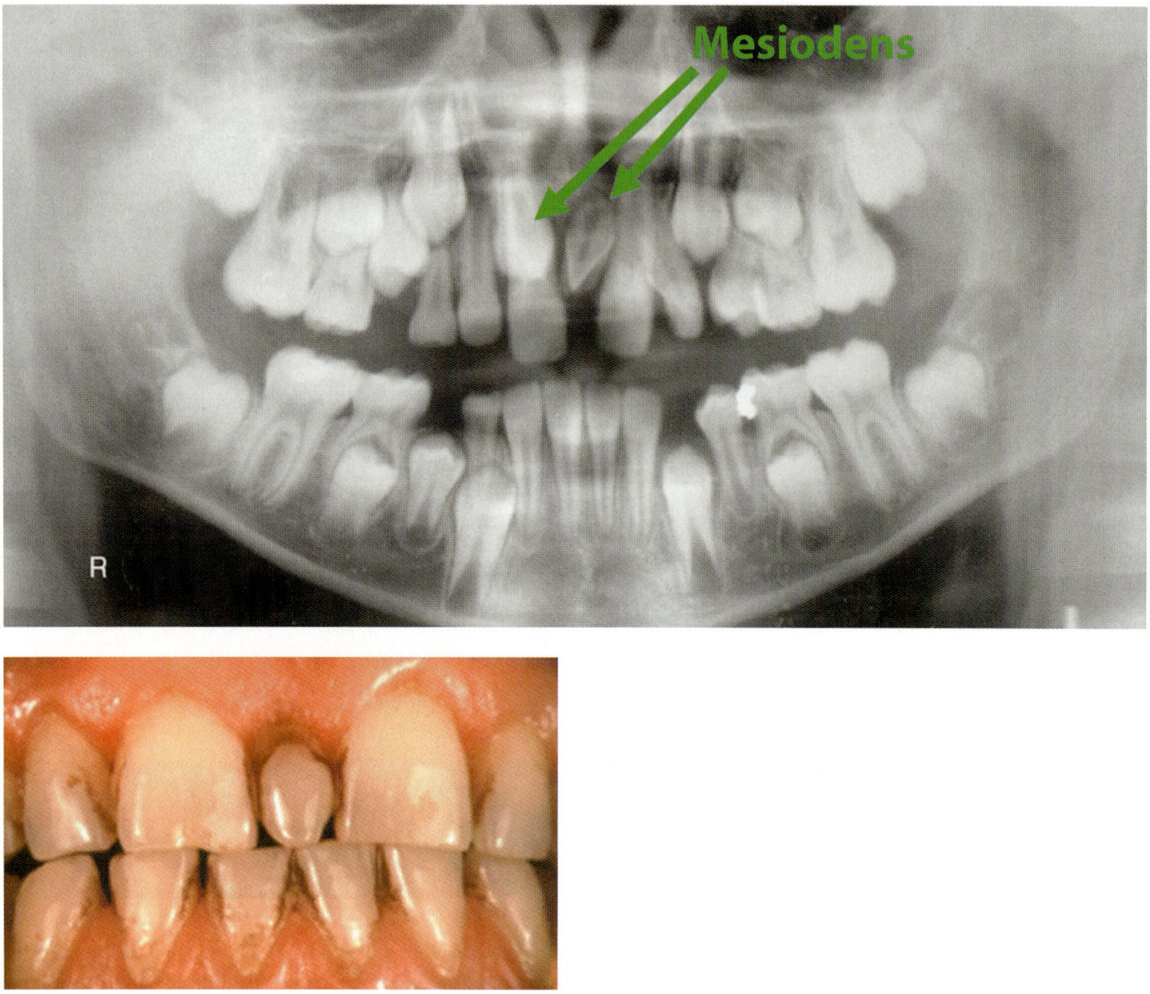

Fig. 6.4 Unerupted mesiodens (*arrow* on panoramic radiograph) is causing displacement of the adjacent regular central incisors. Uncommonly (photograph) there is room for the mesiodens to erupt and "function"

The maxillary central incisors, maxillary first molars, mandibular first molars, and maxillary canines are the most conserved teeth in hypodontia associated with ectodermal dysplasias. Successful use of osseointegrated implants in the anterior mandibles of most of these patients suggests that rehabilitation of the mandible with dental implant-supported prostheses is a reasonable option. This does not negate the need for the patient to receive instructions from a physician regarding such issues as thermal regulation and genetic consultation.

Teeth are essentially ectodermal appendages so dysplasia of ectoderm can affect tooth development.

Supernumerary Teeth

Supernumeraries are present when there is a greater than normal complement of teeth or tooth follicles. This condition is also termed hyperdontia. The frequency of supernumerary teeth in a normal population is around 3% [14]. Most supernumeraries are found in the anterior maxilla (mesiodens) or occur as para- and distomolars in that jaw (see Fig. 6.4). These are followed in frequency by premolars in both jaws (Figs. 6.5, 6.6). Pre-, post-, or paradentition supernumeraries are possible depending on the timing of development of the supernumerary teeth in relation to that of the regular teeth. Most supernumeraries are rudimentary or conical in shape; however, some are regular in shape and

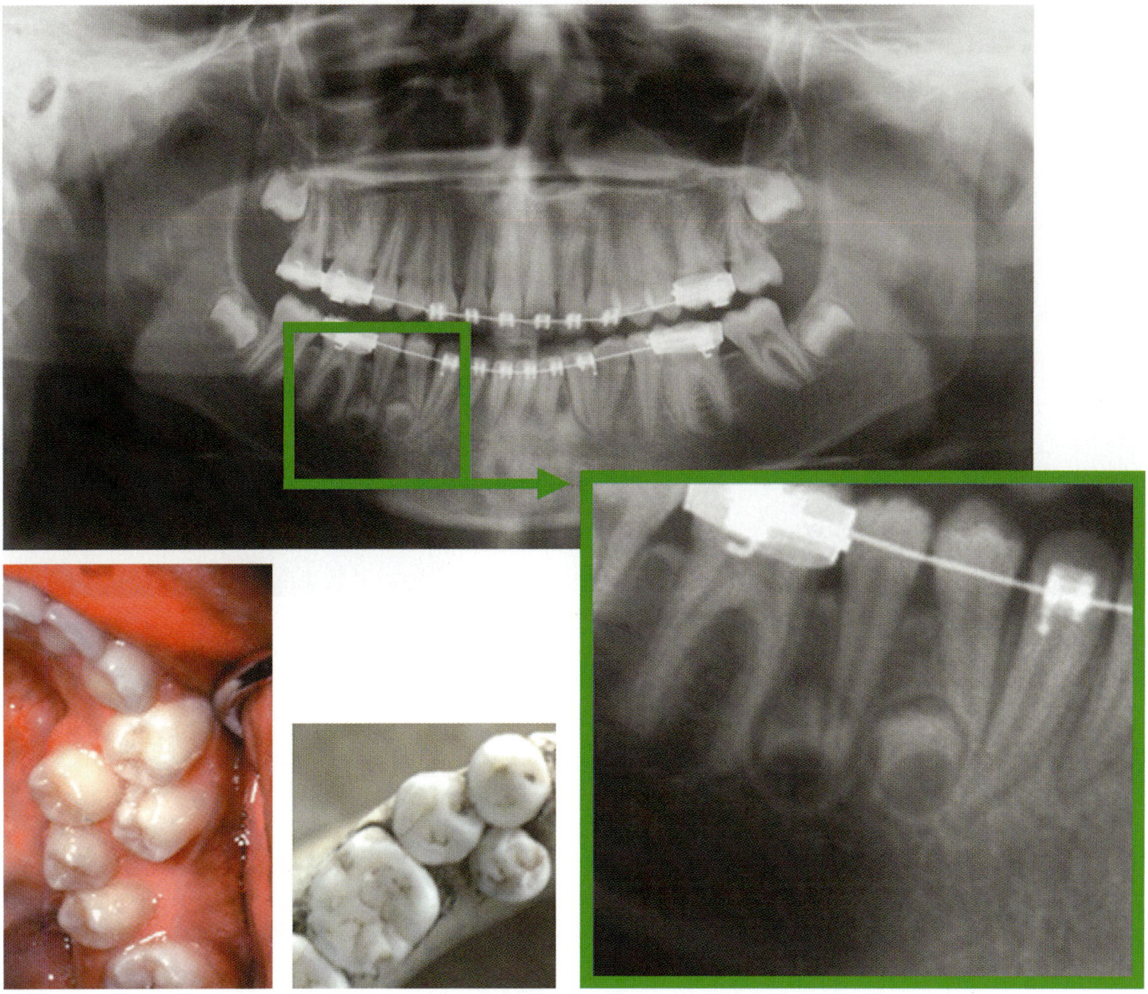

Fig. 6.5 Post-dentition supplemental supernumerary premolars are illustrated in the panoramic radiograph. The clinical photograph shows dental malocclusion occurring in a patient having three such supplemental teeth that have erupted. The dried jaw specimen is of an ancient Indian jaw more than 1,000 years old (Mississippian) showing an erupted supplemental premolar tooth

are then termed supplemental teeth. Supernumerary premolars are frequently supplemental. Complications from supernumerary teeth include impactions and displacement or delayed eruption of regular teeth.

Most individual supernumerary teeth are sporadic in occurrence; however, multiple supernumeraries can occur in association with cleidocranial dysplasia or Gardner syndrome. Multiple supernumeraries should be differentiated from compound odontomas. Compound odontomas are encapsulated discrete hamartomatous collections of denticles. Recognition of supernumerary teeth is essential to determining appropriate treatment [15]. Diagnosis and assessment of the mesiodens is critical in avoiding complications such as impedance in eruption of the maxillary central incisors, cyst formation, and dilaceration of the permanent incisors. Collecting data for diagnostic criteria, utilizing diagnostic radiographs, and determining when to refer to a specialist are important steps in the treatment of mesiodens [15]. Early diagnosis and timely surgical intervention can reduce or eliminate the need for orthodontic treatment and reduce complications to the regular dentition in such cases. As a good rule of thumb, if a permanent tooth is erupted to half its crown height and the contralateral equivalent tooth in the same arch is not seen clinically, a radiograph should be made to investigate the cause.

In a series of ten cases of supernumerary premolars treated in Barcelona: only one case altered the normal eruption of the regular premolars; in two cases fol-

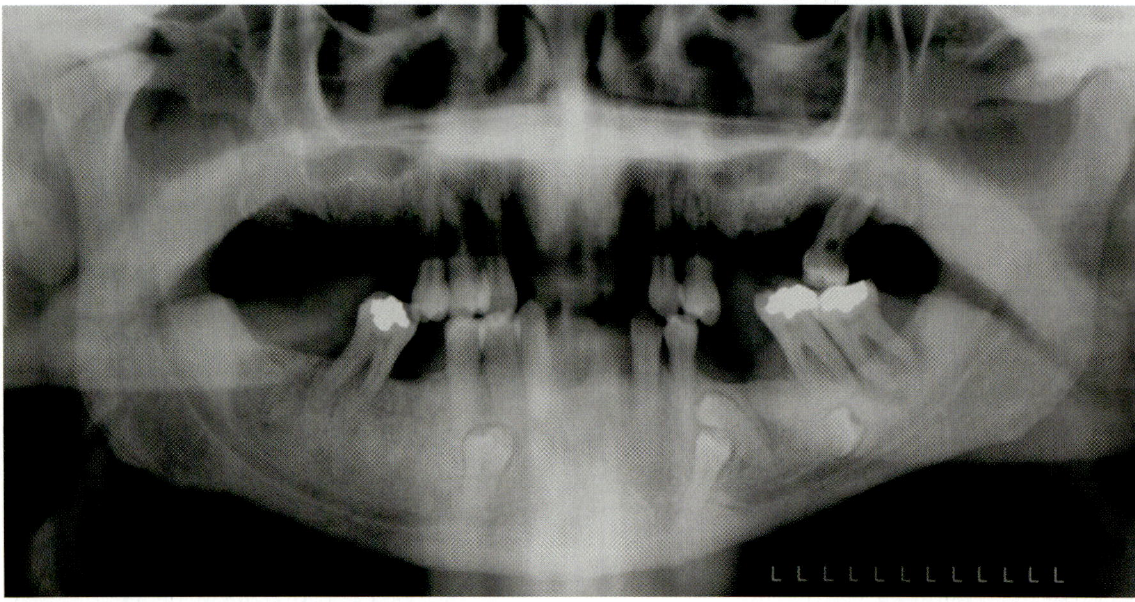

Fig. 6.6 Multiple unerupted supernumerary teeth in the mandible that are not interfering with the regular dentition. In such cases a syndrome such as cleidocranial dysplasia should be ruled out

licular cysts developed [16]. This is consistent with the supernumerary premolars commonly being post-dentition in onset and being impeded from eruption by the regular teeth. Panoramic radiography is an important step toward the identification, localization and surgical removal of such supernumerary teeth [17].

Cleidocranial Dysplasia

Cleidocranial dysplasia is an autosomally dominant condition characterized by defective ossification of cranial bones and clavicles.

Cleidocranial dysplasia is an autosomally dominant condition characterized by defective ossification of cranial bones and clavicles. It is associated with multiple supernumerary teeth, especially anterior to the first permanent molars, retained primary teeth and unerupted permanent teeth (Fig. 6.7). There is also delayed fontanel closure, and hypoplasia or aplasia of the clavicles [18].

McNamara et al. (1999) reported the effectiveness of dental panoramic radiography in identifying features pathognomonic for cleidocranial dysplasia [19]. In addition to the established dental complications of failure of eruption of the permanent dentition and multiple supernumerary teeth, morphological abnormalities of the maxilla and mandible, particularly in the ascending ramus and coronoid process are present. While there often are numerous supernumerary teeth present in cleidocranial dysplasia this might not be apparent clinically. Failures in tooth eruption often results in apparent hypodontia. It is often necessary to fabricate overdentures for the prosthodontic treatment of such patients. Dentigerous cysts may form around the crowns of unerupted regular and supernumerary teeth weakening the structure of the jaw and predisposing it to pathologic fracture. Dental panoramic radiography is a valuable adjunct in confirming the diagnosis of cleidocranial dysplasia and in subsequently checking for dentigerous cyst formation.

Gardner Syndrome

Gardner syndrome (familial adenomatosis coli; intestinal polyposis type II) is characterized by the occurrence of multiple impacted supernumerary teeth, osteomas of

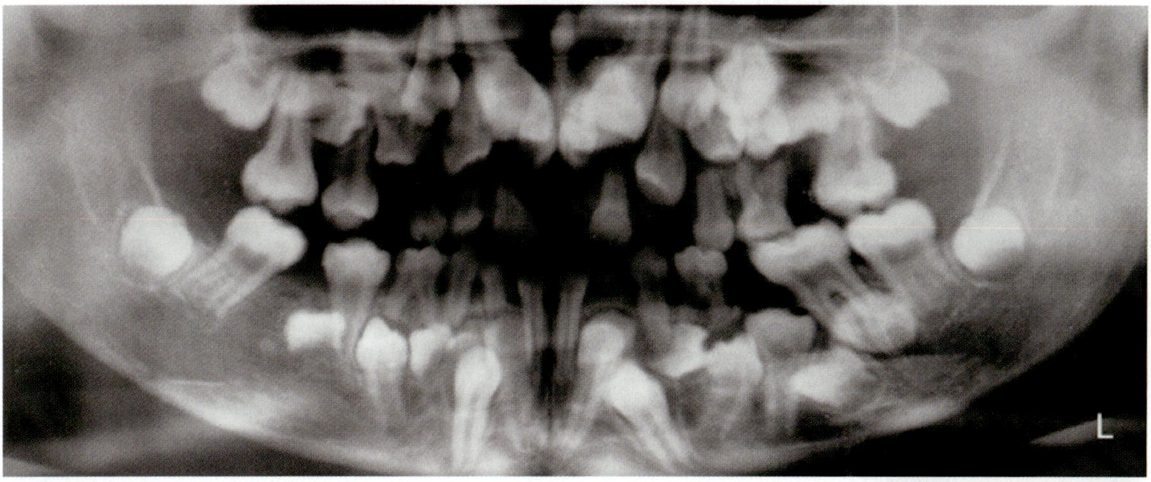

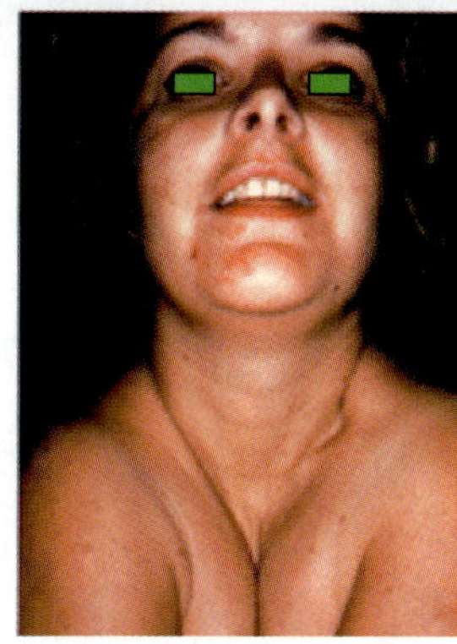

Fig. 6.7 Cleidocranial dysplasia is associated with multiple supernumerary teeth (panoramic radiograph). Affected patients often have hypoplastic or absent clavicles and have the flexibility to bring their shoulders close together in the midline (e.g., photograph)

the long bones, skull and jaws, multiple polyposis of the large intestines and multiple epidermoid or dermoid cysts. The intestinal polyps are premalignant. Detection of osteomas in the jaws and multiple supernumerary teeth (Fig. 6.8) on panoramic radiography can lead to the early determination of the syndrome and preventive management of a potentially fatal malignancy [20]. In a matched study 82% of patients having this syndrome showed osteomatous changes compared to 10% of controls. Supernumerary teeth, compound odontomas and impacted teeth were found in 30% of patients having Gardner syndrome compared to 4% of controls.

Anomalies in Tooth Size

Macrodontia

Macrodontia involves a tooth or teeth being larger than normal in size with proportional enlargement of pulp chamber, crown, and root (Fig. 6.9). This condition can be general or localized. General true macrodontia can be associated with pituitary giantism. Unilateral relative macrodontia can occur in hemifacial hypertrophy. Macrodontia is often sporadic, but can also be a feature of Ekman-Westborg-Julin syndrome and can also occur in association with hemangioma [21, 22].

There is usually a normal complement of teeth. Macrodontia needs to be differentiated from connation (gemination or fusion) and concrescence. In gemination there is division of a tooth with an attempt to make an additional tooth. In fusion there is combination of two or more teeth with a reduction in number. For fusion, this number count presupposes that the combination does not involve a supernumerary tooth or teeth. Concrescence is the joining of adjacent teeth through cementum.

Early detection of macrodontia is of importance for orthodontic planning of space and cosmetic intervention. Certainly if space is not available for eruption of all of the teeth due to macrodontia, impaction or malocclusion is likely to ensue. Panoramic radiology can help in early diagnosis. Caution needs to be applied; however, as the crown of a tooth that is lingually (i.e., palatally) displaced will appear magnified horizontally on standard panoramic views. Moreover care needs to be made to ensure the patient was positioned symmetrically in the cephalostat. Rotation or lateral displace-

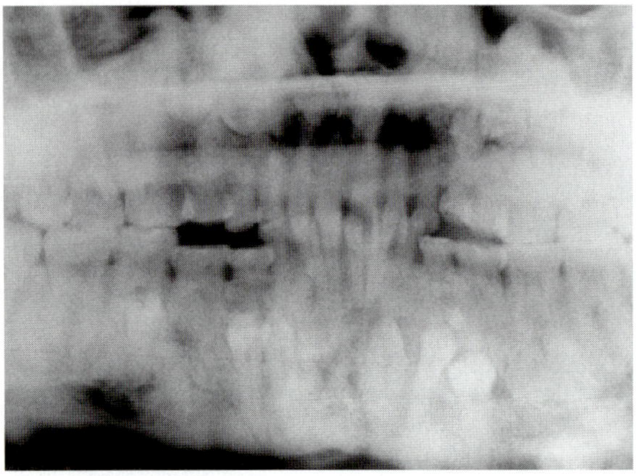

Fig. 6.8 Gardner syndrome: multiple osteomas are present in both jaws and there are also retained primary teeth and multiple impacted permanent teeth. Such patients are also prone to develop intestinal cancer

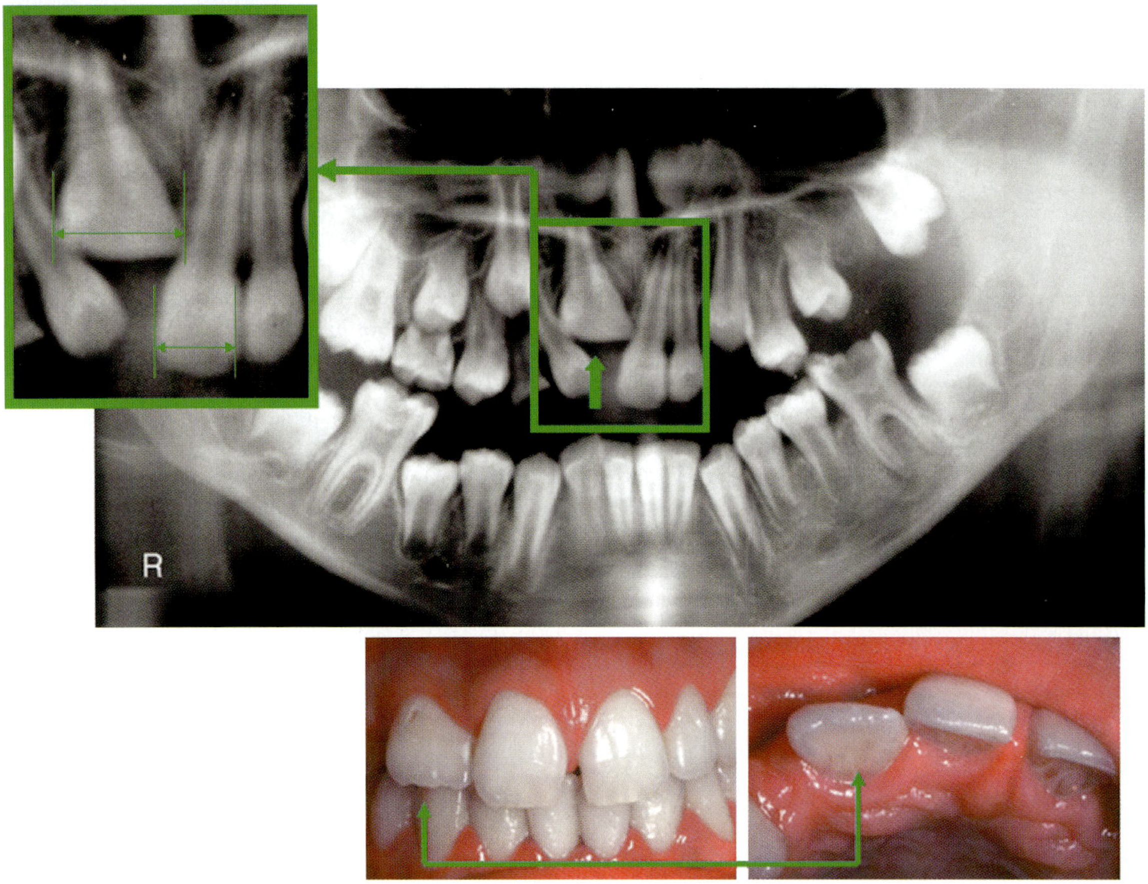

Fig. 6.9 Sporadic macrodontia results in a disproportionately large tooth crown in comparison with the contralateral counterpart tooth (radiograph). The photograph illustrates a case of macrodont lateral incisor in which the tooth was similar in size to a maxillary central incisor tooth

ment of the head during panoramic radiology can cause one side of the jaws and teeth to be minified, while the other side is magnified.

Microdontia

Microdontia implies the abnormal smallness of a single or multiple teeth. This is most commonly an isolated anomaly such as a peg lateral or diminutive third molar tooth (Fig. 6.10). The diminutive tooth tends to be somewhat conical in shape. Such teeth need to be differentiated from rudimentary supernumerary teeth, and abnormally shaped teeth due to ectodermal dysplasia or radiation in childhood. Early detection of microdontia can be effected by use of panoramic radiology for evaluation of growth and development.

Microdontia implies the abnormal smallness of a single or multiple teeth. This is most commonly an isolated anomaly such as a peg lateral or diminutive third molar tooth.

Baccetti (1998) examined patterns of association among five types of dental anomalies (aplasia of second premolars, small size of maxillary lateral incisors, infraocclusion of primary molars, ectopic eruption of first molars, and palatal displacement of maxillary canines) in an untreated orthodontic population, aged 7–14 years [23]. The prevalence of associated tooth anomalies in five groups of 100 subjects each and characterized by the constant presence of one primarily diagnosed dental anomaly was compared to the prevalence for the examined dental anomalies in a control group of 1,000 subjects, deriving from a common initial sample of 4,850 subjects. Significant reciprocal associations ($p < 0.008$) were found among the dental anomalies studied. The statistically demonstrated existence of associations among different tooth anomalies was felt to be clinically relevant, since the diagnosis of a dental anomaly may indicate an increased chance for later tooth developmental and eruption disturbances.

Anomalies in Root Formation

While morphological dental crown anomalies are most frequently detected without the use of radiographs, anomalies in root morphology are usually not apparent without the assistance of radiography. For this reason,

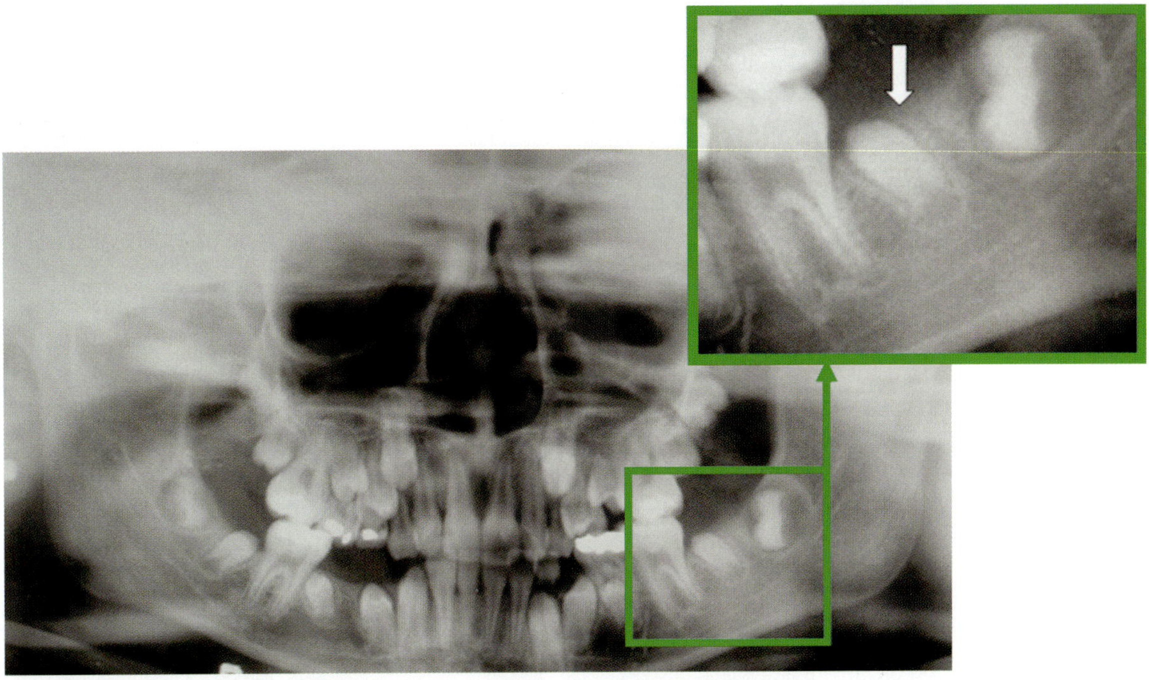

Fig. 6.10 Bilateral microdont mandibular second permanent molar teeth. In such a situation preservation of the third molars should be a consideration

less attention will be made to anomalies in morphology of tooth crowns, especially for conditions affecting the anterior teeth. Nevertheless, such conditions can be frequently encountered in the average private general practice and do affect dental treatment planning.

Dilaceration

Dilaceration is an angulation in the root or crown [18, 24]. The determined prevalence of dilaceration depends largely on the subjective assessment of what is "normal" and what is "excessive" angulation. All tooth roots are curved to some degree, so the term dilaceration is reserved for instances of excess or abnormal root curvature that could complicate endodontic or exodontic treatment (Fig. 6.11). The configuration of the root of a prospective abutment tooth has a significant influence on its potential load bearing capacity; hence, this abnormality can also affect the stability and longevity of an abutment [24]. Dilaceration is most common in the permanent dentition. It is thought to result from prior local infection, trauma or impaction; however, the precise cause has not been elucidated. Clinically, the tooth often appears structurally and positionally normal so the condition is most likely to be discovered radiographically. It should be remembered that conventional radiographs, including panoramic images, are essentially two-dimensional shadows of three-dimensional objects. While mesio-distal dilacerations are relatively easy to determine, bucco-lingual angulations require a little more attention to detail. With dilacerations in a bucco-

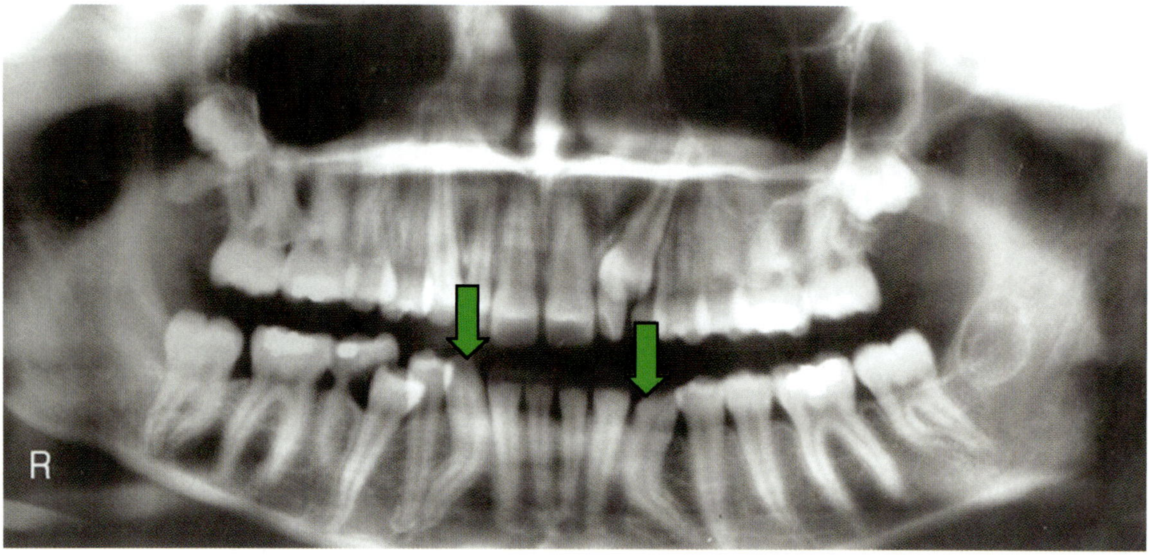

Fig. 6.11 Bilateral dilacerations of mandibular canines was only evident following radiography. This would need to be considered should orthodontic, endodontic, exodontic, or fixed prosthodontic treatment involve these teeth in the future

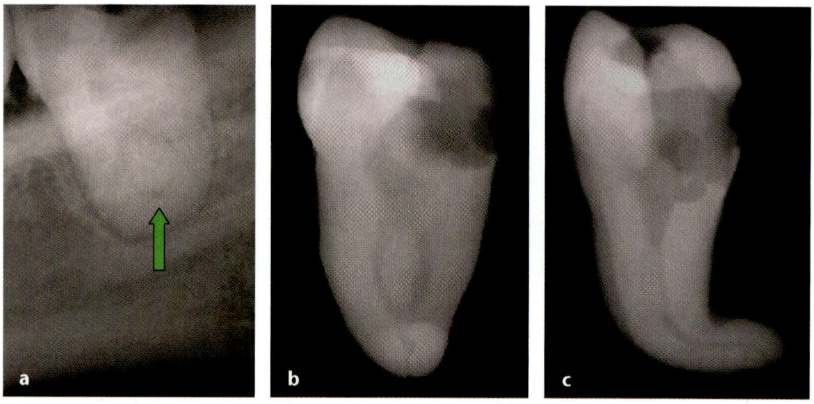

Fig. 6.12 Bucco-lingual dilacerations need careful radiographic scrutiny for the "bull's eye" sign shown in the pre-extraction radiographic detail (**a**). Radiographs of the extracted tooth are shown in a similar orientation to the pre-extraction radiograph (**b**) and rotated through 90° (**c**)

lingual direction, the radiographic appearance is that of a "bull's eye" root (Fig. 6.12) caused by a view down the root axis showing the innermost pulp canal surrounded by tooth structure [18]. Missing these forms of dilacerations has been postulated to be a significant factor in the failure of endodontic treatment due to miscalculation of position of the actual root apex [25].

Taurodontism

Taurodontism is usually bilateral and symmetric in distribution, although involvement of an isolated tooth is not rare.

Taurodontism is an inherited morphological anomaly of multirooted teeth caused by failure of invagination of the Hertwig epithelial root sheath [18]. Taurodontism is usually bilateral and symmetric in distribution, although involvement of an isolated tooth is not rare. Clinical examination of involved teeth fails to reveal any abnormality. Radiologically, affected molar or premolar teeth appear rectangular with an absence of the normal cervical constriction of the root. There is an increased occlusal-apical dimension to the pulp chamber with diminished apical root length (Figs. 6.13, 6.14).

Taurodontism has been reported in association with a number of conditions [26–30]; and is frequently seen in patients having excessive numbers of X chromosomes [31, 32]. However, it can occur in otherwise normal individuals, perhaps as an atavistic memory of prehistoric ancestors. As will be found in most standard texts, the condition has been reported in Neanderthal remains found in various sites in Europe [33, 34]. Neanderthals are known to exhibit enlarged pulp chambers in posterior teeth (taurodontism); however, Bailey (2002) found that they also present a high rate of a mid-trigonid crest in lower molars [35]. Taurodontism is, nonetheless, relatively common in modern man, particularly in Africa [35, 36]. Toure et al. (2000) reported a frequency of 48% in 150 consecutive Senegalese dental patients aged 15–19 years with 18.8% of first and second molars being affected [35]. By way of comparison, the prevalence of taurodontism in Jordanians was determined to be 8%, and 11% in a Saudi population [37, 38]. MacDonald-Jankowski and Li found taurodontism in 56% of female and 36% of male Chinese adolescents who they studied [39]. Hence, in diverse populations, taurodontism can be considered simply a variation of normal.

Regarding the implications of taurodontism for dental treatment, successful endodontic therapy has been documented in such teeth [40]. It has also been reported that taurodonts show increased susceptibility to apical root resorption during orthodontic treatment [41]. Panoramic radiography has been found to be a reliable means of assessing taurodontism [42].

Enamel Pearl

The most common site for enamel pearls is at the cementoenamel junction of multirooted teeth [18]. They are most commonly mesial or distal on maxillary teeth and buccal or lingual on mandibular teeth (Fig. 6.15). Enamel pearls most often occur singly and can be composed exclusively of enamel. They vary in size from microscopic to a few millimeters. Radiologically, they are depicted as dense, smooth radio-opacities overlying any portion of the crown or root of an otherwise unaffected tooth. The major radiologic differential diagnosis is projection geometry causing overlap of root contours in multirooted teeth. In the primary dentition, radiographic interpretation and detection of the enamel pearl can be complicated by the superimposition of the developing permanent tooth [43]. In a study of dental patients, the frequency reported for enamel pearls on molar teeth was 1.6% [44]. It has been reported that enamel pearls can predispose to local periodontal disease and should therefore be removed [45]; however, as they can contain dentin and pulp, caution is advised.

Connation

Connate or "double" teeth include both fusion and gemination. In the case of fusion of adjacent teeth, there should be a reduction in the total number of teeth so long as one of the fused teeth is not a supernumerary. In the case of gemination, there can be the clinical appearance of an added tooth. The result, in either case, is a tooth with an unusually broad crown that may show grooving between elements that are connected by enamel, dentin, pulp, or a combination of these tissues.

Connation is comparatively rare depending on the population, being found in from 0.08% of Saudi children to 1.5% of patients examined in western India [46–49]. Unless there is failure in eruption, connation is often obvious upon clinical inspection (Fig. 6.16). Clinical problems relating to fusion include unacceptable appearance, misalignment of teeth and periodontal disease predisposition [50].

Concrescence

Concrescence is the joining of adjacent teeth through cemental union of their roots [18]. It can either occur during development or be acquired. The cardinal radiologic sign of concrescence is close proximity of adjacent teeth with no detectable intervening periodontal ligament space shadow. When developmental, it might be associated with failed eruption of one or more teeth. When acquired, it can be associated with gross hypercementosis.

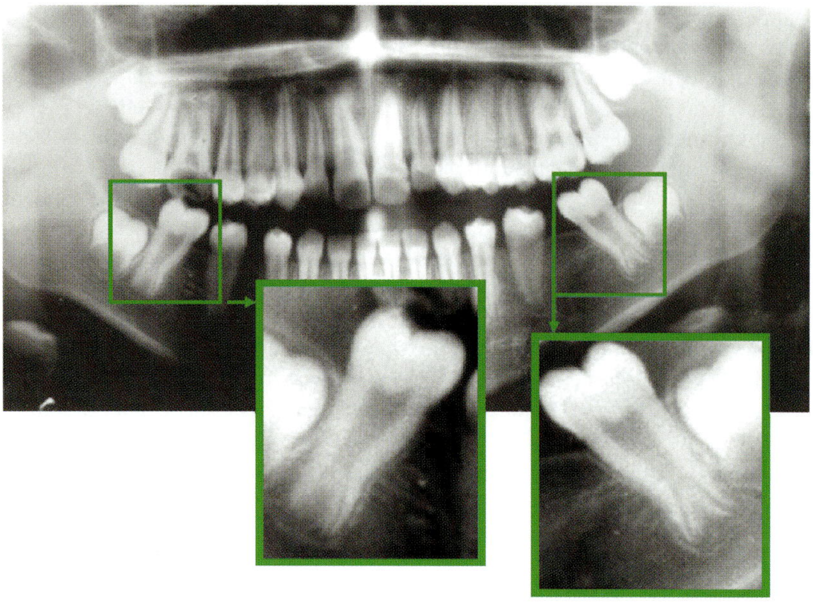

Fig. 6.13 Taurodontism. The mandibular first molar teeth are missing due to extraction in this adolescent patient. The fully formed mandibular second molar teeth show the typical features of taurodontism, namely an extended pulp chamber and very short apical roots

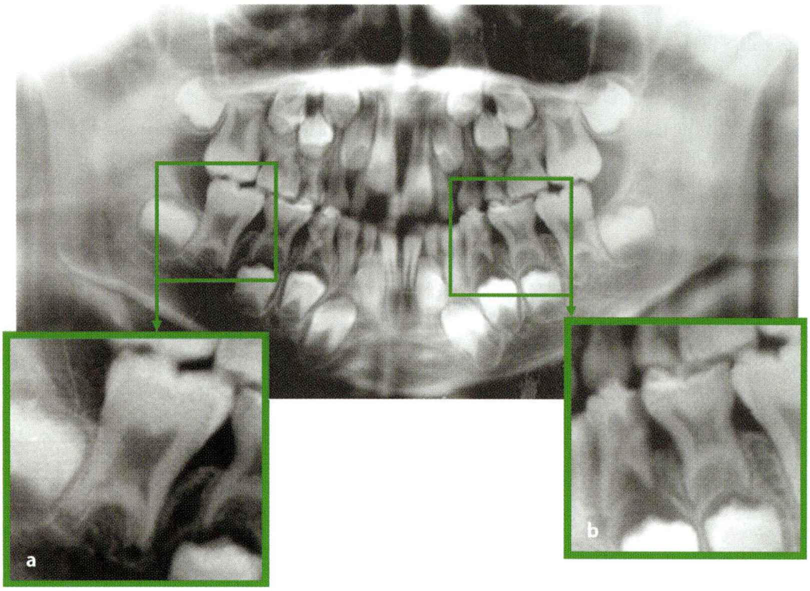

Fig. 6.14 Taurodontism in the mixed dentition showing that this condition can affect both permanent (*enlargement a*) and primary (*enlargement b*) dentitions

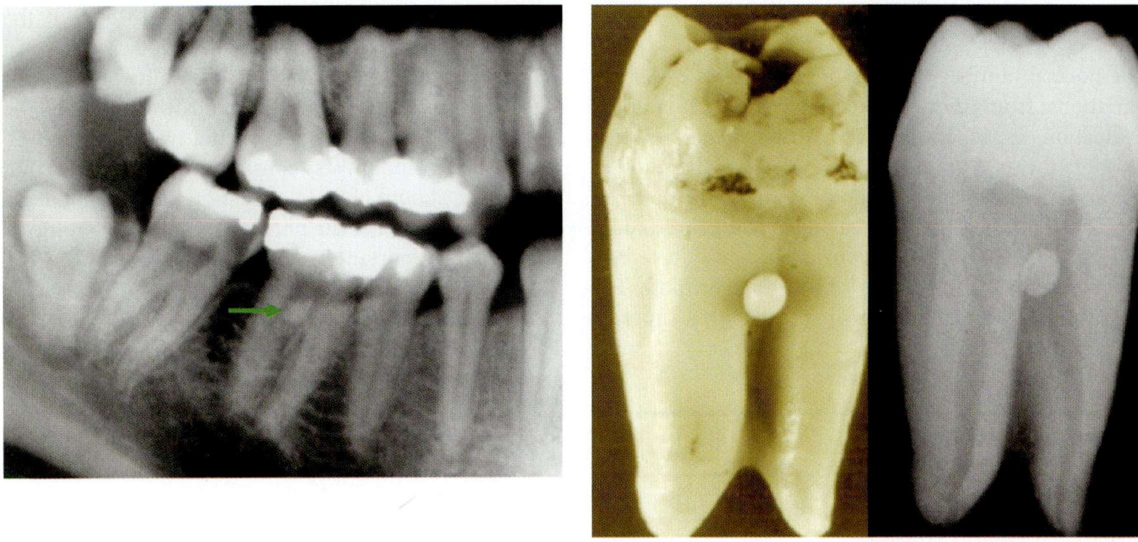

Fig. 6.15 Enamel pearl shown (*arrow*) on the detail of a panoramic radiograph. The photographic appearance of enamel pearl on an extracted molar tooth and the radiograph of this extracted tooth are also illustrated

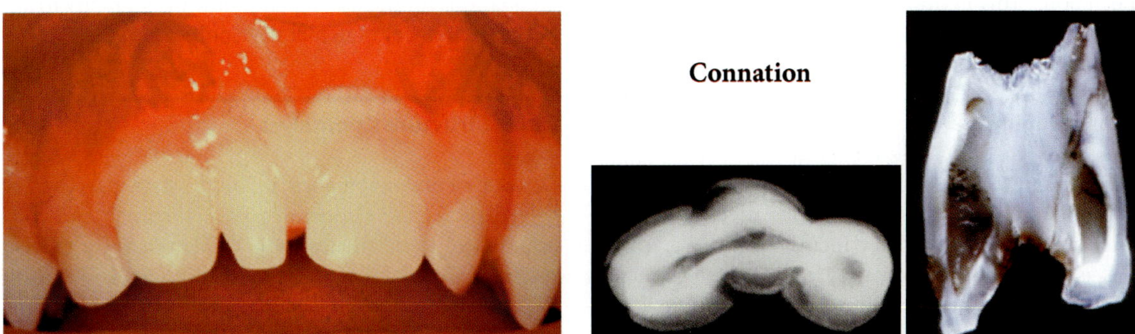

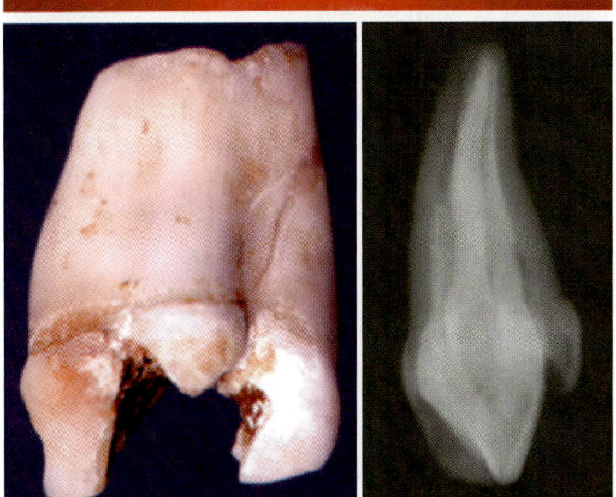

Fig. 6.16 The *upper clinical picture* shows a case of connation (gemination) of a maxillary central incisor complicated by periodontal disease and lateral periodontal abscess. The *lower image sequence* is of a connation specimen where a mesiodens is fused to two primary central incisors

Supernumerary Roots

The normal number of roots or root canals can show variations from the expected, making radiographic evaluation especially relevant when planning endodontic therapy or exodontias [51, 52]. Mandibular molars generally have two roots; however, the detail in Fig. 6.17a shows a mandibular molar with three roots. Similarly, the only premolar to consistently have two separate roots is the maxillary first premolar tooth. Figure 17b shows a mandibular premolar with a supernumerary root.

Anomalies of Tooth Crowns

Talon Cusp

A tooth with a talon cusp generally appears T-shaped (Fig. 6.18a) when viewed from the incisal edge with most additional cusps being lingual and only rare reports of facial "talons" [53, 54]. This condition is clinically obvious and only requires radiographic analysis to determine whether pulpal extensions is present within the "talon." This is best performed using periapical radiography.

Dens Invaginatus

Dens invaginatus (dens in dente) refers to invagination of tooth structure, most commonly affecting the cingular surface of a maxillary incisor tooth (Fig. 6.18b). This is often, but not invariably, suspected clinically. The lesion needs radiographic appraisal, principally using an intraoral radiograph. If no entrance to the invagination can be detected clinically and there are no signs of pulp pathosis, then no treatment is required other than fissure sealing of the invagination [55, 56]. In deep invaginations, it is likely that root-canal treatment will be required. Extensive enamel invaginations can be apparent on panoramic radiography, as will complication sequelae such as an apical dental abscess, cyst, or granuloma.

Dens invaginatus (dens in dente) refers to invagination of tooth structure, most commonly affecting the cingular surface of a maxillary incisor tooth.

Dens Evaginatus

Dens evaginatus (Fig. 6.18c, d) is uncommon in most populations, but occurs in roughly 2% of Asians and AmerIndians [57]. In this dental anomaly, an extra cusp or tubercle protrudes from the occlusal surface of posterior teeth, or occasionally, from the lingual surface of anterior teeth [58]. Complications can arise if the tubercle is worn, ground, or fractured off, resulting in pulpal exposure and possible loss of vitality of the tooth. Radiographs are important to assess the shape of the pulp chamber should dental restorative procedures be required. Orthodontists, considering premolar extraction cases, should include extraction of the anomalous premolars instead of the normal ones. Radiographic assessment is important in such instances.

Panoramic Radiology: An Important Adjunct in the Assessment of Dental Morphology

Panoramic radiography is an important adjunct to clinical inspection for detection of anomalies in dental morphology. Such findings are important in selecting teeth for extraction when needed for orthodontic reasons. Cholitgul and Drummond (2000) studied the panoramic radiographs of 1,608 children and adolescents from New Zealand and found tooth abnormalities in 21% of these radiographs. They concluded that panoramic radiography is valuable for detecting or confirming dental abnormalities, and supported recommendations for the use of panoramic radiography to aid in the assessment of dental development [59].

Tooth Structure Anomalies

Developmental anomalies in tooth structure can involve dental enamel, dentin, pulp, cementum, or a combination of these tissues [60]. While relatively precise typing of some of these anomalies is now possible using techniques in molecular biology, radiography remains important in the assessment of phenotypic manifestations and is often essential in treatment planning for esthetics and function of dental restorations. The panoramic radiograph provides a useful overview of the dentition both for dental anomalies affecting all teeth and for those that are localized to a specific region. The panoramic radiograph might need to be supplemented by selected periapical images when restorative procedures are to be planned.

Enamel Hypoplasia

Enamel hypoplasia is either an inherited imperfect enamel formation (amelogenesis imperfecta), or "environmental hypoplasia" acquired during development due to local or systemic influences (see Fig. 6.19) [61]. Systemic conditions will affect the portion of the crown being formed during the influence of the condition. Systemic conditions associated with enamel hypoplasia include birth-related trauma (Fig. 6.19d), certain chemicals (e.g., excess fluoride, Fig. 6.19c, tetracycline,

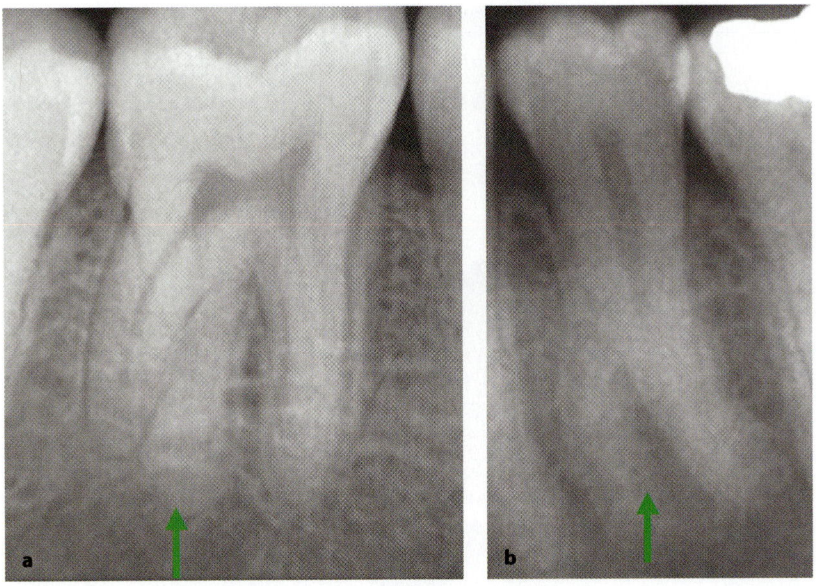

Fig. 6.17 **a** Supernumerary root (*arrow*) on mandibular molar tooth. **b** Supernumerary root (*arrow*) on mandibular premolar tooth

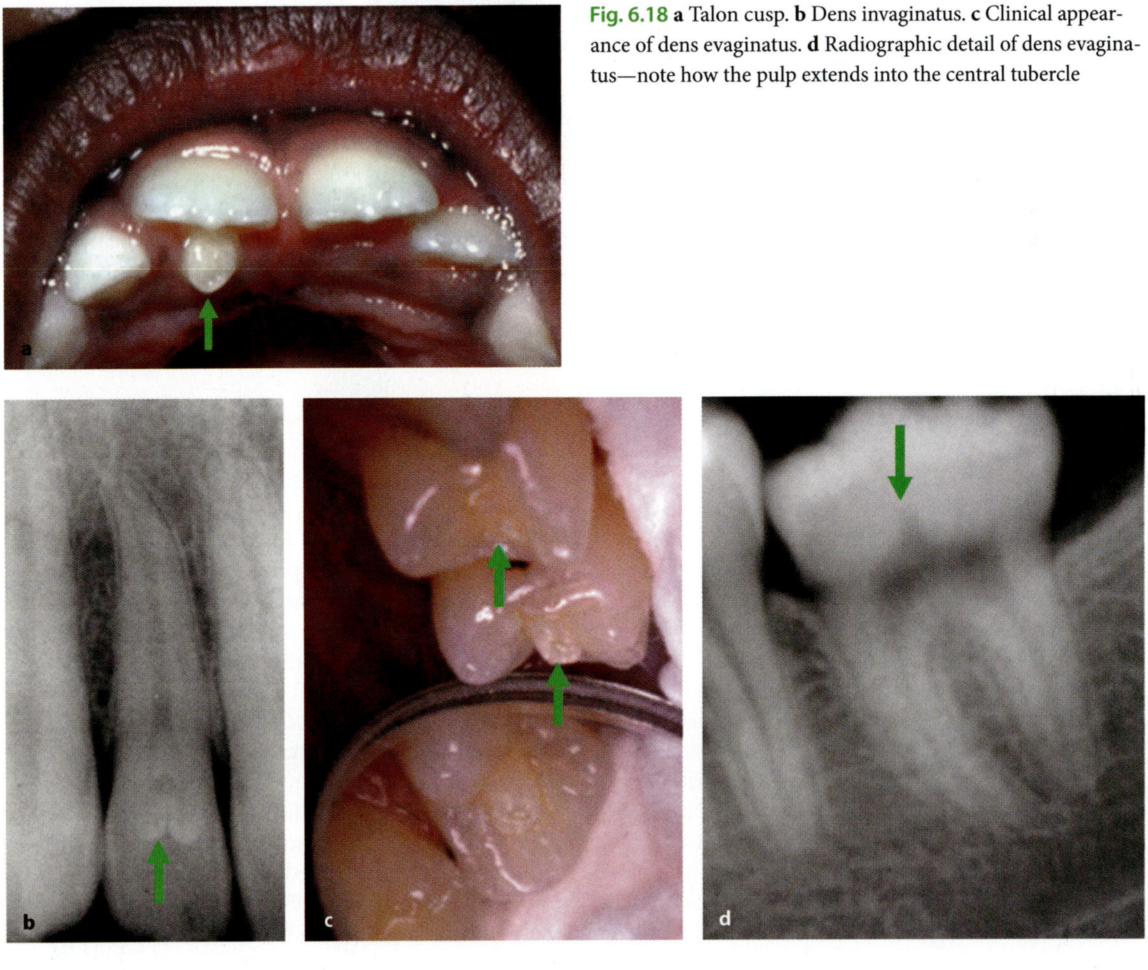

Fig. 6.18 **a** Talon cusp. **b** Dens invaginatus. **c** Clinical appearance of dens evaginatus. **d** Radiographic detail of dens evaginatus—note how the pulp extends into the central tubercle

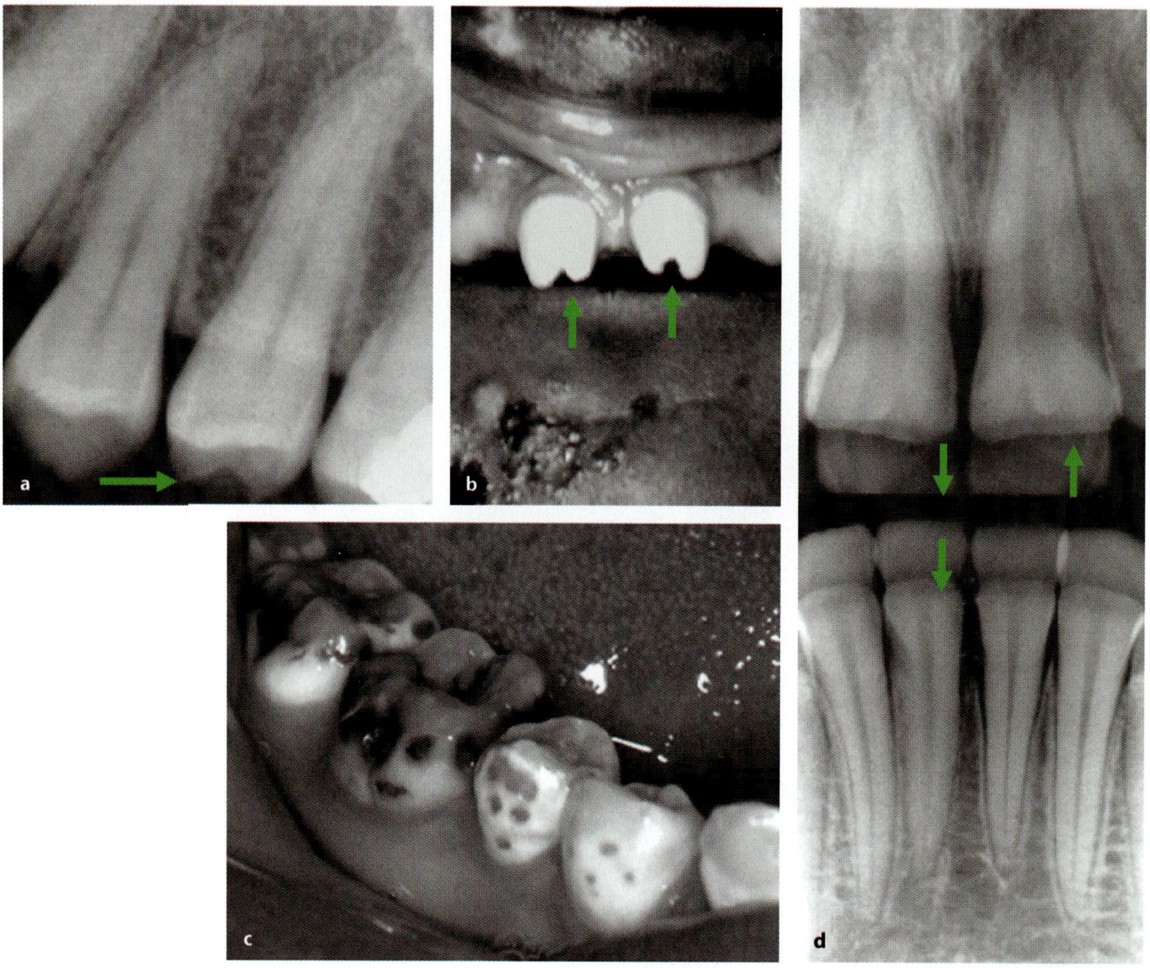

Fig. 6.19 Enamel hypoplasia. **a** The second premolar is a Turner tooth with hypoplasia (*arrow*) likely due to local infection from an abscessed primary second molar. **b** Hutchinson incisors due to congenital syphilis showing typical notching of the incisor edges (*arrow*). **c** Enamel hypoplasia due to dental fluorosis. **d** Enamel hypoplasia in a band (*arrows*) representing the degree of crown formation of the permanent teeth at the time of birth trauma

thalidomide), infections (e.g., chicken pox, measles, rubella, syphilis, Fig. 6.19b), malnutrition, and metabolic disorders [60–63].

Aine et al. (2000) determined that the prevalence of enamel defects in children born prematurely was significantly higher compared with controls in both the primary (78% versus 20%, $p < 0.001$) and permanent (83% versus 36%, $p < 0.001$) dentitions [64]. Low birth weight is also associated with a significantly increased rate of enamel hypoplasia. Ninety-six percent of low birth weight compared to 45% of the normal control children had at least one tooth with enamel defects (a mean of eight teeth were affected per low birth weight child versus a mean of one affected tooth per control child; $p < 0.001$) [65]. Nunn et al. (2000) found 22% of children with renal disease to have enamel hypoplasia [66]. Local causes of enamel hypoplasia include inflammatory disease from a primary tooth with the underlying permanent tooth becoming a Turner tooth (Fig. 6.19a), local infections, local mechanical or electrical trauma, or childhood radiation therapy [60].

Local causes of enamel hypoplasia include inflammatory disease from a primary tooth with the underlying permanent tooth becoming a Turner tooth, local infections, local mechanical or electrical trauma, or childhood radiation therapy.

Amelogenesis Imperfecta

Amelogenesis imperfecta includes a variety of developmental alterations in enamel structure unrelated to systemic disease. The reported prevalence of amelogenesis imperfecta varies from 1:700 to 1:8,000 depending on the population studied [60]. Both primary and perma-

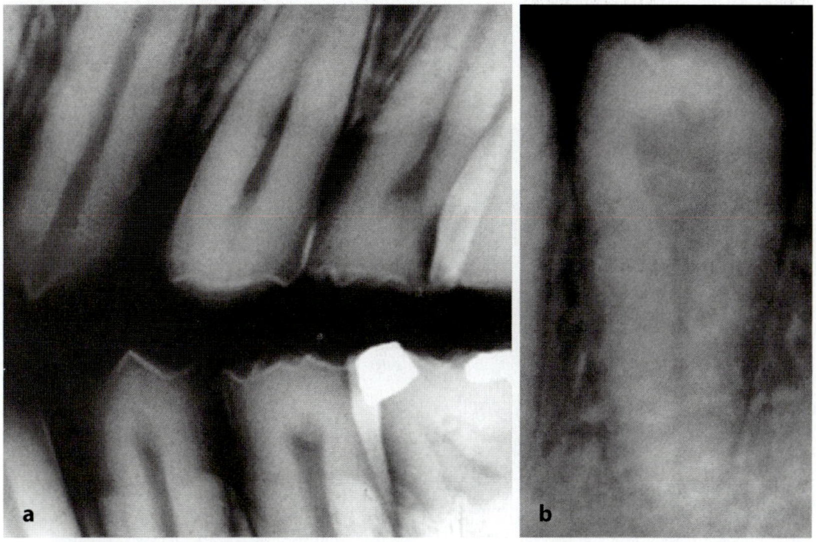

Fig. 6.20 Smooth hypoplastic amelogenesis imperfecta. Two cases (**a**, **b**) where the enamel is much thinner than normal but smooth in surface configuration

nent dentitions are affected. According to Witkop [67] there are at least 14 different varieties of amelogenesis imperfecta, which can be divided according to the enamel development stage affected, namely: elaboration of organic matrix (hypoplastic), mineralization of the matrix (hypocalcified), and maturation of enamel (hypomaturation). Amelogenesis imperfecta has seen much recent publication of findings regarding genetic causations [68–71]. This review will, however, keep to phenotypic signs as is appropriate to a paper concerning radiologic signs.

Hypoplastic Amelogenesis Imperfecta

These conditions are caused by inadequate enamel matrix deposition. Generalized pitted amelogenesis imperfecta (Type IA) is autosomal dominant with affected teeth displaying horizontal rows of pits or linear depressions. Localized pitted amelogenesis imperfecta can be dominant (Type IB) or recessive (Type IC), the latter typically being the more widespread and severe of these localized varieties.

Smooth hypoplastic amelogenesis imperfecta (Fig. 6.20) results in smooth, glossy enamel of less than regular thickness. The tooth color varies from white opaque to brown. It can be inherited as autosomal dominant (Type ID) or X-linked recessive (Type IE). The dominant variety is generalized, whereas the X-linked variety is generalized for males but can show a mosaic for females where there may be one affected and one normal X chromosome present. In such females there can be alternating areas of normal and abnormal enamel.

Rough hypoplastic amelogenesis imperfecta (Type IF) is autosomal dominant. The enamel is thin, hard, rough-surfaced, and can readily become stained (Fig. 6.21). Enamel agenesis (amelogenesis imperfecta Type IG) has teeth that are the color and shape of dentin with crowns tapering toward the rough, occlusal surface.

Hypomaturation Amelogenesis Imperfecta

In hypomaturation varieties (Fig. 6.22a), the enamel matrix is formed normally and initiates mineralization, but the enamel crystals do not mature normally. Radiographically, the affected enamel has a radiodensity approximating that of dentin. Hypomaturation amelogenesis imperfecta can be autosomal recessive and pigmented (Type IIA), X-linked recessive (Type IIB), or X-linked with "snow-capped cusps" (Type IIC). There might also exist an autosomal dominant variety that is present with "snow-capped cusps" (Type IID).

Hypocalcified Amelogenesis Imperfecta

In these types (Fig. 6.22b, c) the enamel matrix is formed normally, but calcification is slight. The teeth are of normal appearance on eruption but the enamel is very soft and rapidly abrades. Radiographically, the radiodensities of the enamel and dentin are similar. Autosomal dominant (Type IIIA) and autosomal recessive (Type IIIB) amelogenesis imperfecta types exist. Combined hypomaturation/hypoplastic amelogenesis

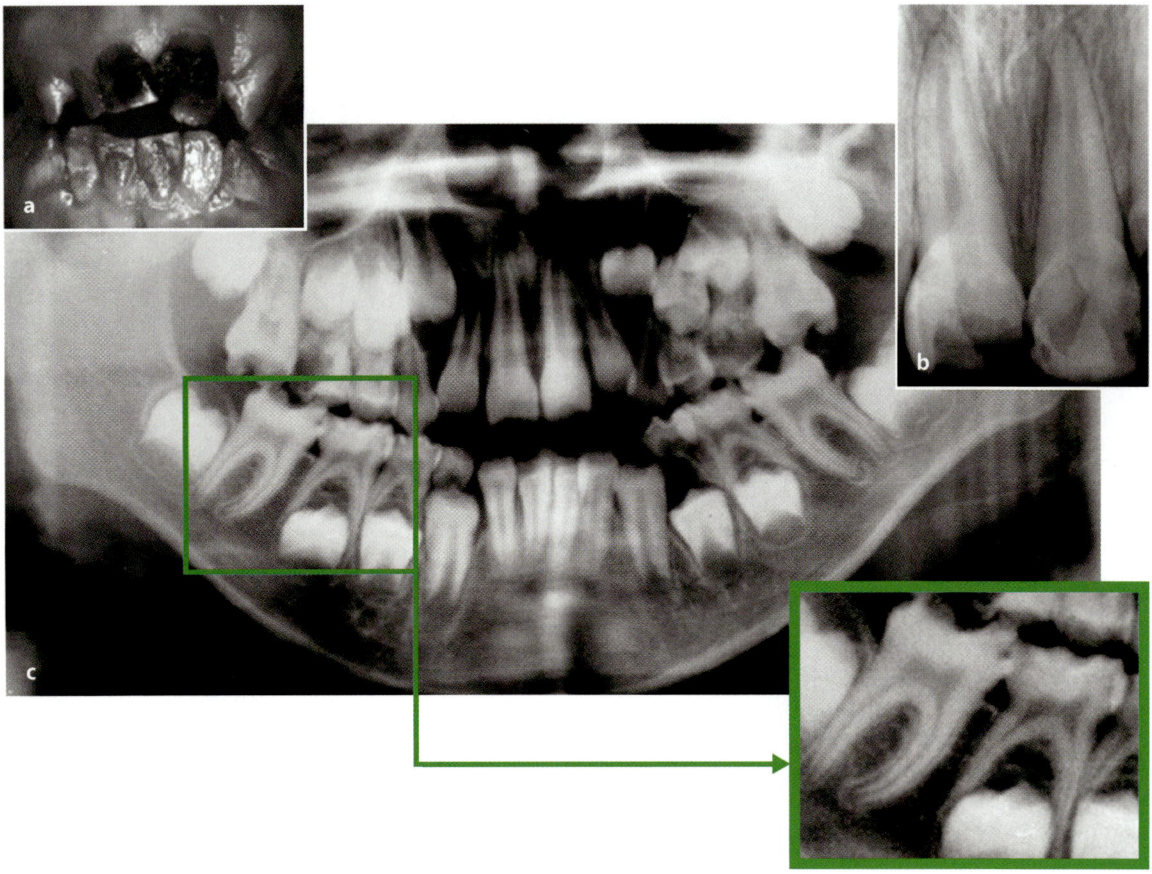

Fig.6.21 Rough hypoplastic amelogenesis imperfecta. **a** Clinical features showing pitting of surface enamel with subsequent extrinsic staining. **b** Periapical radiograph showing the grossly irregular enamel in this condition. **c** Panoramic radiograph showing widespread involvement of teeth from both the primary and permanent dentitions

imperfecta with taurodontism is another type of this condition; amelogenesis imperfecta Type IVA shows predominantly hypomaturation whereas amelogenesis imperfecta Type IVB shows predominantly hypoplasia. Type IV amelogenesis imperfecta is autosomal dominant. Amelogenesis imperfecta with expression of tricho-dento-osseous syndrome [60]. Amelogenesis imperfecta types ID, IE, IG, IIA, IIIA, and IVB have enamel that rapidly abrades if left untreated. These types require full crown coverage as soon as possible. If treatment is delayed there may be a need to resort to overdentures. Other forms of amelogenesis imperfecta are mainly a cosmetic problem and therefore require either anterior crowns or veneers.

Dentinogenesis Imperfecta

The most widely accepted classification of dentinogenesis imperfecta is that of Shields et al. [72]. Shields Type I dentinogenesis imperfecta is associated with a systemic hereditary bone disorder, osteogenesis imperfecta. Osteogenesis imperfecta is a group of closely related inherited diseases characterized by abnormal bone fragility. Present clinical classification delineates six types, one of which (Type II) is so severe that mortality is 100%, either intrauterine or perinatal [73].

Malmgren and Norgren (2002) studied the dental aberrations in a group of non-related individuals with various forms of osteogenesis imperfecta, ages 0.3–20 years, with the aid of panoramic radiographs in

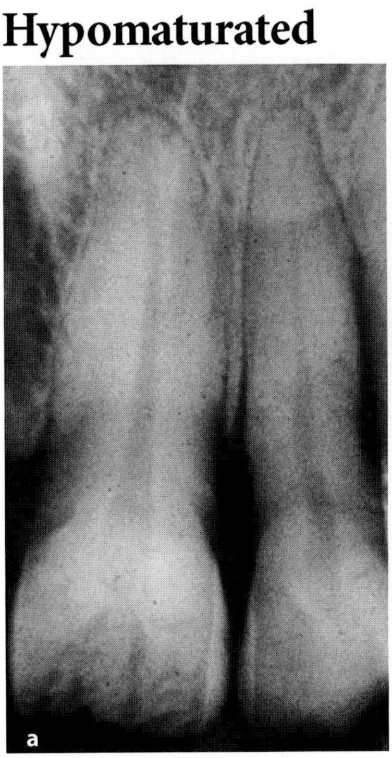

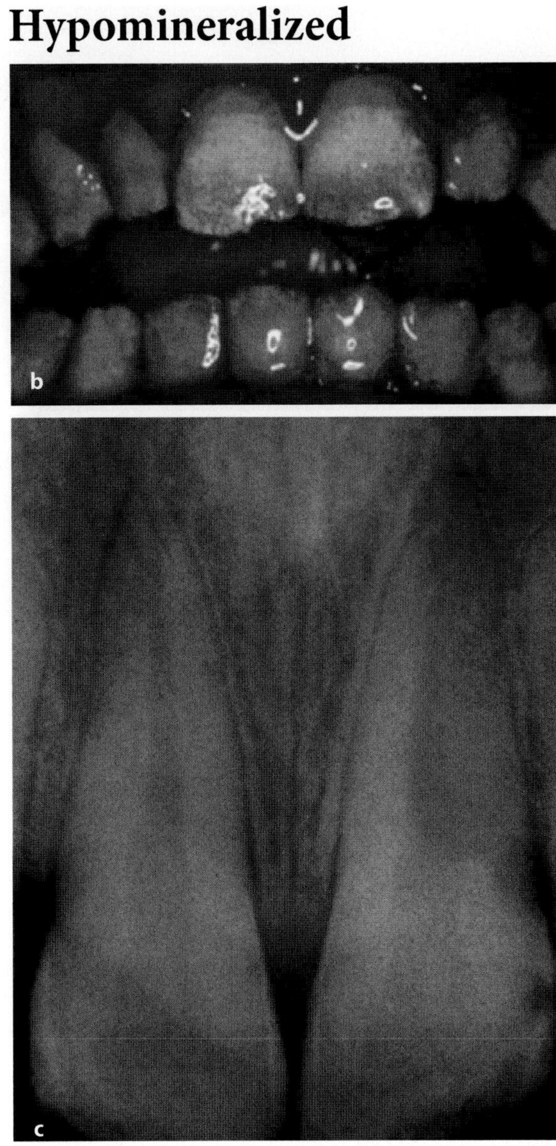

Fig. 6.22 Hypomaturated (**a**) versus hypomineralized (**b**, **c**) amelogenesis imperfecta

most instances [74]. Dentinogenesis imperfecta Type I was present in 27 of 65 patients. The presence or absence of dentinogenesis imperfecta showed almost complete accordance in affected parents and children and in affected siblings. Type II dentinogenesis imperfecta is autosomal dominant hereditary opalescent dentin unassociated with osteogenesis imperfecta (Fig. 6.23). It is found in approximately one in 8,000 US Caucasians. Both dentinogenesis imperfecta Type I and Type II result in teeth that are similar clinically, radiographically, and histopathologically to those encountered in individuals having dentinogenesis imperfecta Type I. The teeth of both dentitions of affected individuals are translucent with a blue to brown hue. High-resolution synchrotron radiation-computed tomography and small-angle X-ray scattering on normal and dentinogenesis imperfecta Type II (dentinogenesis imperfecta -II) teeth showed that the mineral concentration was 33% lower on average in dentinogenesis imperfecta -II dentin than in normal dentin [74, 75]. Radiographically, the teeth have bulbous crowns, cervical construction, narrow roots and early obliteration of the pulp chamber and canals. The enamel is poorly supported by the underlying abnormal dentin, and readily chips away. The enamel-dentin junction when viewed histologically is not normally scalloped. Dentinogenesis imperfecta shows 100% penetrance but variable expressivity. While pulpal obliteration is a common feature, in some cases the dentin is thin with a large pulp and normal enamel thickness. Such teeth are termed "shell teeth." A third

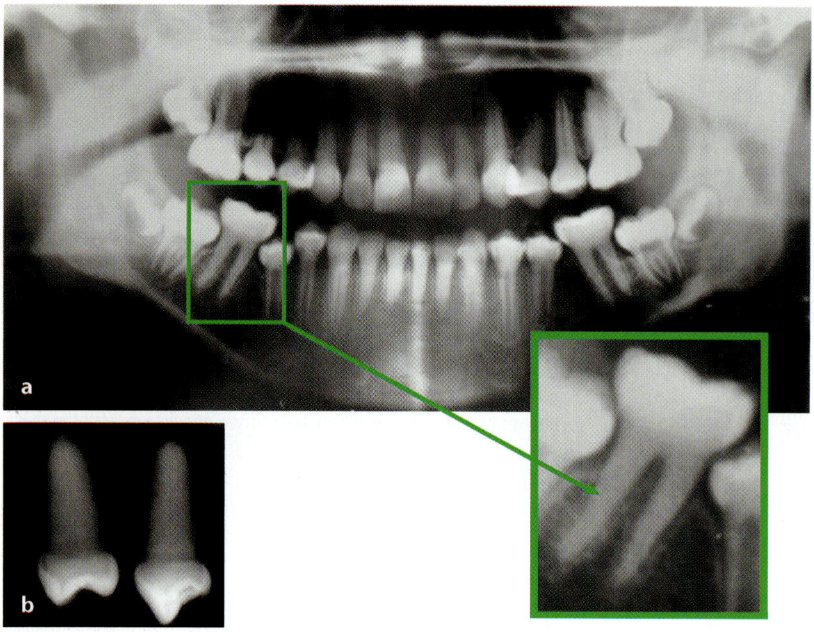

Fig. 6.23 Type II dentinogenesis imperfecta. **a** Panoramic radiograph demonstrates teeth throughout the dentition have narrow spindly root, rapid sclerosis of the pulp chamber and root canals, and bulbous crowns. **b** Radiograph of extracted teeth showing detail of early pulpal sclerosis

type of dentinogenesis imperfecta (Type III) has been described, but this might be nothing more than variable expressivity of dentinogenesis imperfecta Type II [60].

Treatment of choice for DI is full crowning of the teeth before the enamel is lost and the dentin abrades down to gum level.

Genetic linkage studies have identified the critical loci for dentinogenesis imperfecta Types II and III on human chromosome 4q21 [76]. Treatment of choice for dentinogenesis imperfecta is full crowning of the teeth before the enamel is lost and the dentin abrades down to gum level (Fig. 6.24). Alternative treatments are overdentures, full dentures or dental implants [77].

Radicular Dentin Dysplasia

Radicular (Type I) dentin dysplasia (Figs. 6.25, 6.26) is an autosomal dominant condition affecting both dentitions in which the enamel and coronal dentin are normal in appearance, but the root dentin is disorganized and the tooth roots are shortened, sometimes resulting in apparently rootless teeth [78, 79]. Periapical pathoses are frequently encountered. More severely affected teeth may appear to have no pulp chamber or canal. Less severely affected teeth have a crescent-shaped pulp chamber that resembles a finger-nail crimp to an analog film radiograph. Mildly affected teeth may have roots of normal length with a dilated pulp chamber containing a large pulp stone. While dentin dysplasia is not related to systemic disease, dentin dysplasia-like anomalies are sometimes reported in association with calcinosis universalis, tumoral calcinosis and certain rheumatoid or skeletal abnormalities.

Coronal Dentin Dysplasia

Coronal (Type II) dentin dysplasia (Fig. 6.27) is a rare autosomal dominant condition [80]. The chromosomal defect causing this condition is on the same chromosome as that found in dentinogenesis imperfecta Type II [81]. The primary teeth closely resemble dentinogenesis imperfecta; however, the permanent teeth are normal in color and radiographically demonstrate apical extension of the pulp chamber, producing a thistle-tube or flame shape [82]. Pulpal calcifications can be numerous. Teeth have normal root length. This can be differenti-

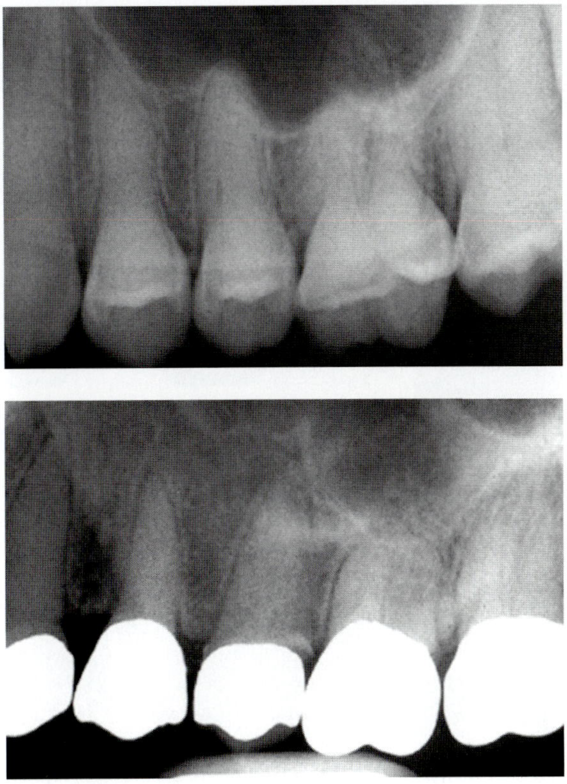

Fig. 6.24 Type II dentinogenesis imperfecta, before and after prosthodontic treatment. Full crowning of all teeth is recommended to prevent rapid attrition of poorly attached enamel and underlying dentin down to gum level. This is especially necessary as pulpal sclerosis will likely make endodontic therapy unachievable

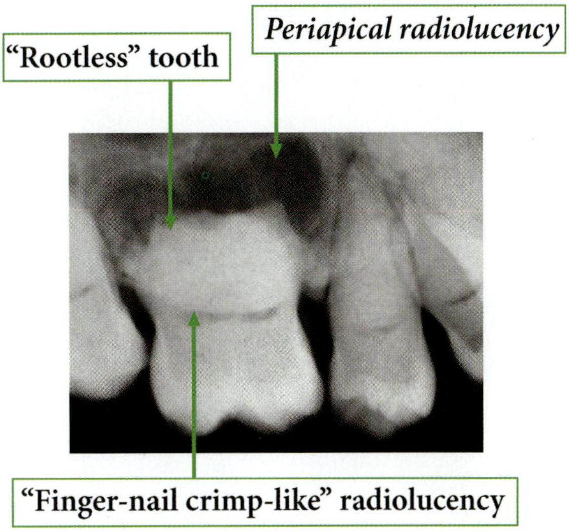

Fig. 6.25 Radicular (Type I) dentin dysplasia. Note typical features of short blunt roots without noticeable pulp canals. Periapical radiolucencies are frequent. Maintenance of such teeth is usually not feasible

ated from pulpal dysplasia in that for the latter, thistle-tube shaped pulps are found in both primary and permanent dentitions.

Odontodysplasia

Regional odontodysplasia is an uncommon non-inherited developmental anomaly that can affect both the primary and the permanent dentition.

Regional odontodysplasia (Fig. 6.28) is an uncommon non-inherited developmental anomaly that can affect both the primary and the permanent dentition [81, 83]. Although it is generally recognized as a localized disorder of dental tissue, its etiology has not yet been well explained [83]. Affected teeth usually are found only in an isolated segment of the dentition in one arch. The involved teeth show anomalous hypoplastic and hypomineralized enamel, dentin, pulp, and cementum resulting in a "ghostlike" appearance radiographically, with correspondingly enlarged pulp chambers and canals. The affected teeth frequently do not erupt. Follicular tissue surrounding the unerupted crown can be thickened and contain discrete calcifications [84, 85]. Rarely the condition may affect more than one dental segment [86] and very occasionally the condition is generalized [87, 88]. Treatment usually involves leaving the unerupted teeth in place to maintain the alveolar ridge. The missing teeth are replaced by a fixed or removable prosthesis. Should the teeth erupt, they are hypoplastic and are often mobile [89]. When affected teeth do erupt, a dentin bonded porcelain bridge can minimize destruction to the hypoplastic tooth tissue if affected teeth are used as abutments [90].

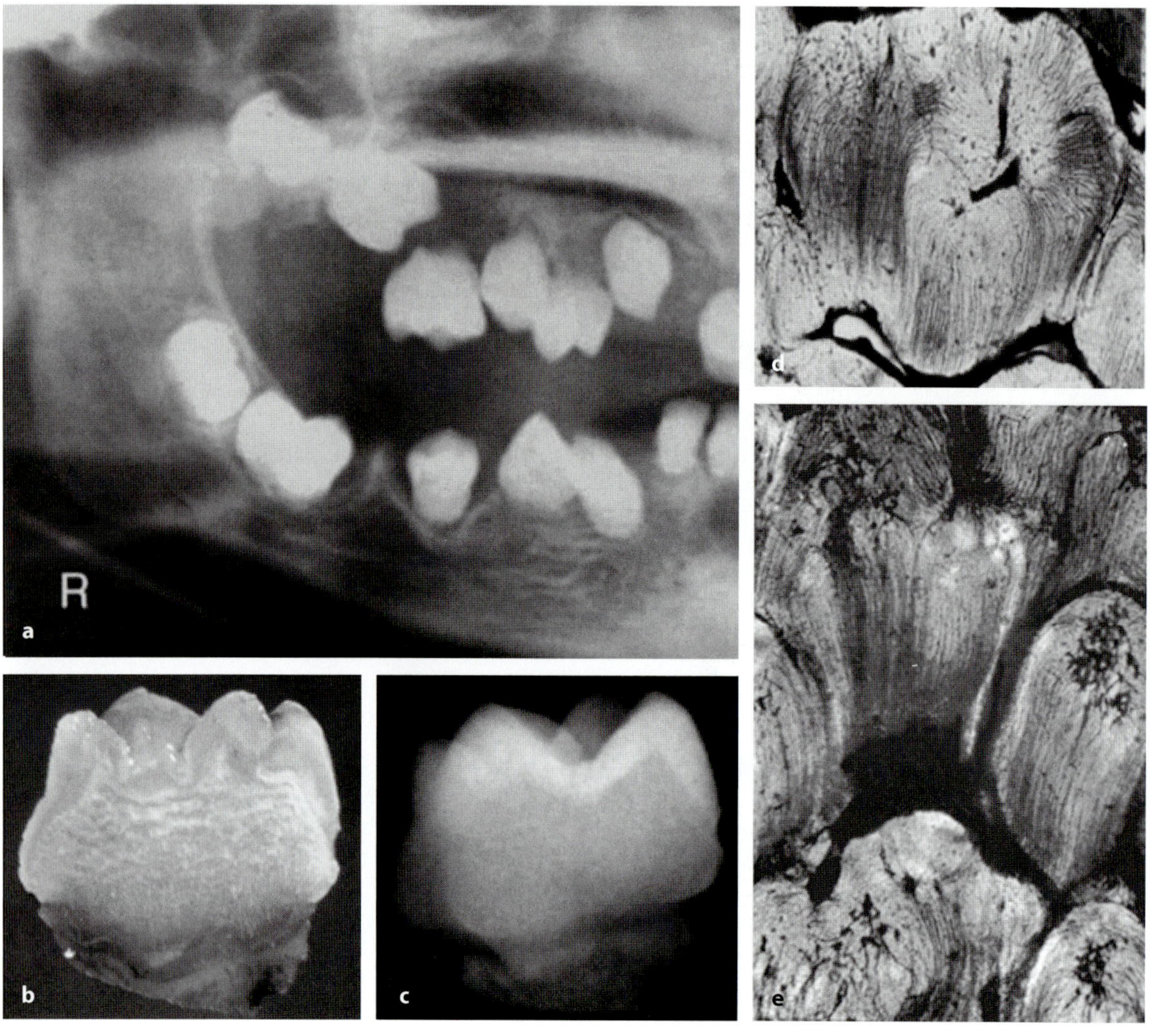

Fig. 6.26 Radicular (Type I) dentin dysplasia. **a** Panoramic radiograph showing generalized nature of this condition. Note the "pulpless" "rootless" teeth throughout. **b** Hemisected tooth from same case showing normal enamel over wavelike abnormal dentin. **c** Radiograph of extracted tooth. **d**, **e** Undemineralized histological sections showing the dentin to resemble the osteodentin found in certain fish species

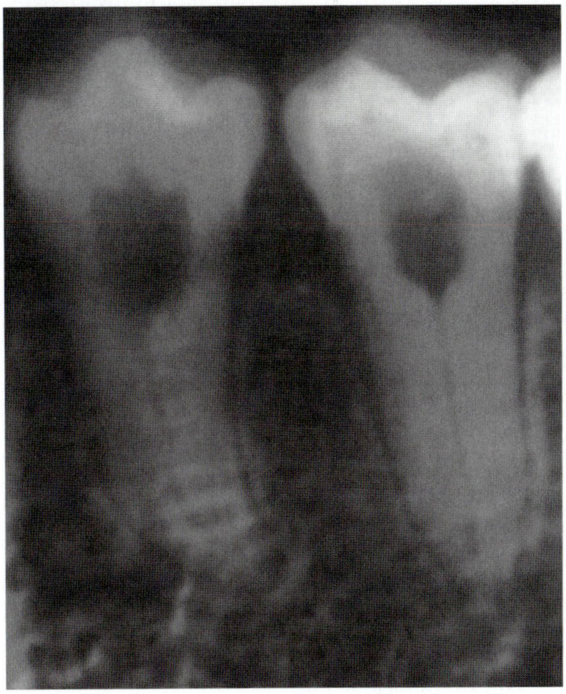

Fig. 6.27 Coronal (Type II) dentin dysplasia. The permanent teeth radiographically demonstrate apical extension of the pulp chamber producing a thistle-tube or flame shape

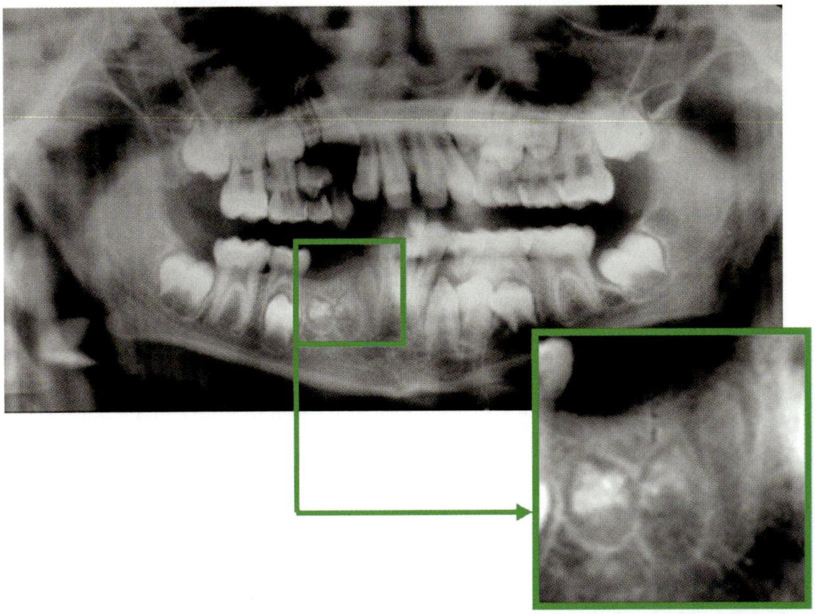

Fig. 6.28 Regional odontodysplasia (right mandibular canine and premolar region)

Concluding Remarks

Developmental anomalies of the dentition are of importance for patient esthetics—and consequently can affect perceptions of self-worth. Early detection of dental anomalies is of importance for planning timely orthodontic intervention to assure optimal function dental occlusion and stomatognathic function. The panoramic radiograph is an important adjunct in the assessment of normal growth and development. Panoramic radiographs are also important in planning dental coronal restorations and endodontic therapy.

References

1. American Academy of Pediatric Dentistry. Guidelines for prescribing dental radiographs (Reviewed and reaffirmed May 1997). AAPD Reference Manual 2000-2001. http://www.aapd.org/pdf/radiograph.pdf
2. Whittington BR, Durward CS. Survey of anomalies in primary teeth and their correlation with the permanent dentition. N Z Dent J 1996;92:4–8
3. Locht S. Panoramic radiographic examination of 704 Danish children aged 9–10 years. Community Dent Oral Epidemiol 1980;8:375–380
4. Neal JJ, Bowden DE. The diagnostic value of panoramic radiographs in children aged nine to ten years. Br J Orthod 1988;15:193–197
5. Cholitgul W, Drummond BK. Jaw and tooth abnormalities detected on panoramic radiographs in New Zealand children aged 10–15 years. N Z Dent J 2000;96:10–13
6. Ith-Hansen K, Kjaer I. Persistence of deciduous molars in subjects with agenesis of the second premolars. Eur J Orthod 2000;22:239–243
7. Yanagida I, Mori S. Statistical studies on numerical anomalies of teeth in children using orthopantomograms-congenital hypodontia. Osaka Daigaku Shigaku Zasshi 1990;35:580–593
8. Peltola JS, Wolf J, Mannik A, Russak S, Seedre T, Sirkel M, Vink M. Radiographic findings in the teeth and jaws of 14- to 17-year-old Estonian schoolchildren in Tartu and Tallinn. Acta Odontol Scand 1997;55:31–35
9. Lynham A. Panoramic radiographic survey of hypodontia in Australian Defense Force recruits. Aust Dent J 1990;35:19–22
10. Shapira Y, Lubit E, Kuftinec MM. Congenitally missing second premolars in cleft lip and cleft palate children. Am J Orthod Dentofacial Orthop 1999;115:396–400
11. Kumasaka S, Miyagi A, Sakai N, Shindo J, Kashima I. Oligodontia: a radiographic comparison of subjects with Down syndrome and normal subjects. Spec Care Dentist 1997;17:137–141
12. Shapira J, Chaushu S, Becker A. Prevalence of tooth transposition, third molar agenesis, and maxillary canine impaction in individuals with Down syndrome. Angle Orthod 2000;70:290–296
13. Guckes AD, Roberts MW, McCarthy GR. Pattern of permanent teeth present in individuals with ectodermal dysplasia and severe hypodontia suggests treatment with dental implants. Pediatr Dent 1998;20:278–280
14. Yanagida I, Mori S. Statistical studies on numerical anomalies of teeth in children using orthopantomograms-congenital hypodontia. Osaka Daigaku Shigaku Zasshi 1990;35:580–593
15. Atwan SM, Turner D, Khalid A. Early intervention to remove mesiodens and avoid orthodontic therapy. Gen Dent 2000;48:166–169
16. Valmaseda-Castellon E, Berini-Aytes L, Gay-Escoda C. Supernumerary premolars. Report of 10 cases. Bull Group Int Rech Sci Stomatol Odontol 2001;43:19–25
17. Yeung KH, Lau YW, Lee KH. Mandibular supernumerary premolars: orthodontic and surgical considerations. Prim Dent Care 1997;4:115–117
18. Farman AG, Nortjé CJ, Wood R. Oral and Maxillofacial Diagnostic Imaging. 1993; Mosby: St Louis
19. McNamara CM, O'Riordan BC, Blake M, Sandy JR. Cleidocranial dysplasia: radiological appearances on dental panoramic radiography. Dentomaxillofac Radiol 1999;28:89–97
20. Wolf J, Jarvinen HJ, Hietanen J. Gardner's dento-maxillary stigmas in patients with familial adenomatosis coli. Br J Oral Maxillofac Surg 1986;24:410–416
21. Ekman-Westborg B, Julin P. Multiple anomalies in dental morphology: macrodontia, multituberculism, central cusps, and pulp invaginations. Oral Surg Oral Med Oral Pathol 1974;38:217–222
22. Yoda T, Ishii Y, Honma Y, Sakai E, Enomoto S. Multiple macrodonts with odontoma in a mother and son: a variant of Ekman-Westborg-Julin syndrome. Oral Surg Oral Med Oral Pathol Oral Radiol Endod 1998;85:301–303
23. Baccetti T. A clinical and statistical study of etiologic aspects related to associated tooth anomalies in number, size, and position. Minerva Stomatol 1998;47:655–663
24. Celik E, Aydinlik E. Effect of a dilacerated root on stress distribution to the tooth and supporting tissues. J Prosthet Dent 1991;65:771–777
25. Chohayeb AA. Dilaceration of permanent upper lateral incisors: frequency, direction, and endodontic treatment implications. Oral Surg Oral Med Oral Pathol 1983;55:519–520
26. Seow WK, Needleman HL, Holm IA. Effect of familial hypophosphatemic rickets on dental development: a controlled, longitudinal study. Pediatr Dent 1995;17:346–350
27. Kaste SC, Hopkins KP, Jones D, Crom D, Greenwald CA, Santana VM. Dental abnormalities in children treated for acute lymphoblastic leukemia. Leukemia 1997;11:792–796
28. Rajic Z, Mestrovic SR. Taurodontism in Down's syndrome. Coll Antropol 1998;22(Suppl):63–67
29. Melnick M, Shields ED, El-Kafrawy AH. Tricho-dento-osseous syndrome: a scanning electron microscopic analysis. Clin Genet 1977;12:17–27
30. Aldred MJ, Savarirayan R, Lamande SR, Crawford PJ. Clinical and radiographic features of a family with autosomal dominant amelogenesis imperfecta with taurodontism. Oral Dis 2002;8:62–68
31. Varrela J, Alvesalo L, Mayhall J. Taurodontism in 45, X females. J Dent Res 1990;69:494–495
32. Hillebrand U, Mohr C, Plewa G. Taurodontism in patients with sex chromosome anomalies. Dtsch Z Mund Kiefer Gesichtschir 1990;14:187–189
33. Lebel S, Trinkaus E. Middle Pleistocene human remains from the Bau de l'Aubesier. J Hum Evol 2002;43:659–685

34. Bailey SE. A closer look at Neanderthal postcanine dental morphology: the mandibular dentition. Anat Rec 2002;269:148–156
35. Toure B, Kane AW, Sarr M, Wone MM, Fall F. Prevalence of taurodontism at the level of the molar in the black Senegalese population 15 to 19 years of age. Odontostomatol Trop 2000;23:36–39
36. Constant DA, Grine FE. A review of taurodontism with new data on indigenous southern African populations. Arch Oral Biol 2001;46:1021–1029
37. Darwazeh AM, Hamasha AA, Pillai K. Prevalence of taurodontism in Jordanian dental patients. Dentomaxillofac Radiol 1998;27:163–165
38. Ruprecht A, Batniji S, el-Neweihi E. The incidence of taurodontism in dental patients. Oral Surg Oral Med Oral Pathol 1987;63:743–747
39. MacDonald-Jankowski DS, Li TT. Taurodontism in a young adult Chinese population. Dentomaxillofac Radiol 1993;22:140–144
40. Hayashi Y. Endodontic treatment in taurodontism. J Endod 1994;20:357–358
41. Kjaer I. Morphological characteristics of dentitions developing excessive root resorption during orthodontic treatment. Eur J Orthod 1995;17:25–34
42. Tulensalo T, Ranta R, Kataja M. Reliability in estimating taurodontism of permanent molars from orthopantomograms. Community Dent Oral Epidemiol 1989;17:258–262
43. Kupietzky A, Rozenfarb N. Enamel pearls in the primary dentition: report of two cases. ASDC J Dent Child 1993;60:63–66
44. Darwazeh A, Hamasha AA. Radiographic evidence of enamel pearls in Jordanian dental patients. Oral Surg Oral Med Oral Pathol Oral Radiol Endod 2000;89:255–258
45. Goldstein AR. Enamel pearls as contributing factor in periodontal breakdown. J Am Dent Assoc 1979;99:210–211
46. Salem G. Prevalence of selected dental anomalies in Saudi children from Gizan region. Community Dent Oral Epidemiol 1989;17:162–163
47. Backman B, Wahlin BY. Variations in number and morphology of permanent teeth in 7-year-old Swedish children. Int J Paediatr Dent 2001;11:11–17
48. Knezevic A, Travan S, Tarle Z, Sutalo J, Jankovic B, Ciglar I. Double tooth. Coll Antropol 2002;26:667–672
49. Tasa GL, Lukacs JR. The prevalence and expression of primary double teeth in western India. ASDC J Dent Child 2001;68:196–200
50. Mader CL. Fusion of teeth. J Am Dent Assoc 1979;98:62–64
51. Kannan SK, Suganya, Santharam H. Supernumerary roots. Indian J Dent Res 2002;13:116–119
52. Morrow JW, Hylin DL. Supernumerary rooted primary central incisors: report of seven cases. ASDC J Dent Child 1993;60:337–338
53. Nadkarni UM, Munshi A, Damle SG. Unusual presentation of talon cusp: two case reports. Int J Paediatr Dent 2002;12:332–335
54. McNamara T, Haeussler AM, Keane J. Facial talon cusps. Int J Paediatr Dent 1997;7:259–262
55. Goncalves A, Goncalves M, Oliveira DP, Goncalves N. Dens invaginatus type III: report of a case and 10-year radiographic follow-up. Int Endod J 2002;35:873–879
56. Gound TG. Dens invaginatus: a pathway to pulpal pathology: a literature review. Pract Periodontics Aesthet Dent 1997;9:585–594
57. McCulloch KJ, Mills CM, Greenfeld RS, Coil JM. Dens evaginatus from an orthodontic perspective: report of several clinical cases and review of the literature. Am J Orthod Dentofacial Orthop 1997;112:670–675
58. Stecker S, DiAngelis AJ. Dens evaginatus: a diagnostic and treatment challenge. J Am Dent Assoc 2002;133:190–193
59. Cholitgul W, Drummond BK. Jaw and tooth abnormalities detected on panoramic radiographs in New Zealand children aged 10–15 years. N Z Dent J 2000;96:10–13
60. Neville BW, Damm DD, Allen CM, Bouquot JE. Abnormalities of the Teeth. In: Oral and Maxillofacial Pathology. 1995; Philadelphia: Saunders, pp 44–95
61. Atasu M, Genc A, Ercalik S. Enamel hypoplasia and essential staining of teeth from erythroblastosis fetalis. J Clin Pediatr Dent 1998;22:249–252
62. Giunta JL. Dental changes in hypervitaminosis D. Oral Surg Oral Med Oral Pathol Oral Radiol Endod 1998;85:410–413
63. Pavithran K. Acquired syphilis in a patient with late congenital syphilis. Sex Transm Dis 1987;14:119–121
64. Aine L, Backstrom MC, Maki R, Kuusela AL, Koivisto AM, Ikonen RS, Maki M. Enamel defects in primary and permanent teeth of children born prematurely. J Oral Pathol Med 2000;29:403–409
65. Lai PY, Seow WK, Tudehope DI, Rogers Y. Enamel hypoplasia and dental caries in very-low birthweight children: a case-controlled, longitudinal study. Pediatr Dent 1997;19:42–49
66. Nunn JH, Sharp J, Lambert HJ, Plant ND, Coulthard MG. Oral health in children with renal disease. Pediatr Nephrol 2000;14:997–1001
67. Witkop CJ Jr. Amelogenesis imperfecta, dentinogenesis imperfecta and dentin dysplasia revisited: problems in classification. J Oral Pathol 1988;17:547–553
68. Kida M, Ariga T, Shirakawa T, Oguchi H, Sakiyama Y. Autosomal-dominant hypoplastic form of amelogenesis imperfecta caused by an enameling gene mutation at the exon-intron boundary. J Dent Res 2002;81:738–742
69. Mardh CK, Backman B, Holmgren G, Hu JC, Simmer JP, Forsman-Semb K. A nonsense mutation in the enamelin gene causes local hypoplastic autosomal dominant amelogenesis imperfecta (AIH2). Hum Mol Genet 2002;11:1069–1074
70. Hart PS, Aldred MJ, Crawford PJ, Wright NJ, Hart TC, Wright JT. Amelogenesis imperfecta phenotype-genotype correlations with two amelogenin gene mutations. Arch Oral Biol 2002;47:261–265
71. Klingberg G, Oskarsdottir S, Johannesson EL, Noren JG. Oral manifestations in 22q11 deletion syndrome. Int J Paediatr Dent 2002;12:14–23
72. Shields ED, Bixler D, El-Kafrawy AM. A proposed classification for hereditable human dentine defects with a description of a new entity. Arch Oral Biol 1973;18:543–553
73. Singer RB, Ogston SA, Paterson CR. Mortality in various types of osteogenesis imperfecta. J Insur Med 2001;33:216–220
74. Malmgren B, Norgren S. Dental aberrations in children and adolescents with osteogenesis imperfecta. Acta Odontol Scand 2002;60:65–71

75. Kinney JH, Pople JA, Driessen CH, Breunig TM, Marshall GW, Marshall SJ. Intrafibrillar mineral may be absent in dentinogenesis imperfecta type II (DI-II). J Dent Res 2001;80:1555–1559
76. MacDougall M, Simmons D, Gu TT, Dong J. MEPE/OF45, a new dentin/bone matrix protein and candidate gene for dentin diseases mapping to chromosome 4q21. Connect Tissue Res 2002;43:320–330
77. Tanaka T, Murakami T. Radiological features of hereditary opalescent dentin. Dentomaxillofac Radiol 1998;27:251–253
78. Perl T, Farman AG. Radicular (type I) dentin dysplasia. Oral Surg Oral Med Oral Pathol 1977;43:746–753
79. Seow WK, Shusterman S. Spectrum of dentin dysplasia in a family: case report and literature review. Pediatr Dent 1994;16:437–442
80. Dean JA, Hartsfield JK Jr, Wright JT, Hart TC. Dentin dysplasia, Type II linkage to chromosome 4q. J Craniofac Genet Dev Biol 1997;17:172–177
81. Melamed Y, Harnik J, Becker A, Shapira J. Conservative multidisciplinary treatment approach in an unusual odontodysplasia. ASDC J Dent Child 1994;61:119–124
82. Brenneise CV, Conway KR. Dentin dysplasia, type II: report of 2 new families and review of the literature. Oral Surg Oral Med Oral Pathol Oral Radiol Endod 1999;87:752–755
83. Fujiwara T, Nakano K, Sobue S, Ooshima T. Simultaneous occurrence of unusual odontodysplasia and oligodontia in the permanent dentition: report of a case. Int J Paediatr Dent 2000;10:341–347
84. Gould AR, Farman AG, Marks ID. Pericoronal features of regional odontodysplasia. J Oral Med 1984;39:236–242
85. Courson F, Bdeoui F, Danan M, Degrange M, Gogly B. Regional odontodysplasia: expression of matrix metalloproteinases and their natural inhibitors. Oral Surg Oral Med Oral Pathol Oral Radiol Endod 2003;95:60–66
86. Gomes MP, Modesto A, Cardoso AS, Hespanhol W. Regional odontodysplasia: report of a case involving two separate affected areas. ASDC J Dent Child 1999;66:203–207
87. Russell K, Yacobi R. Generalized odontodysplasia concomitant with mild hypophosphatasia: a case report. J Can Dent Assoc 1993;59:187–190
88. Shah N, Gupta YK. Generalized odontodysplasia: a case report. J Indian Soc Pedod Prev Dent 1998;16:40–43
89. Ansari G, Reid JS, Fung DE, Creanor SL. Regional odontodysplasia: report of four cases. Int J Paediatr Dent 1997;7:107–113
90. Wilson PH, Ali A. Case report: restorative options in regional odontodysplasia. Eur J Prosthodont Restor Dent 2002;10:5–8

TEST: Panoramic radiologic appraisal of anomalies of dentition

1. Oligodontia is synonymous with:
   (a) Hyperdontia
   (b) Macrodontia
   (c) Cleidocranial dysplasia
   (d) None of the above

2. Ectodermal dysplasias are frequently associated with all BUT one of the following. What is the one EXCEPTION?
   (a) Absence of eyebrows and eyelashes
   (b) Difficulty in thermal regulation
   (c) Hypoplasia of the clavicles
   (d) Multiple missing teeth

3. Significant movement in the positioning of impacted third molar teeth can be observed late into the third decade of life.

   True ☐ **False** ☐

4. The most common congenitally missing teeth are:
   (a) Maxillary and mandibular premolars
   (b) Maxillary lateral incisors and third molars in both jaws
   (c) Primary canines and incisors
   (d) Mandibular first molars

5. In the study by Kumasaka what percentage of Down syndrome patients experienced hypodontia?
   (a) 15
   (b) 47
   (c) 63
   (d) 92

6. 6. The permanent teeth most likely to be present in ectodermal dysplasia are:
   (a) Maxillary central incisors
   (b) Maxillary canines
   (c) Mandibular premolars
   (d) Mandibular first permanent molars

7. According to the work of Shapiro et al., what percentage of patients with clefts also had one or more missing premolars?
   (a) 7.7
   (b) 18
   (c) 34
   (d) 54

8. Hypodontia in the primary dentition is unlikely to be followed by hypodontia in the permanent dentition.

   True ☐ **False** ☐

9. The correct sequence for tooth development is: (1) proliferation; (2) morphodifferentiation; (3) initiation; (4) histodifferentiation; (5) mineralization.

True ☐ **False** ☐

10. The percentage of the normal population likely to have a supernumerary tooth or teeth is:
a) 0.03
b) 0.30
c) 3.00
d) 30.0

11 Supernumerary teeth occur in the mandible in which site most frequently?
(a) Molar
(b) Premolar
(c) Canine
(d) Incisor

12 Which of the following syndromes is most likely to be associated with microdontia?
(a) Ectodermal dysplasias
(b) Gardner syndrome
(c) Cleidocranial dysplasia
(d) Ekman-Westborg-Julin syndrome

13. Which of the following syndromes is most likely associated with macrodontia?
(a) Ectodermal dysplasias
(b) Gardner syndrome
(c) Cleidocranial dysplasia
(d) Ekman-Westborg-Julin syndrome

14 In cleidocranial dysplasia, all BUT one of the following is likely to be found. Which is the one exception?
(a) Hypoplastic clavicles
(b) Intestinal polyposis
(c) Clinical appearance of hypodontia
(d) Open fontanel

15. Detection on panoramic radiology of multiple osteomas in the jaws may be a clue to a premalignant condition of the large intestines.

True ☐ **False** ☐

16. Mesiodens are found with equal frequency in the mandible and the maxilla.

True ☐ **False** ☐

17. Taurodontism can be found in almost half of certain normal populations from Africa.

True ☐ **False** ☐

18. The "bull's eye" radiographic sign is classically found for which of the following?
(a) Concrescence
(b) Dilaceration
(c) Taurodontism
(d) Dens evaginatus

19. Dens evaginatus is found in roughly what percentage of Native Americans?
(a) 0.02
(b) 0.20
(c) 2.00
(d) 20.0

20. Teeth that are connate may be either fused or geminated.

True ☐ **False** ☐

21 Panoramic radiography is important in the detection and diagnosis of talon cusps.

True ☐ **False** ☐

22. For maxillary molars, the enamel pearl is most frequently found on the mesial or distal surface.

True ☐ **False** ☐

23. Taurodonts are associated with short pulp chambers and elongated apical root canals.

True ☐ **False** ☐

24. Coronal (Type II) dentin dysplasia often results in "pulpless" and "rootless teeth."

True ☐ **False** ☐

25. Dentinogenesis imperfecta found in association with osteogenesis imperfecta can appear radiographically identical to that unassociated with this systemic bone condition.

True ☐ **False** ☐

26. Smooth hypoplastic amelogenesis imperfecta may be inherited as either autosomal dominant or X-linked.

True ☐ **False** ☐

27. Which of the following is not usually associated with an increased frequency of enamel hypoplasia?
(a) Low birth weight
(b) Excess fluoride in drinking water
(c) Radicular (Type I) dentin dysplasia
(d) Birth-related trauma

28. The prevalence ratio of dentinogenesis imperfecta Type II in the general population is approximately?
(a) 1:80,000
(b) 1:8,000
(c) 1:800
(d) 1:80

29. Teeth in Type II amelogenesis imperfecta invariably show taurodontism

True ☐ **False** ☐

30. Amelogenesis imperfecta varieties wherein the enamel matrix is formed normally and initiates mineralization, but the enamel crystals do not mature normally, includes which of the following?
(a) Type IIA
(b) Type IB
(c) Type IVA
(d) Type IIIB

31. Shields Type II dentinogenesis imperfecta is usually inherited in which of the following manners?
(a) Sex-linked dominant
(b) Sex-linked recessive
(c) Autosomal recessive
(d) Autosomal dominant

32. "Ghost-like" teeth are typically found in which of the following conditions?
(a) Amelogenesis imperfecta Type IG
(b) Osteogenesis imperfecta Type 3
(c) Congenital syphilis
(d) Odontodysplasia

33. Due to the inherent weakness of the affected dentin, it is not possible to restore teeth with dentinogenesis imperfecta.

True ☐ **False** ☐

Chapter

Tooth Eruption and Dental Impaction

7

Allan G. Farman

Learning Objectives

- Gain understanding of the role of radiography in determining the normality of tooth eruption with regard to positions and time sequence
- Learn about the role of panoramic radiography in identifying and monitoring premature eruption, retarded eruption, and dental impactions
- Learn the proper use of panoramic radiography, its benefits and limitations, in reviewing impactions

A broad range of variation exists in the normal eruption times for primary and permanent teeth in humans. However, normality is usually associated with bilateral symmetry. Furthermore, cases where eruption time is grossly beyond the extremes of normalcy might be considered to represent a pathological state [1]. Radiography plays an important part in determining the normality of tooth eruption with regard to position and time sequence. This is particularly important in patients whose teeth are undetectable by clinical means, such as those with delayed eruption or impaction. Impaction is the impedance of dental eruption by adjacent or overlying tooth, bone, or pathosis.

Premature Eruption

Occasionally, one or two primary teeth—natal teeth—are present at birth or, in the case of neonatal teeth, erupt within the first month of life [2]. Eighty-five percent of such prematurely erupting teeth are mandibular primary central incisors, 11% are primary maxillary incisors, and 4% are primary posterior teeth [2]. Such teeth are generally well-formed and normal in all respects. They should be retained despite nursing difficulties [3]. Although anecdotally there may be a familial occurrence, most cases defy explanation [4]. A study of 34,457 infants born in southern Finland (1997–2000) determined an incidence of 1:1,000 for natal and neonatal teeth and found no association with environmental pollutants [5]. Other studies have put the incidence of natal and neonatal at between 1:700 and 1:3,500 live births with a predilection for occurrence in females [6]. Natal and neonatal teeth are occasionally reported in patients having syndromes such as pachyonychia congenita, Hallerman-Streiff syndrome, and Wiedemann-Rautenstrauch syndrome, the latter being associated with premature aging [7–14]. Radiographic inspection is not necessary.

Premature eruption of a permanent tooth can follow premature loss of the overlying primary tooth. This can readily be assessed using panoramic radiographs [15]. Caries and restorations in primary teeth have also been associated with premature eruption of their successors [16]. A study of 4,468 Flemish children indicate that the emergence of the maxillary and mandibular premolars was accelerated by 2–8 months when its predecessor had been decayed or restored but had not been extracted. Very early eruption of a permanent tooth following agenesis of its primary predecessor has also been reported [17]. Cases of premature eruption involving the whole permanent dentition have been associated with Proteus syndrome [18].

Retarded Eruption

Where there is a systemic cause to delayed eruption, lack of eruptive force can be permanent, and there is no known remedy. Such unimpeded unerupted teeth are termed embedded.

Delay in dental eruption affecting the whole of one or both dentitions has been associated with various systemic conditions, including rickets, cretinism, and cleidocranial dysplasia [1]. Neonatal illness and postnatal nutrition as well as degree of premature birth have been found to affect the timing of primary tooth eruption [19].

Fibromatosis gingivae can either slow or camouflage eruption due to enlarged hyperplastic gingival tissues containing dense connective tissue [20]. If the cause is local (e.g., fibromatosis gingivae, supernumerary tooth, or odontoma), early treatment of the primary condition should promote eruption. Excessive delay in eruption should be evaluated using either panoramic or intraoral radiographs. Panoramic radiology will provide the best overview so long as the patient can cooperate for the full exposure time.

Where there is a systemic cause to delayed eruption (e.g., cleidocranial dysplasia), lack of eruptive force can be permanent, and there is no known remedy [21, 22]. Such unimpeded unerupted teeth are termed embedded (Fig. 7.1). In such cases, periodic panoramic radiography is useful to evaluate the possible development of associated pathoses, including dentigerous cysts.

A variety of conditions have been associated with temporary delayed eruption—or delayed dental development. These include low birth weight [23], HIV infection in childhood [24, 25], Silver-Russell syndrome [26], Kabuki syndrome [27], osteopetrosis [28], and pycnodysostosis [29]. A study of 70 HIV-infected children aged 5 months to 13 years found that delay in tooth eruption is most closely linked to severity of symptoms rather than to CD4 depletion [25].

Dental Impactions

Impacted teeth may be defined as those teeth prevented from eruption due to a physical barrier within the path of eruption. Any tooth can be impacted; however, teeth in the regular permanent dentition or supernumerary teeth are usually affected. A study of radiographs from 3,874 dental patients aged over 20 years determined the prevalence of impaction to be 17% [30]; hence, this condition can be considered among the most common affecting dental care. The most frequently affected regular teeth are the third molars (especially in the mandible) and the permanent maxillary canines. Cases can occur simply due to dental crowding, to space reduction following premature loss of primary teeth, or to an errant path of eruption.

Impacted Third Molars

Impacted mandibular third molar teeth are traditionally classified according to position following the method of Winter (Fig. 7.2) [31]. The most common type of impaction for mandibular molars is mesioangular. Mesioangularly impacted mandibular third molars lie obliquely in bone with the crown slanted in a mesial direction, generally in contact with the distal surface of the ipsilateral second permanent molar tooth. Distoangular impacted third molars lie obliquely in bone with the crown slanted in a distal direction toward the ramus, the roots abutting the distal root of the second molar. Vertical impaction sees the third molar in normal angulation, but prevented from eruption through impingement on the anterior ramus or distal surface of the second permanent molar tooth. With horizontal impaction, the third molar is positioned horizontally within the mandible with the crown directed toward the distal surface of the second molar. In each of these angular impactions, the third molar can be positioned at various depths within bone, and in relation to the mandibular canal. Panoramic radiographs clearly demonstrate the mesiodistal and vertical position of the impacted tooth, but do not provide details of the

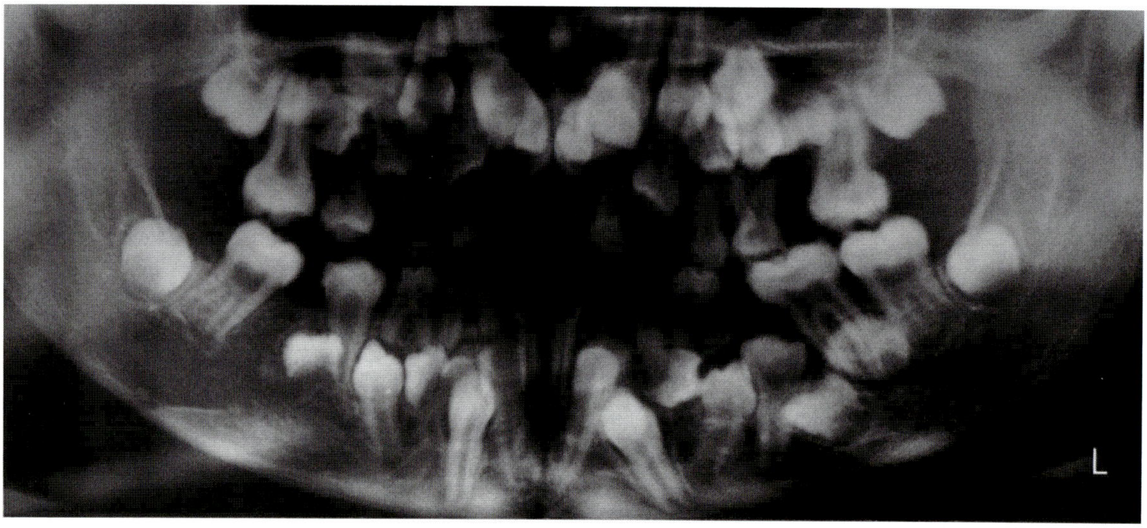

Fig. 7.1 Multiple unerupted regular permanent and supernumerary teeth in a patient having cleidocranial dysplasia

bucco-lingual positioning or bucco-lingual angulation. This can be remedied in most cases by exposing a true occlusal radiograph using a size No. 2 intraoral X-ray film or digital intraoral detector to provide details in the third orthogonal plane. This will be sufficient if the tooth is not superimposed over the mandibular canal or intimately associated with that structure. In the cases where this occurs and extraction is deemed necessary, the case may warrant more advanced imaging using conventional tomography, computed tomography, or cone beam volumetric CT with 3-D reconstruction.

Panoramic radiographs do not show bucco-lingual dimensions, so they should be supplemented where needed because this dimension is often critical for appropriate treatment planning. Damage to the contents of the mandibular canal can lead to temporary or permanent paresthesia of the ipsilateral side of the lower lip. While this complication is perhaps sometimes unavoidable, it is less likely to occur given appropriate radiographic assessment prior to surgery.

A prospective cohort study was performed in Sweden to measure the prevalence of disease in conjunction with mandibular third molars referred for removal [32]. Pericoronitis was found in 64% of cases, caries in the third molar in 31%, periodontitis associated with 8%, caries in the second molar in 5%, and root resorption of the second molar in one per cent of the impacted third molar teeth deemed to be associated with additional pathosis. The odds ratio for disease was highest for distoangular molars (5.8) and for impactions partially covered by soft tissue (6.7). The odds ratio for associated pathoses was between 22 and 34 times higher for molars partially covered by soft tissue than for impactions completely covered by soft or bone tissue. For distoangular molars the odds ratio for associated pathoses was 5–12 times higher than for molars in other positions.

Impacted maxillary third molars (e.g., Fig. 7.3) can also be mesioangular, distoangular, vertical, or horizontal in position. In the maxilla, no structure as critical to surgical success as the mandibular canal is present; hence, pre-surgical assessment using panoramic and true occlusal radiography is almost invariably sufficient. Concerning the treatment of impacted third molars, systematic reviews have generally concluded that, in the absence of association with definite pathosis, it is best not to extract these teeth [33, 34]. Further, there is little evidence that retention of third molars has any effect on anterior crowding that might undermine orthodontic treatment [35]. Nevertheless, univariate analysis based on removal of 354 mandibular third molars identi-

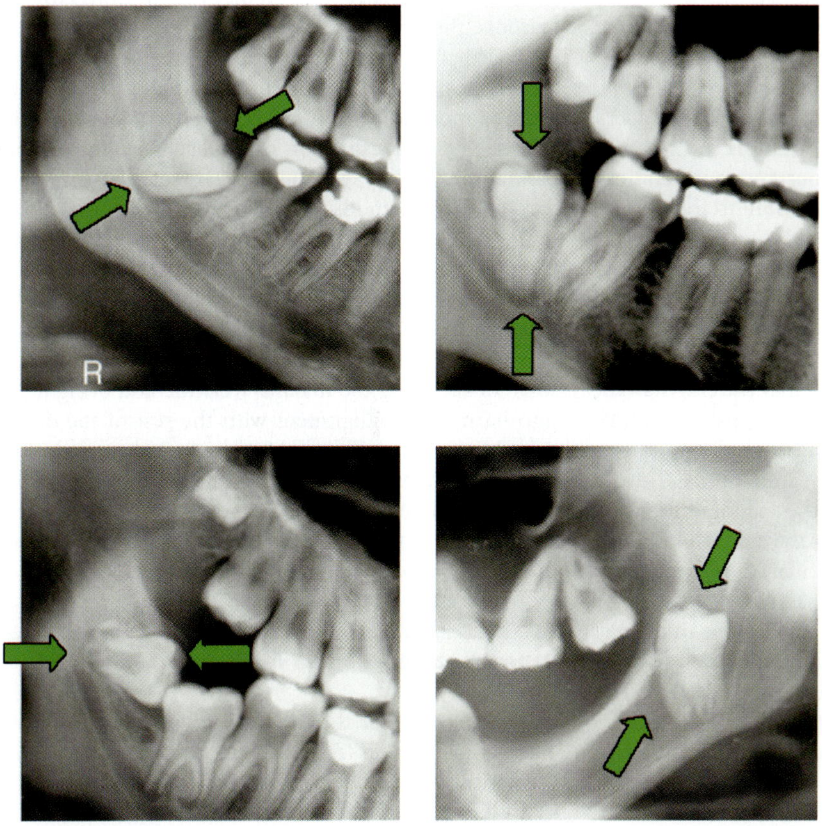

Fig. 7.2 Molar impaction classification according to angulation of the impacted third (and in the case of the horizontal impaction illustrated here—supernumerary/fourth) molar tooth. *Upper left* mesioangular, *upper right* vertical, *lower left* horizontal, *lower right* distoangular

fied increased patient age as a factor that predicted the surgical difficulty of third molar extractions, so delay could have a price if extraction is eventually needed [36]. Other factors ascribed to increased surgical difficulty include bony impaction, depth of tooth within bone, horizontal angulation, proximity to the inferior alveolar canal, male sex, and obesity [36]. When it is decided not to extract impacted third molars, periodic panoramic radiographs should be made to assure that no conditions develop that warrant subsequent surgical intervention.

That periodic re-evaluation is preferred to extraction of third molars in adolescents is supported by a study of 2,857 third molars assessed at age 18 years, where 93% were able to be clinically followed up at age 26 years [37]. Approximately 55% of the teeth that were not considered impacted by age 18 years had erupted by age 26 years. Of the teeth considered impacted at age 18 years, 34% had fully erupted by age 26 years. Of the maxillary teeth that were categorized as "impacted" at age 18 years, 36% had fully erupted by age 26 years, whereas 26% of the mandibular teeth had done so ($p < 0.01$). Excluding horizontally impacted third molars, a substantial proportion of impacted teeth did erupt fully. It can be concluded that radiographically apparent impaction in late adolescence should not be sufficient grounds for their prophylactic removal in the absence of other clinical indications.

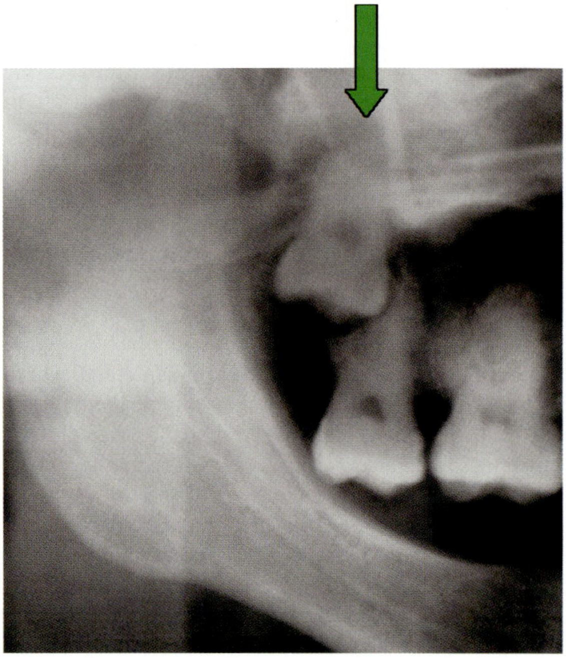

Fig. 7.3 Vertically impacted maxillary third molar tooth

Impacted Canines

Impacted permanent maxillary canines occur in 1–2% of the population [38]. These impactions can occur in different locations. The most important considerations are the relationship of the affected tooth to the erupted regular teeth, especially whether the positions of the crown and roots of the impacted tooth are palatal or facial. This determines the surgical access to the impacted maxillary canine for surgical orthodontics or extraction. In more than 60% of cases of impacted maxillary canines it is possible to decide whether the crown of the impacted tooth is facial or palatal using palpation [39]; however, for the remaining one-third, radiographic assessment is needed to effect localization [40].

As emphasized previously, the panoramic radiograph should not be relied on for the assessment of the facio-lingual position of mandibular third molars. In the anterior maxilla, however, it is possible, by using a single panoramic radiograph, to make some inferences regarding the facio-palatal positioning of the impacted tooth with respect to the erupted regular dentition. This is due to panoramic image layer theory. Objects that are displaced facially with respect to the regular dentition will appear narrowed horizontally, whereas those that are palatally displaced will appear magnified in horizontal dimension (Fig. 7.4). Hence, if the crown or root of the impacted canine appears broader horizontally in the panoramic image than do the regular tooth crowns or roots, the affected impacted canine tooth portion is displaced palatally, whereas if it appears narrowed, it is facially positioned. This presupposes that the impacted tooth is morphologically normal in terms of size. It is suggested that localization of impacted canines using panoramic radiographs be supplemented using standard parallax methods employing periapical or occlusal radiographs made at different vertical beam angulations for the purpose of verification [41, 42]. Cone-beam volumetric computed tomography can also be used to precisely locate impacted maxillary canines. Unlike the case of the third molar, there are important esthetic reasons for retaining the maxillary canine and bringing it into harmonious alignment with the rest of the dentition. Most cases will be treated by forced orthodontic eruption, often following surgical exposure [42, 43]. Treatment time is usually 2–3 years with severely impacted teeth, with younger patients requiring the most time [42]. Successful outcome is typical [43].

Other Impacted Regular Teeth

Regular teeth other than the mandibular third molars and canines are less frequently impacted (Fig. 7.5). The third most commonly impacted teeth are the premolars in both the mandible and maxilla.

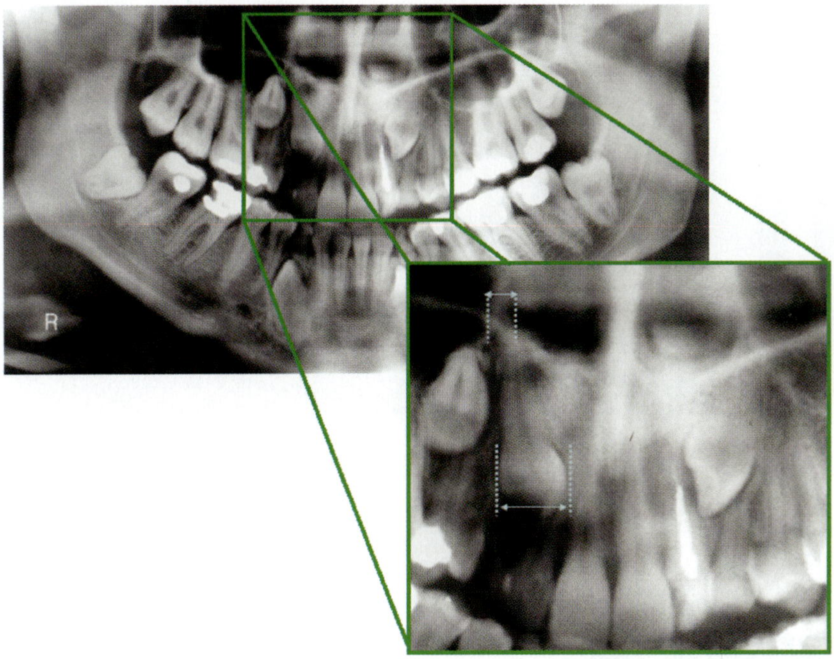

Fig. 7.4 Impacted maxillary canines. Note that the right canine appears to have a relatively wide crown indicating palatal location of the crown; however, the root appears relatively narrow in comparison with those of the regular teeth indicating a facial/labial location. All bets are off for the impacted left canine due to its rotation

Impacted Supernumerary Teeth

A detailed overview of supernumerary teeth is made in Chapter 6 that concerns developmental anomalies of the dentition. Many supernumerary teeth are impacted or lead to impaction of regular teeth. While these can be detected using panoramic radiography even in the anterior segment the panoramic radiograph does not provide a means of determining the facio-lingual relationship of such teeth to the regular dentition. Supernumerary teeth vary too widely in size and morphology for any panoramic assessment of position counting on the effects of tooth magnification with panoramic radiographs.

Both regular and supernumerary teeth completely impacted and embedded in bone can occasionally undergo resorption of the root, or crown, or both.

Resorption of Impacted Teeth

Both regular and supernumerary teeth completely impacted and embedded in bone can occasionally undergo resorption of the root, or crown, or both. In a study of 226 impacted teeth showing resorption, 78% were in the maxilla, and of the maxillary cases, 60% were canines [44]. Examination of panoramic radiographs of 11,598 subjects (average age 47 years) revealed 1,756 subjects had 3,702 impacted teeth with an average retention period of 27 years. Internal resorption was found in 16 (0.43%) of these cases (Fig. 7.6) [45].

Pathoses and Impaction

A retrospective study of patients hospitalized for infections associated with partially-erupted third molars from 1985–94 showed the incidence of serious orofacial infections associated with partially-erupted third molars to be 0.016 cases per year per 1,000 patients at risk [46]. The same investigators determined the incidence of large third-molar associated cystic lesions requiring hospitalization to be 0.016 cases per year per 1,000 patients at risk [47].

Within the jaws, teeth are occasionally displaced so that they are malpositioned in the dental arch (transposition), or erupt into even more dramatically anomalous positions.

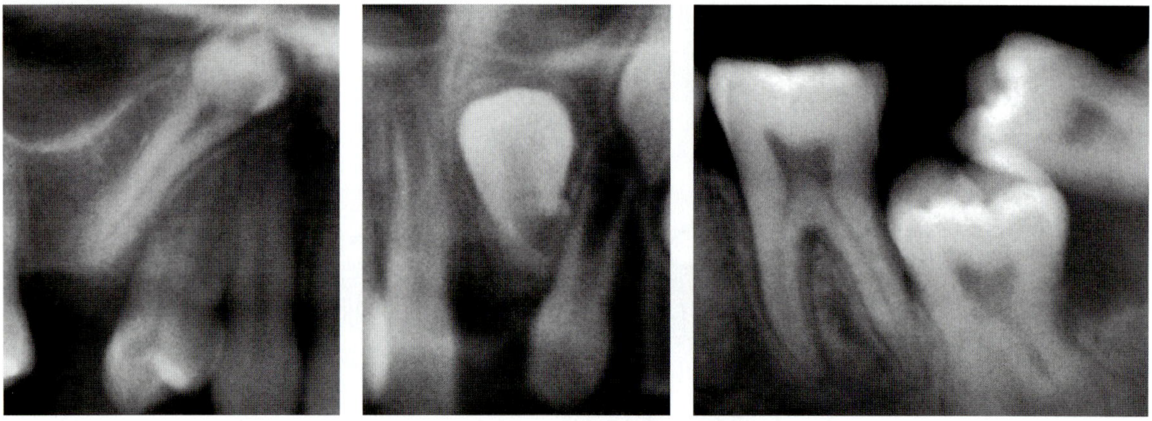

Fig. 7.5 Any tooth can be impacted. *Left* impacted premolar, *middle* impacted incisor, *right* impacted second molar

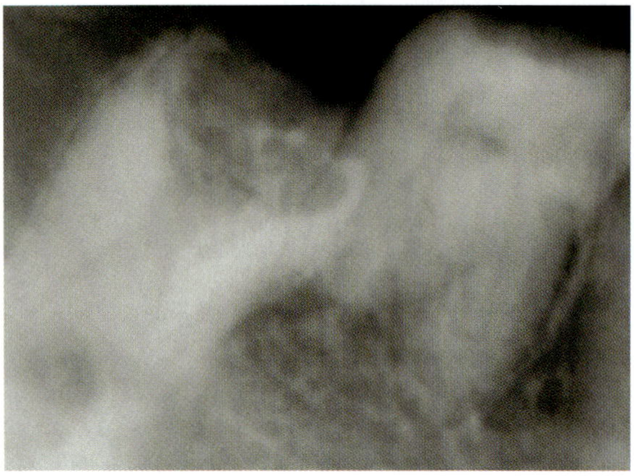

Fig. 7.6 Detail of resorption of an impacted mandibular third molar tooth

The presence of mandibular third molar impactions has also been found to be a significant predisposing factor for mandibular angle fractures during injury [48].

Cause-and-effect, or sequence of events, can be difficult to determine. In some cases, impacted teeth develop dentigerous cysts (Fig. 7.7) [45, 49, 50]. Upon panoramic follow-up, these have been reported to have regressed, only infrequently [49]. Surgical removal of the cystic lesion is the current treatment of choice. Following formation of the cyst, the affected tooth can be displaced considerably as the cyst grows. Of 3,702 impacted teeth retained over an average period of approximately 27 years, dentigerous cystic changes occurred in about 30 (0.81%) [45]. A variety of additional pathoses can cause—or be associated with—impaction and displacement of teeth (Fig. 7.8). These include the ameloblastoma, keratocystic odontogenic tumor (previously termed odontogenic keratocyst), odontomas, adenomatoid odontogenic tumor [50–53], and, less commonly, ameloblastic fibroma [54] and other cysts and neoplasms.

Ectopic Dental Eruption

Within the jaws, teeth are occasionally displaced so that they are malpositioned in the dental arch (transposition), or erupt into even more dramatically anomalous positions. The prevalence of ectopic eruption of the first permanent molars in a group of 4,232 Thai students, ages 6–9 years, was found to be 0.75% [55].

Transposition has been reported also in the anterior arches [56, 57]. Teeth appearing perfectly normal can also be formed at distant sites in the body, such as the ovaries in teratomas [58], but, needless to state, dental panoramic radiography does not work in such situations!

Concluding Remarks

While there is some controversy concerning the correct strategy to follow in watching or removing apparently impacted third molars, it is indisputable that the panoramic radiograph provides a valuable means of assessing these teeth. The panoramic radiograph provides information only in the vertical and mesiodistal planes, so additional radiographs might be necessary to establish bucco-lingual relationships between teeth and associated anatomic structures.

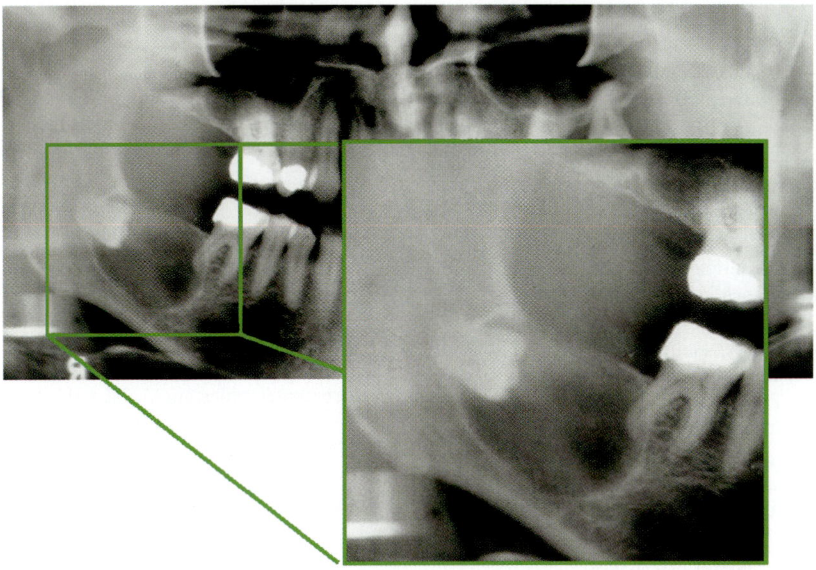

Fig. 7.7 Dentigerous cyst associated with horizontally positioned impacted mandibular third molar. The dentigerous cyst forms within the dental follicle space and shows attachment at the enamel-cemental junction

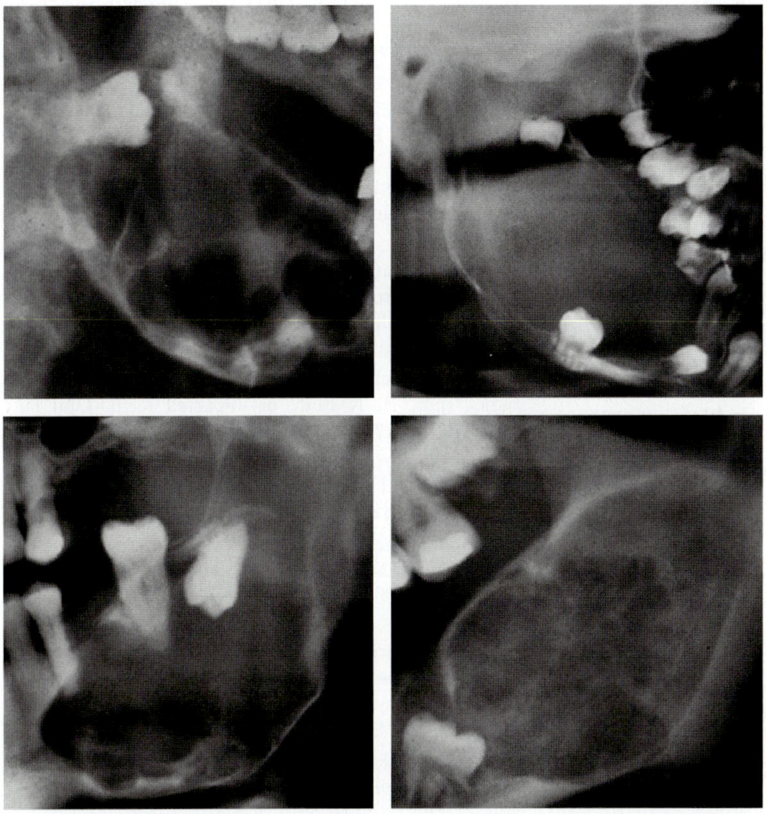

Fig. 7.8 Several different pathoses can be associated with dental impactions and tooth displacement. Examples shown here are of ameloblastoma (*upper left*), ameloblastic fibroma (*upper right*), keratocystic odontogenic tumor (*lower left*), and a malignant neoplasm, mesenchymal chondrosarcoma (*lower right*). All four of these examples displaced unerupted teeth. All four needed histologic analysis of tissue specimens to derive the correct diagnosis

References

1. Shafer WG, Hine MK, Levy BM. A Textbook of Oral Pathology, 4th edn. Philadelphia: Saunders, 1983; pp 59, 64
2. Neville BW, Damm DD, Allen CM, Bouquot JE. Oral and Maxillofacial Pathology. Philadelphia: Saunders, 1995; p 63
3. Kaur P, Sharma A, Bhuller N. Conservative management of a complication of neonatal teeth: a case report. J Indian Soc Pedod Prev Dent 2003;21:27–29
4. Asquinazi ML, Pouezat JA, Jasmin JR. Multiple natal teeth and oligodontia: a case report. Refuat Hapeh Vehashinayim 2001;18:102–107
5. Alaluusua S, Kiviranta H, Leppaniemi A, Holtta P, Lukinmaa PL, Lope L, Jarvenpaa AL, Renlund M, Toppari J, Virtanen H, Kaleva M, Vartiainen T. Natal and neonatal teeth in relation to environmental toxicants. Pediatr Res 2002;52:652–655
6. Groeneveld X, van Damme P. (Neo)natal tooth in perspective. Literature review and report of two cases. Ned Tijdschr Tandheelkd 1993;100:49–51
7. Strober BE. Pachyonychia congenita, type II. Dermatol Online J 2003;9:12
8. Koenig R. Teebi hypertelorism syndrome. Clin Dysmorphol 2003;12:187–189
9. Hou JW. Hallermann-Streiff syndrome associated with small cerebellum, endocrinopathy and increased chromosomal breakage. Acta Paediatr 2003;92:869–871
10. Nicholson AD, Menon S. Hallerman-Streiff syndrome. J Postgrad Med 1995;41:22–23
11. Korniszewski L, Nowak R, Okninska-Hoffmann E, Skorka A, Gieruszczak-Bialek D, Sawadro-Rochowska M. Wiedemann-Rautenstrauch (neonatal progeroid) syndrome: new case with normal telomere length in skin fibroblasts. Am J Med Genet 2001;103:144–148
12. Pivnick EK, Angle B, Kaufman RA, Hall BD, Pitukcheewanont P, Hersh JH, Fowlkes JL, Sanders LP, O'Brien JM, Carroll GS, Gunther WM, Morrow HG, Burghen GA, Ward JC. Neonatal progeroid (Wiedemann-Rautenstrauch) syndrome: report of five new cases and review. Am J Med Genet 2000;17;90:131–140
13. Mandal AK. Primary congenital glaucoma and erupted teeth (natal teeth) in the newborn: a report of two cases. Ophthalmic Surg Lasers 2001;32:419–421
14. Balci S, Guler G, Kale G, Soylemezoglu F, Besim A. Mohr syndrome in two sisters: prenatal diagnosis in a 22-week-old fetus with post-mortem findings in both. Prenat Diagn 1999;19:827–831
15. Czecholinski JA, Kahl B, Schwarze CW. Early deciduous tooth loss: the mature or immature eruption of their permanent successors. Fortschr Kieferorthop 1994;55:54–60
16. Leroy R, Bogaerts K, Lesaffre E, Declerck D. Impact of caries experience in the deciduous molars on the emergence of the successors. Eur J Oral Sci 2003;111:106–110
17. Turnbull NR, Lai NN. Eruption of a permanent mandibular canine in a 5-year-old boy. Int J Paediatr Dent 2003;13:117–120
18. Becktor KB, Becktor JP, Karnes PS, Keller EE. Craniofacial and dental manifestations of Proteus syndrome: a case report. Cleft Palate Craniofac J 2002;39:233–245
19. Viscardi RM, Romberg E, Abrams RG. Delayed primary tooth eruption in premature infants: relationship to neonatal factors. Pediatr Dent 1994;16:23–28
20. Huang JS, Ho KY, Chen CC, Wu YM, Wang CC, Ho YP, Liu CS. Collagen synthesis in idiopathic and dilantin-induced gingival fibromatosis. Kaohsiung J Med Sci 1997;13:141–148
21. Unger S, Mornet E, Mundlos S, Blaser S, Cole DE. Severe cleidocranial dysplasia can mimic hypophosphatasia. Eur J Pediatr 2002;161:623–626
22. Seow WK, Hertzberg J. Dental development and molar root length in children with cleidocranial dysplasia. Pediatr Dent 1995;17:101–105
23. Liu X, Sun Z, Neiderhiser JM, Uchiyama M, Okawa M. Low birth weight, developmental milestones, and behavioral problems in Chinese children and adolescents. Psychiatry Res 2001;101:115–129
24. Fine DH, Tofsky N, Nelson EM, Schoen D, Barasch A. Clinical implications of the oral manifestations of HIV infection in children. Dent Clin North Am 2003;47:159–174
25. Hauk MJ, Moss ME, Weinberg GA, Berkowitz RJ. Delayed tooth eruption: association with severity of HIV infection. Pediatr Dent 2001;23:260–262
26. Bergman A, Kjellberg H, Dahlgren J. Craniofacial morphology and dental age in children with Silver-Russell syndrome. Orthod Craniofac Res 2003;6:54–62
27. Petzold D, Kratzsch E, Opitz Ch, Tinschert S. The Kabuki syndrome: four patients with oral abnormalities. Eur J Orthod 2003;25:13–19
28. Dupuis-Girod S, Corradini N, Hadj-Rabia S, Fournet JC, Faivre L, Le Deist F, Durand P, Doffinger R, Smahi A, Israel A, Courtois G, Brousse N, Blanche S, Munnich A, Fischer A, Casanova JL, Bodemer C. Osteopetrosis, lymphedema, anhidrotic ectodermal dysplasia, and immunodeficiency in a boy and incontinentia pigmenti in his mother. Pediatrics 2002;109:e97
29. Soliman AT, Ramadan MA, Sherif A, Aziz Bedair ES, Rizk MM. Pycnodysostosis: clinical, radiologic, and endocrine evaluation and linear growth after growth hormone therapy. Metabolism 2001;50:905–911
30. Dachi SF, Howell FV. A survey of 3,874 routine full-month radiographs. II. A study of impacted teeth. Oral Surg 1961;14:1165–1169
31. Winter GB. Principles of Exodontia as Applied to the Impacted Third Molar. St Louis: American Medical Book Company, 1926
32. Knutsson K, Brehmer B, Lysell L, Rohlin M. Pathoses associated with mandibular third molars subjected to removal. Oral Surg Oral Med Oral Pathol Oral Radiol Endod 1996;82:10–17
33. Edwards MJ, Brickley MR, Goodey RD, Shepherd JP. The cost, effectiveness and cost effectiveness of removal and retention of asymptomatic, disease free third molars. Br Dent J 1999;187:380–384
34. Hicks EP. Third molar management: a case against routine removal in adolescent and young adult orthodontic patients. J Oral Maxillofac Surg 1999;57:831–836
35. Song F, O'Meara S, Wilson P, Golder S, Kleijnen J. The effectiveness and cost-effectiveness of prophylactic removal of wisdom teeth. Health Technol Assess 2000;4:1–55

36. Renton T, Smeeton N, McGurk M. Factors predictive of difficulty of mandibular third molar surgery. Br Dent J 2001;190:607–610
37. Kruger E, Thomson WM, Konthasinghe P. Third molar outcomes from age 18 to 26: findings from a population-based New Zealand longitudinal study. Oral Surg Oral Med Oral Pathol Oral Radiol Endod 2001;92:150–155
38. Richardson G, Russell KA. A review of impacted permanent maxillary cuspids: diagnosis and prevention. J Can Dent Assoc 2000;66:497–501
39. Smailiene D. Localization of impacted maxillary canines by palpation and orthopantomography. Medicina (Kaunas) 2002;38:825–829
40. Mason C, Papadakou P, Roberts GJ. The radiographic localization of impacted maxillary canines: a comparison of methods. Eur J Orthod 2001;23:25–34
41. Jacobs SG. Radiographic localization of unerupted teeth: further findings about the vertical tube shift method and other localization techniques. Am J Orthod Dentofacial Orthop 2000;118:439–447
42. Stewart JA, Heo G, Glover KE, Williamson PC, Lam EW, Major PW. Factors that relate to treatment duration for patients with palatally impacted maxillary canines. Am J Orthod Dentofacial Orthop 2001;119:216–225
43. Caminiti MF, Sandor GK, Giambattistini C, Tompson B. Outcomes of the surgical exposure, bonding and eruption of 82 impacted maxillary canines. J Can Dent Assoc 1998;64:572–579
44. Stafne EC, Austin LT. Resorption of embedded teeth. J Am Dent Assoc 1945;32:1003–1009
45. Stanley HR, Alattar M, Collett WK, Stringfellow HR Jr, Spiegel EH. Pathological sequelae of "neglected" impacted third molars. J Oral Pathol 1988;17:113–117
46. Berge TI. Incidence of infections requiring hospitalization associated with partially erupted third molars. Acta Odontol Scand 1996;54:309–313
47. Berge TI. Incidence of large third-molar-associated cystic lesions requiring hospitalization. Acta Odontol Scand 1996;54:327–331
48. Yamada T, Sawaki Y, Tohnai I, Takeuchi M, Ueda M. A study of sports-related mandibular angle fracture: relation to the position of the third molars. Scand J Med Sci Sports 1998;8:116–119
49. Shah N, Thuau H, Beale I. Spontaneous regression of bilateral dentigerous cysts associated with impacted mandibular third molars. Br Dent J 2002;192:75–76
50. Ikeshima A, Tamura Y. Differential diagnosis between dentigerous cyst and benign tumor with an embedded tooth. J Oral Sci 2002;44:13–17
51. Philipsen H-P, Reichart PA. Unicystic ameloblastoma. A review of 193 cases from the literature. Oral Oncol 1998;34:317–325
52. Tsukamoto G, Makino T, Kikuchi T, Kishimoto K, Nishiyama A, Sasaki A, Matsumura T. A comparative study of keratocystic odontogenic tumors associated with and not associated with an impacted mandibular third molar. Oral Surg Oral Med Oral Pathol Oral Radiol Endod 2002;94:272–275
53. Liu JK, Hsiao CK, Chen HA, Tsai MY. Orthodontic correction of a mandibular first molar deeply impacted by an odontoma: a case report. Quintessence Int 1997;28:381–385
54. McGuinness NJ, Faughnan T, Bennani F, Connolly CE. Ameloblastic fibroma of the anterior maxilla presenting as a complication of tooth eruption: a case report. J Orthod 2001;28:115–118
55. Chintakanon K, Boonpinon P. Ectopic eruption of the first permanent molars: prevalence and etiologic factors. Angle Orthod 1998;68:153–160
56. Alaejos-Algarra C, Berini-Aytes L, Gay-Escoda C. Transmigration of mandibular canines: report of six cases and review of the literature. Quintessence Int 1998;29:395–398
57. Shapira Y, Kuftinec MM. Maxillary tooth transpositions: characteristic features and accompanying dental anomalies. Am J Orthod Dentofacial Orthop 2001;119:127–134
58. Main DM. Tooth identity in ovarian teratomas. Br Dent J 1970;129:328–332

TEST: Eruption and dental impaction

1. Natal teeth are not present at birth but appear during the first month after birth.

   True ☐ **False** ☐

2. An impacted maxillary canine with the crown situated palatally to the dental arch will appear magnified horizontally (proportionately wider than reality) in the panoramic radiograph.

   True ☐ **False** ☐

3. Internal resorption of impacted teeth has been reported to occur in less than 0.5% of long standing impactions.

   True ☐ **False** ☐

4. Teeth retarded in eruption due to cleidocranial dysplasia are readily brought into place by standard orthodontic procedures.

   True ☐ **False** ☐

5. Systematic reviews have generally concluded that, in the absence of association with definite pathoses, it is best not to extract impacted third molars teeth.

   True ☐ **False** ☐

6. Supernumerary teeth vary too widely in size and morphology for any assessment in position due to the effects of tooth magnification in panoramic radiographs.

   True ☐ **False** ☐

7. Distoangular impacted third molars lie obliquely in bone with the root slanted in a distal direction toward the ramus.

   True ☐ **False** ☐

8. Male sex and obesity have been found to be factors, among others, that influence surgical difficulty of third molar extractions.

   True ☐ **False** ☐

9. The odds for associated pathoses are the same for molars partially covered by soft tissue as for molars completely covered by soft or bone tissue.

   True ☐ **False** ☐

10. Pathoses reported in association with impacted teeth include the ameloblastoma, keratocystic odontogenic tumor, odontomas, and adenomatoid odontogenic tumor.

    True ☐ **False** ☐

Chapter

Panoramic Radiographic Assessment in Orthodontics

8

Anibal M. Silveira
in association with Allan G. Farman

Learning Objectives

After studying this article, the reader should be able to:

- Define the roles of panoramic radiology in orthodontic practice
- Explain the importance of root parallelism for assessing orthodontic treatment success
- Describe the advantages and disadvantages of panoramic radiography for assessment of form distance and angulations

Panoramic radiography has a role in support of orthodontic assessment both in pre-treatment planning and also in post-treatment evaluation of success or failure. Panoramic radiographs are important in assessing the presence or absence of specific teeth, their morphology and structure, and their eruption sequence and spatial relationships. Panoramic radiographs are also required by the American Board of Orthodontics for examination of treatment success of cases presented by candidates for Diplomate status. In particular the panoramic radiograph is used in the assessment of tooth root parallelism.

The panoramic radiograph is an expedient and efficient diagnostic imaging projection that provides a representation of both dental arches and their surrounding structures. It provides an image useful for identifying anomalies of the dentition, alveolar bone morphology, and the relationships of maxillofacial structures to one another. Graber (1967) advocated periodic panoramic radiographic examination during orthodontic treatment to achieve the optimal treatment goals [1].

Pros and Cons

Panoramic imaging is an excellent technique if used with the realization that it has greater value for observations rather than for making precise measurements. Panoramic radiographs provide valuable information about present, missing, or supernumerary teeth along with dental age and the tooth eruption sequence. They are also used for detection of dental anomalies and for the evaluation of general dental health including advanced dental caries and periodontal disease. A panoramic projection can reveal the presence of pathologic conditions and variations from normal. However, it provides more limited information about mandibular symmetry, paranasal sinuses, space availability in the dental arch, root parallelism, and the temporomandibular joints.

Advantages of panoramic radiography include low radiation dose, low operator time usage, relatively short patient exposure time, and excellent patient comfort. A point to stress, however, is that panoramic radiography has many shortcomings related to the reliability and accuracy in the assessment of size, location, and form. Discrepancies arise because the panoramic image is made by creating an image layer or region of focus to conform to a "generic" (average) jaw form and size [2]. Panoramic radiographic projections provide the best images when the anatomy being imaged approximates this "generic," or "ideal," maxillofacial complex.

Previous chapters have detailed the use of panoramic radiography for detection of anomalies of the dentition [3–6] and dental impactions [7]. The use of panoramic radiographs in determining dental age and jaw growth potential will follow in the next chapter [8]. All of these uses of panoramic radiography are very important for the orthodontist. Perhaps the most important role assigned to panoramic radiography by orthodontics that is not covered elsewhere in this book is the determination of tooth root parallelism.

Root Parallelism

One of the goals of orthodontic treatment is to ensure that each tooth is in a biologically and mechanically favorable position in the jaw. Over the years, various authors have emphasized the importance of achieving root parallelism as one of the final goals of orthodontic treatment and the use of panoramic radiographs to verify this proper root position [9–13]. In 1972, Andrews published *The Six Keys to Normal Occlusion* and *The Six Keys to Optimal Occlusion*, establishing the standard of care to which clinicians aim their treatment [14]. Since then, other researchers and clinicians have added to Andrews' guidelines using their own criteria. The ultimate goal of all has been that the position of the dentition is made compatible with the patient's skeletal and soft tissue of the face and jaws. In 1998, the American Board of Orthodontics (ABO) established an Objective Grading System to evaluate dental casts and panoramic radiographs [12]. The ABO criteria represent the current standard of care to which all patients should be treated.

There are seven criteria categories that are graded for cases presented by candidates for Board Diplomate Status in the ABO: root angulation, marginal ridges, bucco-lingual inclination, overjet, occlusal contacts, occlusal relationship, and interproximal contacts. Root angulation is used to assess the position of the teeth in relation to one another. While the ABO recognizes that the panoramic radiograph is not the "perfect record for evaluating root angulation, it is probably the best means possible for making this assessment" [12]. Root parallelism is assessed on the panoramic image for each tooth by examining its deviation with respect to the adjacent teeth and its orientation perpendicular to a constructed arbitrary occlusal plane.

As explained above, the traditional panoramic radiograph does not provide an undistorted image of the jaws and the dentition. Various investigators have studied image layer (or focal trough) [15–22], projection angle [23, 24], horizontal and vertical magnification [25–28], angular distortion [9, 10, 17, 27–29], and patient positioning and their effects on the dimensional accuracy of panoramic images [10, 30]. Distortion on panoramic radiographs of the angle between inclined teeth is the result of the combined distortions in the vertical and horizontal dimensions [13, 31]. Inherent distortion effects exist within this type radiograph for assessing "root parallelism," but currently it remains the most efficient imaging modality available within clinical orthodontic practice.

Philipp and Hurst (1978) noted the increasing usage of panoramic radiographs by orthodontists to determine root parallelism and the axial relationship of these same teeth to the occlusal plane [27]. They evaluated these relationships and the type, amount and place of distortion occurring in the posterior buccal segments. The effect of varying the cant of the occlusal plane on this distortion was also determined. The test device used was a protractor stabilized to a plastic base with mounted rectangular wires—one placed horizontally with five vertical wires spot welded at equal intervals perpendicular to the horizontal wire. While collecting the data, the angular settings of the test device were varied from −4° to +20° perpendicular to a line parallel to the floor. They reached the following conclusions for the system tested: (a) as the occlusal plane was tipped from −4° to +20° in parallel with the floor, the maxillary tooth roots converged away from the occlusal plane and the mandibular tooth roots diverged away from the occlusal plane; (b) the largest amount of distortion in parallelism was in the canine-premolar region of both arches; (c) the largest amount of distortion of the tooth long axis to the occlusal plane was in the molar region with maxillary teeth angulated to the mesial and the mandibular teeth angulated to the distal; (d) there was the least amount of distortion when the occlusal plane was located at +6°; (d) elongation was more pronounced in the maxilla and increased in the molar region; and (e) magnification ranged from 23% to 28%. They, nevertheless, concluded that the clinical significance of the distortion was not important so long as the clinician understands that there is distortion that varies with the cant of the occlusal plane [27].

Mayoral (1982) reported that few studies had been performed up to that time point to evaluate root "parallelism" by means of panoramic radiography [32]. He stated that root parallelism is of prime importance if one wishes to obtain a correct alignment of the teeth within their apical bases, a normal occlusion, and maintenance of a stable treatment result. In his study, 53 patients planned for first premolar extraction were treated with light continuous wire therapy. Panoramic radiographs were made before and after active treatment and one year out of retention. The long axes of the upper and lower canines and second premolars were traced and the angulation between them was measured to evaluate root "parallelism" [32]. The end results were classified as follows into four groups according to the angulation of the roots (Table 8.1).

Lucchesi et al. (1988) investigated the suitability of the panoramic radiograph for the assessment of the mesiodistal angulation of teeth [10]. They used a mandibular phantom constructed of Plexiglas with steel pins at known mesiodistal angulations ranging from −20° to +20° and bucco-lingual inclinations ranging from 0° (perpendicular to the Plexiglas base) to 25° (with the crown directed lingually). Panoramic and plain film (lateral-oblique) radiographs were made of the model.

Table 8.1 Classification of root parallelism

Mayoral parallelism criteria	Arch	
	Maxilla	Mandible
Good	−5° to +5°	0° to +12°
Acceptable	+6° to +10°	+13° to +18°
Poor	> +11°	> +19°
Overtreatment	< −6°	< 0°

The results obtained during this study indicated that the plain-film technique was more accurate than the panoramic technique employed for assessing mesiodistal root angulations. The authors stated, though, that the beam-receptor angulation in the plain-film technique could not be controlled as well in a clinical situation as it was in this experiment with the stationary, transparent phantom.

Burson et al. (1994) reported on the accuracy of four panoramic radiographic systems in determining tooth angulations [29]. A dry skull with stainless steel orthodontic wires glued to the buccal surfaces of the teeth was used as the test model to simulate the long axis of the teeth (from canine to second molar). An additional, four wires were glued to the occlusal plane to be used as horizontal reference lines. For each of the four systems employed, panoramic radiographs were made using the following six patient positions: (1) correct position, (2) 5 mm forward position, (3) 5 mm backward position, (4) 10° head up position, (5) 10° head down position, and (6) 5 mm left position. All of the machines studied showed a significant correlation between the mean radiographic estimates and the actual measurements regardless of positioning. This study evaluated the accuracy of the tooth angulations in the correct skull position with three different degrees of error tolerances (±2°, 3°, and 5°). The results were reported in this manner so that orthodontists could choose the degree of error that they are willing to accept as clinically acceptable. All systems tested were accurate at a 5° tolerance.

Wyatt et al. (1995) also investigated the accuracy of dimensional and angular measurements from panoramic and lateral oblique radiographs [30]. Three panoramic systems were used. Acrylic test models had wires positioned to represent the position and angulations of the teeth. This study reported that there were not any statistically significant differences in the angular measurement accuracy of the radiographs produced by the panoramic versus the lateral oblique radiographic techniques.

McKee et al. (2002) studied the accuracy of four panoramic systems with regard to mesiodistal tooth angulations [13]. A constructed "typodont" tooth inserted into a dry skull was radiographed on five different occasions for each of the panoramic systems evaluated. Custom designed software and a three-dimensional coordinate-measuring device were used to determine the true tooth angulations. Seventy-four percent of the maxillary and mandibular image mesiodistal angulations were significantly different from the true angulations. Inaccuracy was evenly distributed among the four panoramic systems. In the maxilla, the largest angular difference between adjacent teeth occurred between the canine and first premolar with measurements ranging from 5.4° to 7.0° depending on the tested system. Generally, the anterior roots were displayed more mesially and the posterior roots more distally. In the mandible, the largest angular difference of adjacent teeth occurred between the lateral incisor and the canine with measurements ranging between 3.7° and 5.7°. All roots were projected more mesially, but this was especially the case for the canines and premolars. McKee et al. noted that if the object is positioned within the image layer and does not have an extreme bucco-lingual inclination, the mesiodistal inclination may be measured in panoramic radiography with a moderate error (±5°) [13]. With the clinically relevant tolerance limit of 2.5° (in either direction), they showed a significant difference from the truth in 61% of measurements. In conclusion, the authors stated that panoramic radiographs should be examined with an understanding of the inherent image distortions.

Quality Control

In addition to the inherent distortion of panoramic radiographs, human technique error can have a significant effect on clinical image quality. Rushton et al. (1999) sampled the quality of 1,813 panoramic radiographs made in 41 general dental practices in England [33]. Radiographs were judged based on correct technique and film processing and 33% were determined to be of "unacceptable" quality. Poor anterior-posterior positioning was responsible for over half of the 33% of "failing" radiographs and occlusal plane errors were also responsible for almost a third. Patient positioning errors appeared in over 85% of the radiographs judged as failing. The limited dimensions of the image layer—perhaps with older vintage panoramic machines—translated into positioning errors.

Akarslan et al. (2003) evaluated 460 panoramic radiographs for the 20 most common errors—and only 38% were found to be technique error-free [34]. They found that positioning errors were responsible for over 38% of the errors. Errors included improper occlusal plane tilt, blurring, narrowing, and widening of anterior teeth, effects that are largely a result of careless anterior-posterior head positioning. Practitioners and their assistants evidently need better training in how to use panoramic X-ray systems to produce optimal images.

American Board of Orthodontics Panoramic Requirement

The ABO requires the use of the panoramic radiograph in an Objective Grading System that includes evaluation of "tooth root parallelism"—the deviation of tooth root axes from "ideal"—as part of the fulfillment of the clinical portion of the Orthodontic Board certification examination [35].

Root angulation is but one of the seven categories graded by the ABO and is used to assess the position of the teeth in relation to one another. In theory, root parallelism ensures sufficient bone between adjacent teeth, helping to protect against future periodontal bone loss. While the ABO recognizes that the panoramic radiograph is not the perfect record for evaluating root angulation, it is still considered the best practical means for making this assessment [12]. The ABO instructions for determining root parallelism using the panoramic radiograph are that the deviation of each tooth is to be assessed with respect to its deviation from adjacent teeth, and its orientation perpendicular to a constructed occlusal plane perpendicular to an arbitrary midsagittal line.

As part of the clinical examination, ABO candidates must supply six to ten completed clinical cases and defend each case. Panoramic radiographs are required for each of the presented cases. A total deduction of 20 points from a total of 380 is allowable for each case from an assessment of each patient's models and panoramic radiograph. Deviations of 1–2 mm from the "ideal" result in a one point deduction. Deviations greater than 2 mm result in a two point deduction.

The ABO reports on four internal field tests to validate their Objective Grading System [12]; however, there are no published peer-reviewed data to support the accuracy of this assessment system. In the instructional compact disc (ABO 2002) supplied to ABO candidates [35], the ideal orientation for a particular tooth is determined by drawing a line parallel to the midline through the middle of the incisal edge of the tooth (Fig. 8.1). This quantitative technique does not relate the tooth axis to the occlusal plane. The occlusal plane can vary significantly with respect to patient head position and panoramic equipment used; therefore these variables could influence the assessment of root angulation using this system. Perhaps a better approach would be to follow the method displayed in Fig. 8.2.

Conclusions

The panoramic radiograph has become an indispensable diagnostic image considered of importance in determining success or failure of orthodontic treatment. It provides information concerning the presence or absence of teeth, their morphological and structural variations, orientation and pattern of eruption. From the dental development it is possible to estimate dental maturity. Further, the panoramic radiograph has become the standard for assessing tooth root parallelism, a feature considered of importance in determining success or failure of orthodontic treatment.

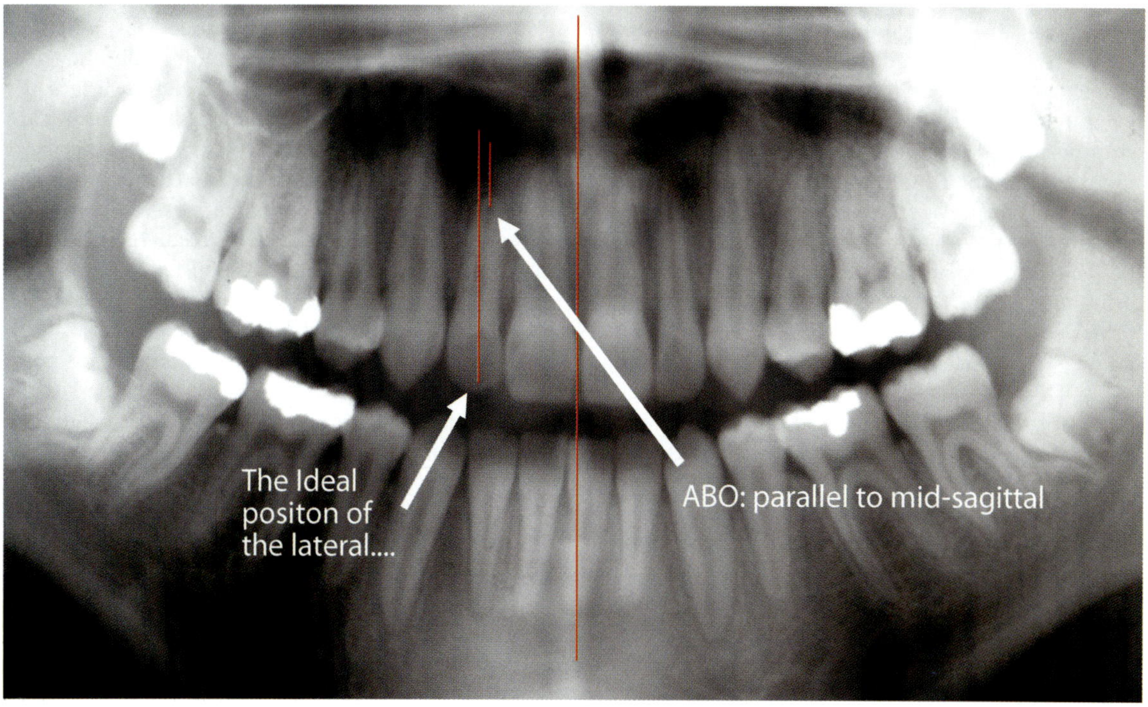

Fig. 8.1 First method for assessing root parallelism. An arbitrary vertical line is drawn to which is used as a reference for the ideal position of root angulation. The distance between the ideal and the actual location of the root apex is measured in millimeters

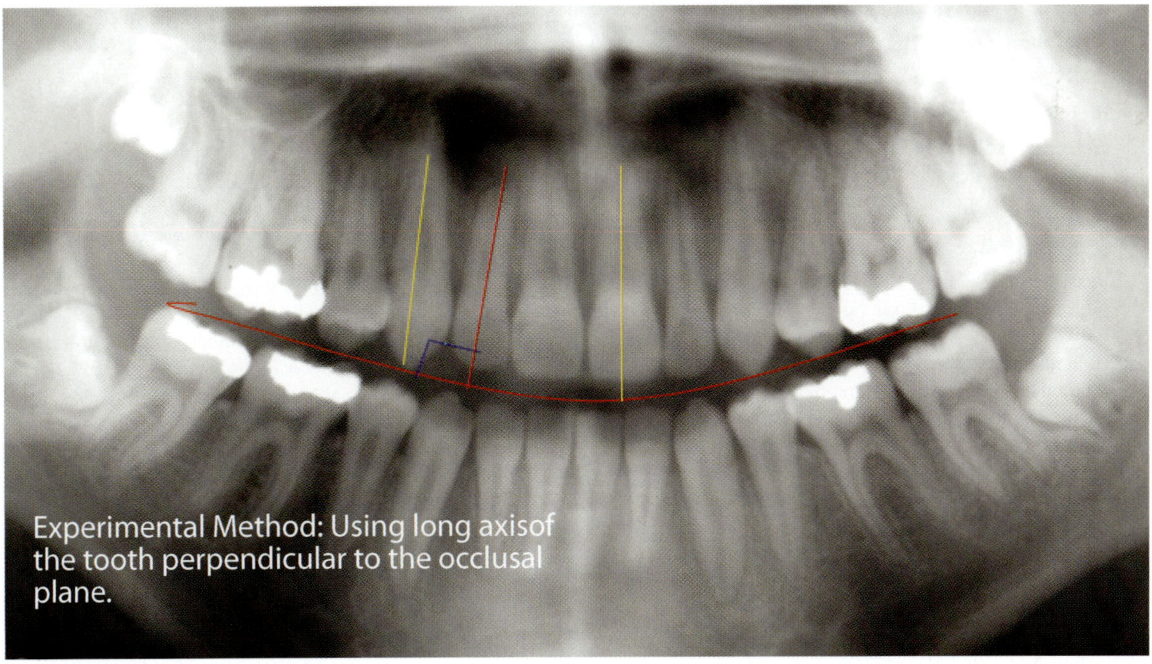

Fig. 8.2 Second method for assessing root parallelism. With this method the ideal position of the long axis of the root is perpendicular to the occlusal plane. The distance between the ideal and the actual is measured in millimeters

References

1. Graber TM. Panoramic radiography in orthodontic diagnosis. Am J Orthod 1967;53:799–821
2. Welander U, Nummikoski P, Tronje G, McDavid WD, Legrell PE, Langlais RP. Standard forms of dentition and mandible for applications in rotational panoramic radiography. Dentomaxillofac Radiol 1989;18:60–67
3. Farman AG. Panoramic radiologic appraisal of anomalies of dentition: Chapter #1. Panoramic Imaging News 2003;3(1):1–7
4. Farman AG. Panoramic radiologic appraisal of anomalies of dentition: Chapter #2. Panoramic Imaging News 2003;3(2):1–5
5. Farman AG. Panoramic radiologic appraisal of anomalies of dentition: Chapter #3 – Tooth morphology. Panoramic Imaging News 2003;3(3):1–6
6. Farman AG. Panoramic radiologic appraisal of anomalies of dentition: Chapter #4 – Tooth structure. Panoramic Imaging News 2004;4(1):1–7
7. Farman AG. Tooth eruption and dental impactions. Panoramic Imaging News 2004;4(2):1–7
8. Farman AG. Assessing growth and development with panoramic radiographs and cephalometric attachments: a critical tool for dental diagnosis and treatment planning. Panoramic Imaging News 2004;4(4):1–11
9. Samfors KA, Welander U. Angle distortion in narrow beam rotation radiography. Acta Radiol Diagn 1974;15:570–576
10. Lucchesi MV, Wood RE, Nortjé CJ. Suitability of the panoramic radiograph for assessment of mesiodistal angulation of teeth in the buccal segments of the mandible. Am J Orthod Dentofacial Orthop1988;94:303–310
11. Ursi WJ, Almeida RR, Tavano O, Henriques JF. Assessment of the mesiodistal axial inclination through panoramic radiography. J Clin Orthod 1990;24:166–173
12. Casko JS, Vaden JL, Kokich VG, Damone J, James RD, Cangialosi TJ, Riolo ML, Owens SE Jr, Bills ED. Objective grading system for dental casts and panoramic radiographs. American Board of Orthodontics. Am J Orthod Dentofacial Orthop 1998;114:589–599
13. McKee IW, Williamson PC, Lam EW, Heo G, Glover KE, Major PW. The accuracy of 4 panoramic units in the projection of mesiodistal tooth angulations. Am J Orthod 2002;121:166–175
14. Andrews LF. In: Andrews LF (ed) Straight Wire: The Concept and Appliance. Los Angeles: Wells; 1989, p 4
15. Glass BJ, McDavid WD, Welander U, Morris CR. The central plane of the image layer determined experimentally in various rotational panoramic X-ray machines. Oral Surg Oral Med Oral Pathol 1985;60:104–112
16. McDavid WD, Tronje G, Welander U, Morris CR, Nummikoski P. Imaging characteristics of seven panoramic X-ray units. Chapter II: The image layer. Dentomaxillofac Radiol 1985;8(Suppl):5–11

17. Welander U, McDavid WD, Tronje G, Morris CR. VI Inclined objects. In: McDavid WD, Tronje G, Welander U, Morris CR, Nummikoski P (eds) Imaging Characteristics of Seven Panoramic X-ray Units. Dentomaxillofac Radiol 1985;8(Suppl):45–50
18. Welander U, McDavid WD, Tronje G, Morris CR. An analysis of different planes within the image layer in rotational panoramic radiography. Dentomaxillofac Radiol 1987;16:79–84
19. Razmus TF, Glass BJ, McDavid WD. Comparison of image layer location among panoramic machines of the same manufacturer. Oral Surg Oral Med Oral Pathol 1989;67:102–108
20. Welander U, Tronje G, McDavid WD. Layer thickness in rotational panoramic radiography: some specific aspects. Dentomaxillofac Radiol 1989;18:119–124
21. Farman TT, Kelly MS, Farman AG. The OP 100 Digipan: evaluation of the image layer, magnification factors and dosimetry. Oral Surg Oral Med Oral Pathol Oral Radiol Endod 1997;83:281–287
22. Farman TT, Farman AG. TMJ pantomography using CCD, photostimulable phosphor and film receptors: a comparison. J Digit Imaging 1999;12(2Suppl.1):9–13
23. Tronje G, Welander U, McDavid WD, Morris CR III. Projection angle. In: McDavid WD, Tronje G, Welander U, Morris CR, Nummikoski P (eds) Imaging Characteristics of Seven Panoramic X-ray Units. Dentomaxillofac Radiol 1985;8(Suppl):21–28
24. Scarfe WC, Nummoikoski P, McDavid WD, Welander U, Tronje G. Radiographic interproximal angulations: Implications for rotational panoramic radiography. Oral Surg Oral Med Oral Pathol 1993;76:664–672
25. Samfors KA, Welander U. Area distortion in narrow beam rotation radiography. Acta Radiol Diagn (Stockh) 1974;15:650–655
26. Sjoblom A, Samfors KA, Welander U. Form distortion in a narrow beam rotation radiography. Acta Radiol Diagn (Stockh) 1975;16:565–571
27. Philipp RG, Hurst RV. The cant of the occlusal plane and distortion in the panoramic radiograph. Angle Orthod 1978;48:317–323
28. Farman TT, Farman AG, Kelly MS, Firriolo FJ, Yancey JM, Stewart AV. Charge-coupled device panoramic radiography: effect of beam energy on radiation exposure. Dentomaxillofac Radiol 1998;27:36–40
29. Burson SD, Farman AG, Kang B. Comparison of four panoramic dental radiographic systems for tooth angulation measurement accuracy under different tolerances. J Kor Acad Oral Maxillofac Radiol 1994;24:317–324
30. Wyatt DL, Farman AG, Orbell GM, Silveira AM, Scarfe WC. Accuracy of dimensional and angular measurements from panoramic and lateral oblique radiographs. Dentomaxillofac Radiol 1995;24:225–231
31. McDavid WD, Tronje G, Welander U, Morris CR. Dimensional reproduction in rotational panoramic radiography. Oral Surg Oral Med Oral Pathol 1986;62:96–101
32. Mayoral G. Treatment results with light wires studied by panoramic radiography. Am J Orthod 1982;91:489–497
33. Rushton VE, Horner K, Worthington HV. The quality of panoramic radiographs in a sample of general dental practices. Br Dent J 1999;186:630–633
34. Akarslan ZZ, Erten H, Gungor K, Celik I. Common errors on panoramic radiographs taken in a dental school. J Contemp Dent Pract 2003;4:24–34
35. American Board of Orthodontics. Grading System for Dental Casts and Panoramic Radiographs: Microsoft PowerPoint Presentation Windows/Macintosh. CD ROM. ABO, 2002

TEST: Panoramic radiology in orthodontics

1. According to the scientific literature panoramic radiography can be conveniently used to precisely measure distances in the horizontal plane.

   True ☐ **False** ☐

2. Studies of panoramic radiographs made in general dental practice suggest that dentists and their assistants could be better trained to avoid technique errors.

   True ☐ **False** ☐

3. The use of panoramic radiographs by orthodontists to assess tooth root parallelism is approved by the American Board of Orthodontics.

   True ☐ **False** ☐

4. The most common error in panoramic radiology is probably that of incorrect patient positioning.

   True ☐ **False** ☐

5. A study of panoramic radiography using several systems determined that in the panoramic image the anterior roots were displayed more distally and the posterior roots more mesially.

   True ☐ **False** ☐

6. Wyatt's study (1995) found statistically significant differences between panoramic systems in terms of accuracy of angular assessments.

   True ☐ **False** ☐

7. While lateral-oblique radiographs are easy to position with test phantoms, angular accuracy might not be so easy to replicate in a clinical situation.

   True ☐ **False** ☐

8. One method advocated for measuring tooth root parallelism considers the ideal position of the long axis of the root to be perpendicular to the occlusal plane.

   True ☐ **False** ☐

9. The ABO measures parallelism in terms of millimeters of the root apex from the "ideal" position.

   True ☐ **False** ☐

10. Panoramic image measurement accuracy is dependent on the degree to which the individual patient matches the "generic" jaw shape used by the manufacturer of the system concerned.

    True ☐ **False** ☐

Chapter

Assessing Growth and Development with Panoramic Radiographs and Cephalometric Attachments

9

Allan G. Farman

Learning Objectives

- Gain knowledge of the importance of tooth and skeletal maturity determinations as it inputs into dental treatment planning
- Learn the roles of panoramic, cephalometric, and hand-wrist radiographic studies in biological age determinations
- Learn the factors acting as determinants of relative dental and skeletal maturity findings

It is recommended that radiographs be made periodically both during the mixed dentition (8–9 years old) and adolescence (12–14 years old) to evaluate growth and development, and to look for asymptomatic dental disease [1–3]. Substantial differences in the assessed biological and the known chronological age can be indicators of a variety of inherited and congenital conditions. Further, local failure in dental eruption within the normal time range can be evidence of dental impaction and possibly of a pathological process such as a hamartoma, cyst, or tumor. Failure to remove causes of impaction prior to cessation of the normal eruption time can lead to otherwise unnecessary surgical orthodontics, a poorer outcome prognosis, and perhaps to a sequence of time consuming, expensive, and less than ideal replacement strategies [4]. The dental panoramic radiograph is a quick, simple, and relatively safe way to achieve the goal of evaluating the whole dentition in a manner that is easy to explain to the patient or concerned parent.

Eruption Sequence and Timing

There is some controversy as to the precision with which tooth development and eruption predict chronological age; however, most reports suggest that there is a moderately good correlation. One key indicator of age is that the three permanent molar teeth in each quadrant erupt approximately at 6-year intervals. The first permanent molar erupts around 6 years, the second permanent molar around 12 years, and the third molars around 18 years. Root formation for permanent teeth is completed roughly 3 years following eruption. The first major attempt at developing a chronology for human tooth development was that of Logan and Kronfeld (1933) and with minor modification is still usable as a rough and ready guide. Using this table, eruption times for permanent teeth usually are within 2 years of the actual chronological age (Table 9.1; Figs. 9.1–9.5) [5].

Up to 5–6 years of age, no difference was found in the timing of dental development between boys and girls, in contrast to the older ages where girls were always more advanced dentally than boys.

Demirjian and Levesque (1980) studied dental development of a genetically homogeneous French-Canadian group of children ranging in age from 2.5 to 19 years using 5,437 panoramic radiographs [6–8]. The maturity of each mandibular tooth was evaluated individually. For each stage of each tooth, the developmental curves of boys and girls were compared. Up to 5–6 years of age, no difference was found in the timing of dental development between boys and girls, in contrast to at older ages where girls were always more advanced dentally than boys. Elsewhere, Hegde and Sood (2002) evaluated dental age in 197 children of known chronological age (6–13 years) in Belgaum, India [6, 9]. When the method of Demirjian et al. [6–8] was applied to Belgaum children, mean difference between true and assessed age for males showed overestimation of 0.14 years (51 days) and females showed overestimation of 0.04 years (15 days); hence, the method of Demirjian et al. showed high accuracy in this population group.

In contrast, Teivens et al. (1996) studied the developmental stages of the mandibular teeth according to the method by Demirjian et al. and reported discrepancies in staging where children of ages 5 and 12 years were found to fit the same developmental stage [7, 8, 10]. Their study involved analysis of 197 panoramic radiographs of children aged 5, 6, 9, and 12 years collected and examined by each of 13 independent pedodontists, radiologists, and forensic odontologists. It was concluded that any method for age determination of

Table 9.1 Approximate dental maturation schedule (after Logan and Kronfeld [2])

Dentition/arch	Tooth	Calcification commences	Enamel complete	Eruption	Root complete
Primary maxillary	Central incisor	4 months IU	1.5 months	7.5 months	18 months
	Lateral incisor	4.5 months IU	2.5 months	9 months	24 months
	Canine	5 months IU	9 months	18 months	39 months
	First molar	5 months IU	6 months	14 months	2.5 years
	Second molar	6 months IU	11 months	24 months	3 years
Primary mandibular	Central incisor	4.5 months IU	2.5 months	6 months	18 months
	Lateral incisor	4.5 months IU	3 months	7 months	18 months
	Canine	5 months IU	9 months	16 months	39 months
	First molar	5 months IU	5.5 months	12 months	27 months
	Second molar	6 months IU	10 months	20 months	3 years
Permanent maxillary	Central incisor	3–4 months	4–5 years	7–8 years	10 years
	Lateral incisor	10–12 months	4–5 years	8–9 years	11 years
	Canine	4–5 months	6–7 years	11–12 years	13–15 years
	First premolar	18–21 months	5–6 years	10–11 years	12–13 years
	Second premolar	24–27 months	6–7 years	10–12 years	12–14 years
	First molar	At birth	2.5–3 years	6–7 years	9–10 years
	Second molar	2.5–3 years	7–8 years	12–13 years	14–16 years
	Third molar	7–9 years	12–16 years	17–21 years	18–25 years
Permanent mandibular	Central incisor	3–4 months	4–5 years	6–7 years	9 years
	Lateral incisor	3–4 months	4–5 years	7–8 years	10 years
	Canine	4–5 months	6–7 years	9–10 years	12–14 years
	First premolar	21–24 months	5–6 years	10–12 years	12–13 years
	Second premolar	27–30 months	6–7 years	11–12 years	13–14 years
	First molar	at birth	2.5–3 years	6–7 years	9–10 years
	Second molar	2.5–3 years	7–8 years	11–13 years	14–15 years
	Third molar	8–10 years	12–16 years	17–21 years	18–25 years

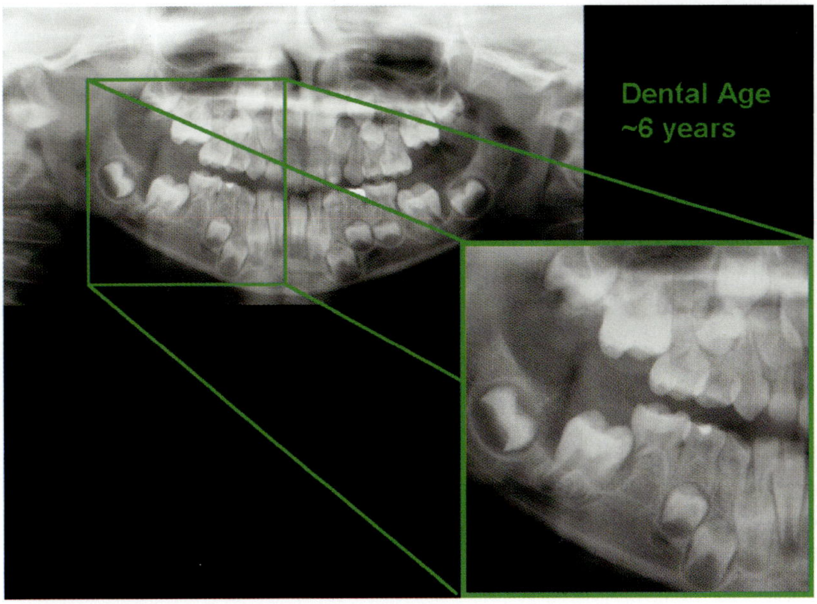

Fig. 9.1 Dental age approximately 6 years. The first permanent molar commences eruption at around 6 years of age. Note that the crown of the second permanent molar is developing at this time

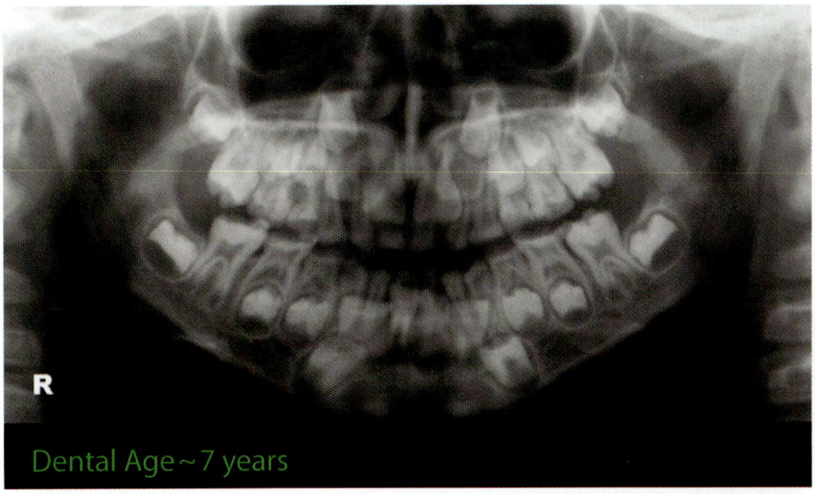

Fig. 9.2 Dental age approximately 7 years. The first permanent molar is generally fully erupted by 7 years; however the roots are still developing. Note that the root apices are wide open ("blunderbuss" shape). Root completion is approximately 3 years following eruption

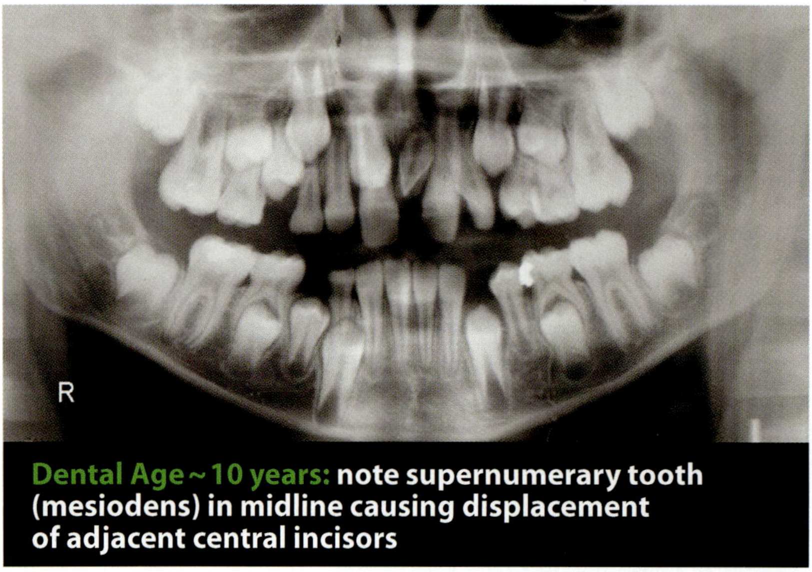

Fig. 9.3 Dental age approximately 10 years. At 10 years in the mixed dentition all permanent first molars and permanent incisors are erupted. The mandibular first premolars are in process of eruption. The roots of the first permanent molars are complete. This case shows a mesiodens (supernumerary tooth) in the maxilla that is displacing the central incisors and, left unattended, might complicate eruption of the permanent maxillary canines due to consequent dental crowding

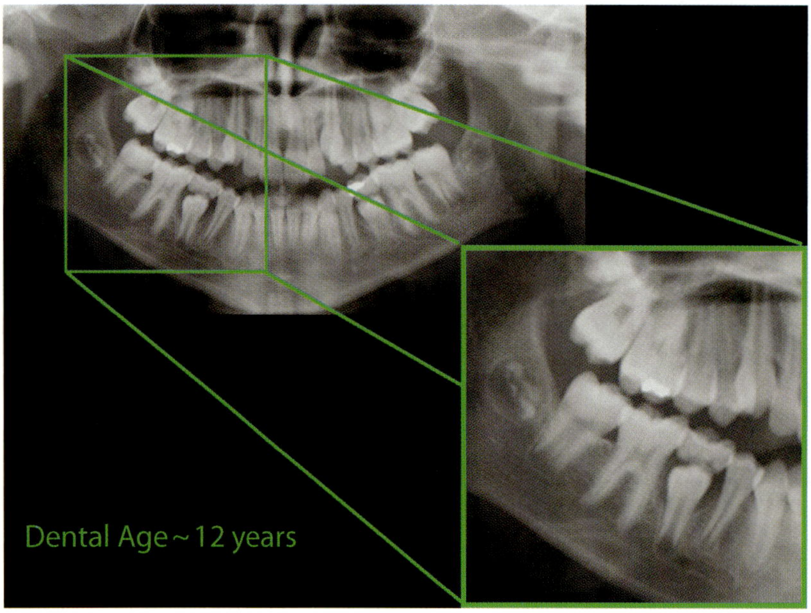

Fig. 9.4 Dental age approximately 12 years. At 12 years, the second permanent molars erupt. All premolars are erupted save for the mandibular second premolars that are still in process of eruption. The permanent maxillary canines are in process of completion of eruption. The mandibular third molars have commenced calcification

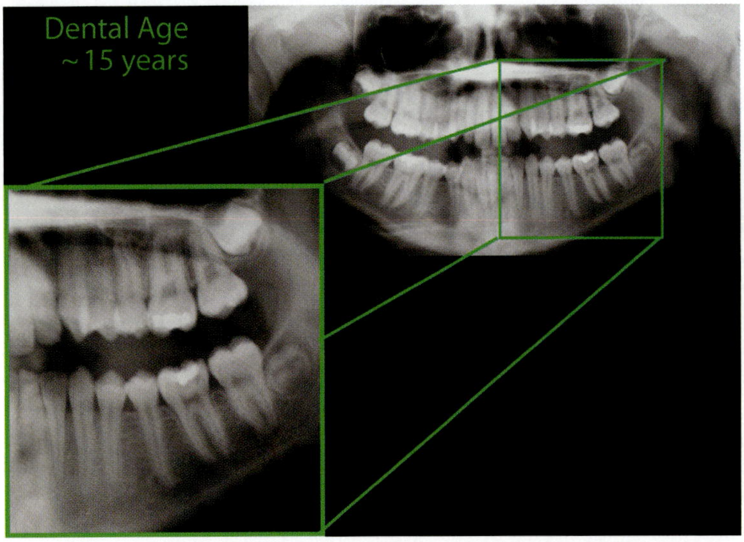

Fig. 9.5 Dental age approximately 15 years. At 15 years the roots of the second permanent molars are complete. All permanent teeth, excepting the third molars, are erupted and completely formed

children with the aid of tooth development will suffer from a rather wide range of uncertainty owing to individual variations. In a separate paper from the same institution, it was found that different observers could vary to an extreme degree in age assessments made on the same radiographs, thus baseline standardization of observers rather than the assessment per se could well have contributed to finding a lack of reliability [11].

Dental age was studied by Nykanen et al. in a sample of 261 Norwegian children (128 boys and 133 girls) by using panoramic radiographs with the same maturity standards [7, 12]. Reliability was analyzed by repeated assessments of 134 of the radiographs, and the overall mean difference between duplicate dental age determinations was 0.5 months for intra- and 1.8 months for inter-examiner comparisons. The Norwegian children were generally somewhat advanced in dental maturity compared with the French-Canadian reference sample. Among the boys the mean difference between dental age and chronological age varied in the different age groups from 1.5 to 4.0 months. Among the girls the difference increased with age, varying from 0 to 3.5 months in the younger age groups (5.5–9.0 years) and from 4.5 to 7.5 months in the age groups 9.5 years and above. The variability in individual dental age was sometimes marked and increased with age. For the older age groups 95% of the individual age estimates were within ±2 years of the real chronological age.

Normal Variations in Eruption Timing

Sex

As indicated earlier, the dental development of a genetically homogeneous French-Canadian group of children ranging in age from 2.5 to 19 years was evaluated from 5,437 panoramic radiographs by the method of Demirjian et al. [7, 8]. Up to 5–6 years of age, no difference was found in the timing of dental development between boys and girls, in contrast to the older ages where girls were always more developed than boys. A close relation was established between the stage of formation of all teeth and their emergence.

In a study of dental maturity in 903 healthy Chinese children (boys: 465, girls: 438) aged 3–16 years, at 3–5 years old, boys had dental maturity slightly more advanced than girls but the sex difference was not statistically significant [13]. In the age range of 7–14 years, girls were more advanced than boys ($p < 0.05$), with girls being on average 0.45 years more mature than boys. The maximum average difference was 0.85 years for the permanent canine tooth. The time that each developmental stage took was shorter in 50% of girls, but longer in 28% of girls compared to the average for boys. There was no difference between boys and girls in the remaining 22% of cases.

In a study of 929 female and 686 male Japanese subjects aged between 12 and 30 years, a total of 1,615 panoramic radiographs were examined [14]. The mineralization stages of third molars were evaluated on the basis of the Demirjian et al. stages, modified in accordance with Mincer's model [7, 8]. No statistically significant differences in the chronology of third molar mineralization between maxilla and mandible and between sides were observed. A comparison between sexes did not reveal any substantial differences with respect to third molar development.

Skeletal Pattern

In a Japanese population, Sasaki et al. (1990) examined variations in dental maturity between girls having skeletal Class II and Class III malocclusions. Using panoramic radiographs and lateral cephalograms, they found that the timing of dental eruption was not significantly affected by jaw skeletal type [15].

In Brazil, Janson et al. carried out a double blind determination of dental maturation, expressed by dental age, for each of 20 subjects (10 male and 10 female for each group) selected from 400 subjects by virtue of representing the extremes in open and deep bite. Given the same chronological age, the open bite group had a mean dental age 6 months greater than that determined for the deep overbite group [16]. This difference proved to be statistically significant ($p < 0.05$) [16].

Ethnicity

Prabhakar et al. (2002) used the standard Demirjian et al. (1973) dental maturation system for 151 healthy Indian children in Davangere and found that this ethnic group was on average more dentally advanced than the standard by slightly more than one year for boys (1.20 ± 1.02 years) and just less than one year for girls (0.90 ± 0.87) [6, 17].

Davidson and Rodd (2001) used a cross-sectional study to compare dental age with chronological age in Somali children under 16 years of age and age- and sex-matched white Caucasian children, resident in Sheffield, England [18]. Dental age was determined for each subject using existing panoramic radiographs. Comparisons of the difference between dental age and chronological age were made for sex and ethnic group, using independent sample t-tests and setting significance at $p = 0.05$. The sample group comprised 162 subjects: 84 Somali and Caucasian boys (mean age 10.6 years) and 78 Somali and Caucasian girls (mean age 11.2 years). The mean difference between dental and chronological age was 1.01 years for Somali boys, 0.19 years for Caucasian boys; 1.22 years for Somali girls, and 0.52 years for Caucasian girls. The difference between dental and chronological age was significantly greater in Somali subjects than in Caucasian children. Somali subjects showed a marked discrepancy between ascribed chronological age and dental age (range −1.75 to +5.42 years), which was most evident in 8- to 12-year-old children. These findings suggest that there is a need for population specific dental development standards to improve the accuracy of dental age assessment.

Local Causes of Delayed Dental Eruption

Individual or multiple teeth in a jaw segment can fail to erupt in a timely manner due to impaction against a "mechanical" obstruction commonly caused by inappropriate tooth orientation during development (especially maxillary permanent canine or third molar teeth in either jaw), crowding (impaction against a regular tooth or teeth), supernumerary tooth or teeth, retained primary teeth, or tooth roots, with or without ankylosis. Primary teeth most likely to be involved are those that have inflamed pulps or periapical lesions, and those that have been treated by pulpotomy. Other fairly common obstructions to dental eruption are follicular cysts (eruption or dentigerous cyst) and hamartomas (complex or compound odontomas) [19]. For tumors or cysts to prevent or delay tooth eruption locally, the lesion needs to arise in childhood or adolescence. Benign tumors that can envelop or overlie a developing tooth include adenomatoid odontogenic tumor, ameloblastoma (usually unicystic), ameloblastic fibroma, ameloblastic fibro-odontoma, odontogenic myxoma, and cementifying-ossifying fibroma. Other conditions that can locally delay tooth eruption include cherubism (usually bilaterally) and fibrous dysplasia (generally unilateral) [19]. Obviously teeth that are absent cannot erupt, so hypodontia also needs to be excluded radiographically. Regional odontodysplasia can also result in failure of eruption of a segment of teeth, and again requires radiographic study. Fibromatosis gingivae may either delay eruption or simply hide the teeth from clinical view.

Systemic Conditions Delaying Dental Eruption

Low Birthweight

Seow (1996) studied the development of the permanent dentition in very low birthweight (< 1,500 g) Caucasian children in Australia [20]. Fifty-five very low birthweight children (mean age at dental examination 7.7 ± 2.2 years, mean birthweight 1.203 ± 240 g, and mean gestational age 29.8 ± 2.4 weeks) were compared to 55 normal birth weight children matched for race, sex, and age. Dental maturity determined from panoramic radiographs found very low birthweight children to experience a delay in dental maturation of 0.29 ± 0.54 years compared with normal birthweight children ($p < 0.02$). Very low birthweight children less than 6 years of age showed the greatest delay of 0.31 ± 0.68 years ($p < 0.001$). In contrast, children aged 9 years and older showed no difference in dental maturity compared to controls ($p > 0.01$), suggesting that "catch-up" growth had occurred. In a separate study carried out in Finland, comparing dental development in preterm versus matched control children, premature birth again had no appreciable late effects on tooth-maturation by age 9 years [21].

Second-hand Smoke

For evaluation of the effects of second-hand smoke on dental development, panoramic radiographs of 203 children between the ages of 7 and 10 years were studied [22]. Four groups were separated: a control group in which neither parent had smoked during the pregnancy, a group exposed to tobacco smoke from the mother only, a group exposed to smoke from the father only, and a group exposed to tobacco smoke from both parents. Maximum differences between chronological and dental ages were found in children subjected to cigarette smoke from both parents (35% reduction in dental maturation).

Syndromes

Several syndromes are associated with delay or failure in dental eruption.

Several syndromes are associated with delay or failure in dental eruption. One of the most common of these is cleidocranial dysplasia, in which there are multiple supernumerary teeth, with delayed or arrested eruption of the permanent teeth (however, the primary dentition erupts normally) [23, 24].

Trisomy 21 (Down syndrome) and juvenile hypothyroidism (cretinism) have also been attributed as causes of delayed eruption. Other, less common, syndromes associated with delayed or failed dental eruption include: hypopituitarism, osteomatosis intestinal polyposis syndrome (Gardner syndrome in which there is a high propensity for development of intestinal cancer), chondroectodermal dysplasia (Ellis-van Crevald syndrome), progeria (Hutchinson-Gilfords syndrome), osteopetrosis, pyknodysostosis, acrocephaly-syndactyly (Apert syndrome), focal dermal hypoplasia (Goltz syndrome), vitamin D deficiency syndromes, and dystrophic epidermolysis bulosa [25, 26]. Drug-induced gingival hyperplasia, such as that related to use of phenytoin (Dilantin) in prevention of seizures, can either delay eruption, or simply hide the teeth from clinical view. Radiation therapy for treating malignancies in childhood has also been associated with failed tooth development and either delayed or premature dental eruption.

Delayed Puberty

Gaethofs et al. (1990) compared the dental age of boys with constitutional delay in growth and puberty with that of normal healthy boys [27]. The Demirjian et al. method was found to be accurate for the Belgium control subjects examined. Boys with delayed puberty had significant delay in dental development ($p < 0.01$).

Factors in Premature Dental Eruption

Individual teeth can erupt in advance as a sporadic variant (i.e., natal teeth). Premature eruption of a permanent tooth quite frequently occurs following early loss of its primary antecedent. More generalized premature eruption has been reported in juvenile rheumatoid arthritis [28], Turner syndrome [29, 30], hyperthyroidism, pituitary giantism, hypergonadism, Cushing syndrome, and adrenogenital syndrome. Local premature dental eruption has been found in association with adjacent benign vascular hemangioma) or neural tumors, or due to pressure from growing subjacent jaw neoplasms (e.g., osteogenic sarcoma).

Hass et al. studied 28 subjects aged 4–19 years having Turner syndrome using serial panoramic and cephalometric radiographs. They found dental development to be advanced in all of the subjects and the administration of growth hormone had no effect on this finding [29].

Kotilainen and Pirinen investigated dental maturity in 28 Fragile X chromosome affected boys and three girl carriers of this condition [31]. The mean relative dental age was advanced in Fragile X males, based both on formation and on emergence, with more pronounced advancement seen in younger children. Dental maturity was advanced in heterozygous carrier girls as well. Height and skeletal maturity did not show a similar trend toward advanced development.

Assessment of Biological Age Using Hand-Wrist Radiographs

Skeletal development is an important maturity indicator during childhood [32]. In clinical practice, determination of skeletal age is helpful for the diagnosis of disorders of growth and development. Typical disharmonic patterns in the appearance of bone centers of hand and wrist have been found in certain disorders of development [32].

Fishman developed a widely-used system of hand-wrist skeletal maturation indicators (SMI), using four stages of bone maturation (initial ossification, width, capping, and fusion) at six anatomical sites [33]. Table 9.2 details specific criteria to be used with the Fishman system. The various anatomical features that need to be recognized are annotated in Fig. 9.6 and detailed in examples in Figs. 9.7 and 9.8. Using this system, it is possible to judge the remaining growth potential of the jaws, an important issue for orthodontic treatment planning (Figs. 9.7, 9.8). Hand-wrist radiographs can be made using a standard cephalometric extension to a panoramic machine.

Skeletal development is an important maturity indicator during childhood.

Assessment of Biological Age Using Lateral Cephalograms

Lateral cephalometric and left hand-wrist radiographs from the Bolton-Brush Growth Center at Case Western Reserve University were reviewed to develop a cervical vertebrae maturation index [34]. By using the lateral profiles of the second, third, and fourth cervical vertebrae, it was possible to develop a reliable ranking of patients in terms of the potential for future adolescent growth (Table 9.3; Figs. 9.9, 9.10). A subsequent study evaluated lateral cephalometric and left hand-wrist radiographs of 180 untreated subjects (99 girls and 81 boys) aged from 8 to 18 years [35]. The results of this study indicated that cervical vertebral maturation and hand-wrist skeletal maturation were significantly related. A study in Italy by Franchi et al. concurred that cervical vertebral maturation is an appropriate method for the appraisal of mandibular skeletal maturity in individual patients on the basis of a single cephalometric observation [36]. They concluded that the accuracy of the cervical vertebral method in the detection of the onset of the pubertal spurt in mandibular growth provides helpful indications for orthodontic treatment timing of patients having mandibular deficiencies. The accuracy of cervical vertebral maturation in determining skeletal age during the circum-pubertal period was found to be valid and reliable in children of Chinese ethnicity [37]. Minars et al. (2003) used repeated evaluations of 30 randomly selected, pretreatment lateral cephalometric radiographs and found the accuracy of determining skeletal maturity and growth potential with lateral cephalograms to be R = 0.98 (highly accurate) [38].

Biological Age and Orthodontic Intervention

In Australia, Grave and Townsend constructed velocity curves for stature and mandibular growth for 47 boys and 27 girls, and plotted maturation events on the curves [39]. For the majority of children, peak velocity in mandibular growth coincided with peak velocity in stature increments. Particular radiologic maturation events occurred consistently before, during, or after the adolescent growth spurt, contributing to a positive, purposeful, and more confident approach to the management of orthodontic patients, particularly those with a Class II malocclusion.

Kopecky and Fishman (1993) treated 41 patients with clinically diagnosed Class II, Division I malocclusions with midface prognathism using Kloehn-type cervical headgear [40]. All cases included longitudinal series both of lateral cephalometric radiographs and of hand-wrist films made before, during, and after treatment. Skeletal and dental changes were related to specific maturational periods and compared with their related chronological age to evaluate optimum timing for maximum treatment response. This study found timing of cervical headgear treatment on the basis of skeletal maturation is preferable to use of chronological age. The most favorable results were demonstrated during maturational periods associated with a high degree of incremental growth velocity.

Baccetti et al. (2001) evaluated the short-term and long-term treatment effects of rapid maxillary expansion in two groups of subjects treated with the Haas appliance [41]. Treatment outcomes were evaluated before and after the peak in skeletal maturation, as assessed by the cervical vertebral maturation method, in a sample of 42 patients compared to a control sample of 20 subjects. The group receiving early treatment had not passed the pubertal peak in skeletal growth when treatment commenced, whereas the late treatment subjects had (see Table 9.3). Rapid maxillary expansion treatment before the peak in skeletal growth velocity was able to induce more pronounced transverse craniofacial changes at the skeletal level. Biological age determination is important in treatment planning effective rapid palatal expansion.

Age and Identity

In Belgium, Van Erum et al. evaluated 48 patients aged 2–32 years with short stature of prenatal origin. They observed tooth development and craniofacial growth using panoramic and cephalometric radiographs [42]. While craniofacial growth was closely related to general growth and skeletal age, dental maturation closely correlated with chronological age.

In the United States, an immigrant's age can be critical to his or her effort to gain entry to and residence in the

Table 9.2 Hand-wrist maturation schedule (after Fishman [30])

Stage	Bone	Age (years)	
		Female	Male
Ossification	Hamate/capitate	0.5	0.5
	Radius distal epiphysis	1	1
	Thumb phalanx distal epiphysis	1	1.5
	Metacarpal epiphysis (all four fingers)	1	1.5
	Thumb metacarpal epiphysis	1.5	2.5
	Triquetral	1.5	2.5
	Thumb phalanx proximal epiphysis	2	3
	Lunate	4	4
	Trapezium	4	5
	Scaphoid	4.5	5.5
	Trapezoid	4	6
	Ulna distal epiphysis	5	6
	Pisiform	9	11
	Adductor sesamoid	11	12
Width	Proximal phalanx middle finger	10	11
	Middle phalanx middle finger	11	12
	Middle phalanx little finger	11	12
Capping	Proximal phalanx middle finger	12	13
	Middle phalanx middle finger	12	14
	Middle phalanx little finger	12	14
Fusion	Proximal phalanx middle finger	13	15
	Middle phalanx middle finger	14	16
	Middle phalanx little finger	15	16
	Radius distal epiphysis	16	17
	Ulna distal epiphysis	17	19

country. Minors who enter the United States illegally are, unlike adults, exempt from immediate deportation. Minors are permitted to remain in the United States if they are granted political asylum or "special immigrant juvenile status," given when a child is the victim of abuse or neglect. If denied asylum, minors cannot be sent home until relatives in their home country are contacted. In the view of the federal immigration authorities, dental and bone radiographs are one of the most reliable ways of determining age [43]. Trager, a US dentist with a practice directly above Customs and Immigration at Kennedy Airport, NY, and another practice in LaGuardia Airport, noted that the eruption of third molars and the fusion of bones in the wrist usually signify that a person is over 18 years of age [43]. Detainee's challenges to this means of age determination have apparently been dismissed in federal court [44]. Nevertheless, there can be no precision in correlation of biological (skeletal or dental) age and the chronological age that is so important in law. One can only specify the likelihood

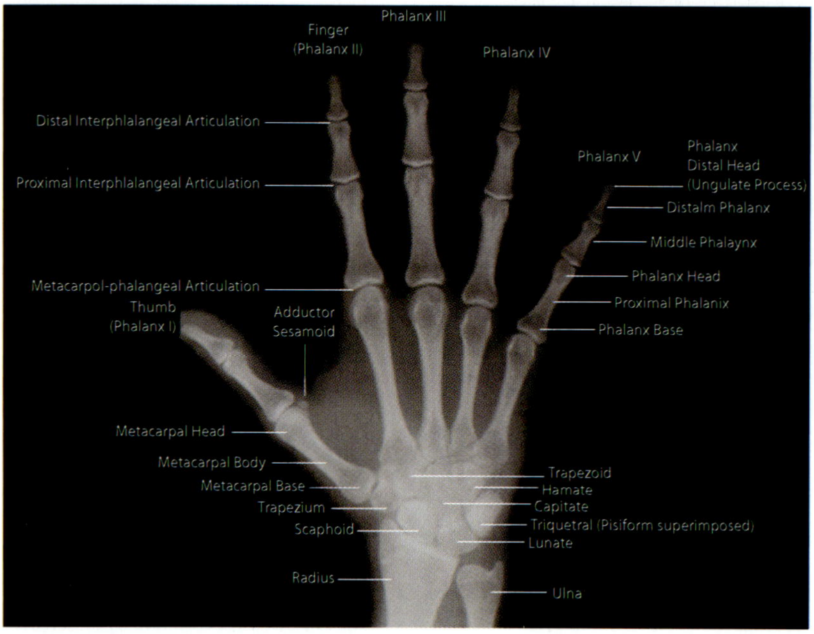

Fig. 9.6 Annotated hand-wrist radiograph indicating the landmarks needed to assess skeletal age using the Fishman method

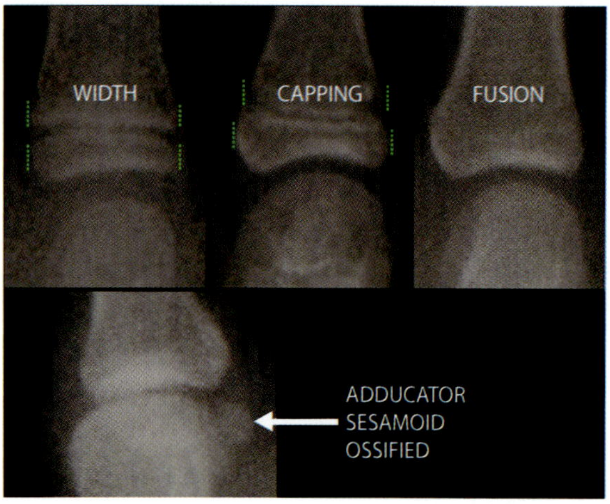

Fig. 9.7 Details of epiphyseal "width," "capping," and "fusion" at phalanx base, and of ossification of the adductor bone. These are key indicators of skeletal age

of age given a population sample, not the exact age of a specific individual. Biological age is important for dental treatment planning and can be assessed with some utility using dental, cephalometric, and hand-wrist radiographs. Precise chronological age correlations can never be guaranteed. The most accurate determinant of being over 18 years of age, however, according to Friedrich et al. is the presence of filled wisdom teeth. The correlation was reported as being 100% [44].

Flores et al. (2006) made similar conclusions for the accuracy of skeletal indices from hand-wrist radiographs and cervical spine assessment using lateral cephalograms for the assessment of chronological age [45]. Correlation values between both skeletal maturation methods were moderately high, high enough to use either for research purposes but not for the assessment of individual patients.

Concluding Remarks

The literature points to there being close correlation between growth potential and skeletal maturity as demonstrated from morphological evaluation of the cervical spine on lateral cephalograms, or of the bones of the hand and wrist. It is this skeletal growth potential that is important for orthodontic assessment. As the lateral cephalogram is standard for orthodontic assessment

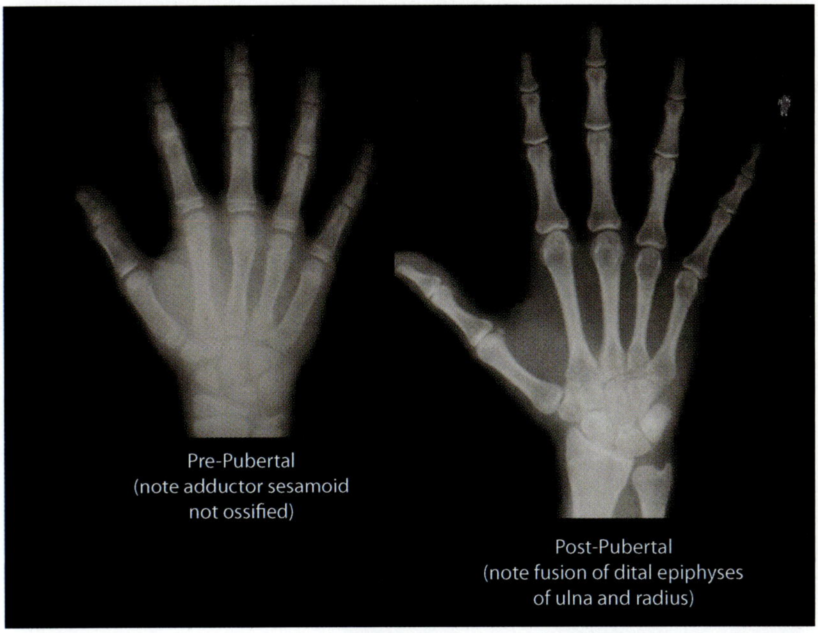

Fig. 9.8 Comparison of hand-wrist radiographs from pre-pubertal patient having significant growth potential (*left*; note adductor sesamoid not ossified), and of post-pubertal individual with little growth potential (*right*; note fusion of distal epiphyses of ulna and radius)

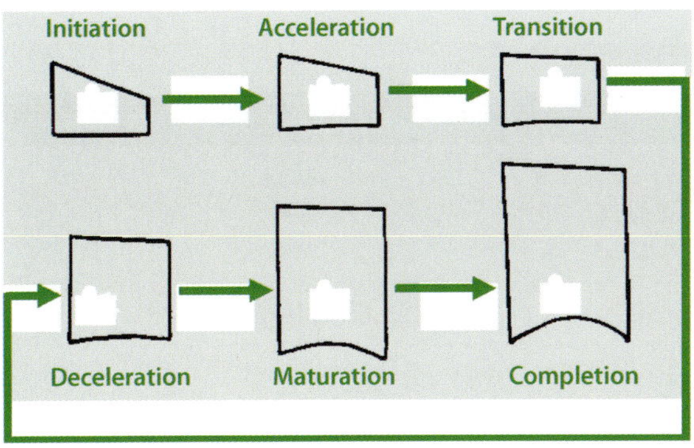

Fig. 9.9. Schematic of maturation sequence of third cervical vertebra (C3) after Hassel and Farman [34]

presently, evaluation of the spine obviates an additional radiograph being made of the hand and wrist. Even when a thyroid shield is worn by the patient, C3 is usually included in the cephalogram [46].

There seems to be a closer association between dental development as viewed on a panoramic radiograph and chronological age, than between chronological age and skeletal maturity.

There seems to be a closer association between dental maturity viewed on a panoramic radiograph and chronological age, than between chronological age and skeletal maturity. This is particularly the case if ethnic variability is taken into account. Nevertheless, population standards are not precise when it comes to evaluation of the individual. Kjaer et al. found that while skeletal maturation was delayed by more than four years in four siblings with Seckel syndrome, tooth maturity progressed normally [47]. While there are many local and systemic causes of delayed and premature dental eruption, tooth development is perhaps the best radiographic indicator of chronological age during childhood and adolescence.

It may be necessary to make adjustments over time to any reference chart as it appears that the rate of dental maturation might be accelerating. Nadler (1998) compared 1970 and 1990 Caucasian patient samples,

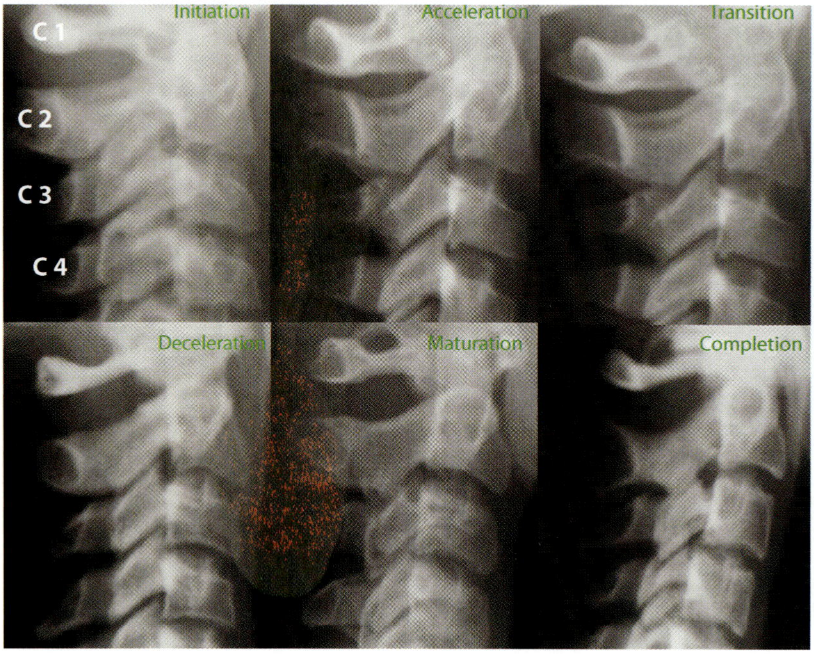

Fig. 9.10 Maturation sequence for cervical vertebra (C2–4) used for skeletal growth potential determination after Hassel and Farman [34]

Table 9.3 Cervical vertebral maturation indicators (after Hassel and Farman [31])

Stage	Vertebral indicators	Growth potential
Initiation	C2, C3, and C4 inferior vertebral body borders flat. Superior vertebral bodies tapered posterior to anterior	Very significant adolescent growth expected
Acceleration	C2 and C3 lower body borders developing concavities. C4 body inferior border flat. C3 and C4 more rectangular in shape	Significant adolescent growth expected
Transition	Distinct concavities in C2 and C3 lower borders. C4 develops concavity in body lower border. C3 and C4 bodies rectangular in shape	Moderate adolescent growth expected
Deceleration	Distinct concavities in lower borders of bodies of C2, C3, and C4. C3 and C4 bodies nearly square in lateral profile	Small amount of adolescent growth expected
Maturation	Accentuated concavities of inferior vertebral body borders of C2, C3, and C4. C3 and C4 vertebra; bodies are square in lateral profile	Insignificant amount of adolescent growth expected
Completion	Deep concavities of inferior vertebral body borders of C2, C3, and C4. C3 and C4 vertebral body heights greater than widths	Adolescent growth completed

age 8.5–14.5 years old, and demonstrated dental age reductions of 1.2 years for males and 1.5 years for females, giving a combined mean reduction of 1.4 years [48]. Further, it has been established that there is a variation of ±15 months at the 95% confidence interval using dental age to estimate chronological age among Chinese children [47]. Perhaps like in aging horses, the use of dental aging for humans is to best be considered as being a "respected imprecise science" [49].

When there is a local cause of failed eruption, early intervention can save much time, effort, cost, and discomfort with respect to the patient.

Knowledge of the normal sequence and timing of dental eruption provides useful information regarding the selection of radiographic procedures to evaluate the patient who falls outside the normal range, or who shows asymmetry in tooth eruption patterns. When there is a local cause of failed eruption, early intervention can save the patient much time, effort, cost, and discomfort. A most comprehensive overview of the dentition, providing ready bilateral comparisons, is the panoramic radiograph. Diligent use of the panoramic radiography at key stages of growth and development is advocated as an appropriate standard of care.

References

1. FDA Dental Radiographic Selection Panel, Joseph LP. The Selection of Patients for X Ray Examinations: Dental Radiographic Examinations. HHS Publication FDA 88-8273; 1987
2. Espelid I, Mejare I, Weerheijm K. EAPD guidelines for use of radiographs in children. Eur J Paediatr Dent 2003;4:40–48
3. Langland OE, Langlais RP, Preece JW. Principles of Dental Imaging, edn 2. Lippincott Williams and Wilkins: Philadelphia; 2002
4. Farman AG, Eloff J, Joubert JJ de V, Nortjé CJ. Clinical absence of the permanent maxillary central incisor: a study of 30 cases. Rhodesian J Dent 1979;8:4–6
5. Logan WH, Kronfeld R. Development of the human jaws and surrounding structures from birth to the age of fifteen years. J Am Dent Assoc 1933;20:379–427
6. Demirjian A, Goldstein H, Tanner JM. A new system of dental age assessment. Hum Biol 1973;45:211–227
7. Demirjian A, Goldstein H. New systems for dental maturity based on seven and four teeth. Ann Hum Biol 1976;3:411–421
8. Demirjian A, Levesque GY. Sexual differences in dental development and prediction of emergence. J Dent Res 1980;59:1110–1122
9. Hegde RJ, Sood PB. Dental maturity as an indicator of chronological age: radiographic evaluation of dental age in 6 to 13 years children of Belgaum using Demirjian methods. J Indian Soc Pedod Prev Dent 2002;20:132–138
10. Teivens A, Mornstad H, Reventlid M. Individual variation of tooth development in Swedish children. Swed Dent J 1996;20:87–93
11. Reventlid M, Mornstad H, Teivens AA. Intra- and inter-examiner variations in four dental methods for age estimation of children. Swed Dent J 1996;20:133–139
12. Nykanen R, Espeland L, Kvaal SI, Krogstad O. Validity of the Demirjian method for dental age estimation when applied to Norwegian children. Acta Odontol Scand 1998;56:238–244
13. Zhao J, Ding L, Li R. Study of dental maturity in children aged 3–16 years in Chengdu. Hua Xi Yi Ke Da Xue Xue Bao 1990;21:242–246
14. Olze A, Taniguchi M, Schmeling A, Zhu BL, Yamada Y, Maeda H, Geserick G. Studies on the chronology of third molar mineralization in a Japanese population. Leg Med (Tokyo) 2004;6:73–79
15. Sasaki M, Sato K, Mitani H. Tooth formation and eruption in skeletal Class II and Class III malocclusions. Nippon Kyosei Shika Gakkai Zasshi 1990;49:435–442
16. Janson GR, Martins DR, Tavano O, Dainesi EA. Dental maturation in subjects with extreme vertical facial types. Eur J Orthod 1998;20:73–78
17. Prabhakar AR, Panda AK, Raju OS. Applicability of Demirjian's method of age assessment in children of Davangere. J Indian Soc Pedod Prev Dent 2002;20:54–62
18. Davidson LE, Rodd HD. Interrelationship between dental age and chronological age in Somali children. Community Dent Health 2001;18:27–30
19. Farman AG, Nortjé CJ, Wood RE. Oral and maxillofacial diagnostic imaging. St Louis: Mosby-Year Book 1993
20. Seow WK. A study of the development of the permanent dentition in very low birthweight children. Pediatr Dent 1996;18:379–384
21. Backstrom MC, Aine L, Maki R, Kuusela AL, Sievanen H, Koivisto AM, Ikonen RS, Maki M. Maturation of primary and permanent teeth in preterm infants. Arch Dis Child Fetal Neonatal Ed 2000;83:F104–F108
22. Kieser JA, Groeneveld HT, da Silva P. Delayed tooth formation in children exposed to tobacco smoke. J Clin Pediatr Dent 1996;20:97–100
23. Jensen BL, Kreiborg S. Development of the dentition in cleidocranial dysplasia. J Oral Pathol Med 1990;19:89–93
24. Shaikh R, Shusterman S. Delayed dental maturation in cleidocranial dysplasia. ASDC J Dent Child 1998;65:325–329, 355
25. Myllarniemi S, Lenko HL, Perheentupa J. Dental maturity in hypopituitarism, and dental response to substitution treatment. Scand J Dent Res 1978;86:307–312
26. Kostara A, Roberts GJ, Gelbier M. Dental maturity in children with dystrophic epidermolysis bullosa. Pediatr Dent 2000;22:385–388
27. Gaethofs M, Verdonck A, Carels C, de Zegher F. Delayed dental age in boys with constitutionally delayed puberty. Eur J Orthod 1999;21:711–715
28. Lehtinen A, Oksa T, Helenius H, Ronning O. Advanced dental maturity in children with juvenile rheumatoid arthritis. Eur J Oral Sci 2000;108:184–188
29. Hass AD, Simmons KE, Davenport ML, Proffit WR. The effect of growth hormone on craniofacial growth and dental maturation in Turner syndrome. Angle Orthod 2001;71:50–59

30. Midtbo M, Halse A. Skeletal maturity, dental maturity, and eruption in young patients with Turner syndrome. Acta Odontol Scand 1992;50:303–312
31. Kotilainen J, Pirinen S. Dental maturity is advanced in Fragile X syndrome. Am J Med Genet 1999;83:298–301
32. Heinrich UE. Significance of radiologic skeletal age determination in clinical practice. Radiologe 1986;26:212–215
33. Fishman LS. Maturational patterns and prediction during adolescence. Angle Orthod 1987;57:178–193
34. Hassel B, Farman AG. Skeletal maturation evaluation using cervical vertebrae. Am J Orthod Dentofacial Orthop 1995;107:58–66
35. Kucukkeles N, Acar A, Biren S, Arun T. Comparisons between cervical vertebrae and hand-wrist maturation for the assessment of skeletal maturity. J Clin Pediatr Dent 1999;24:47–52
36. Franchi L, Baccetti T, McNamara JA Jr. Mandibular growth as related to cervical vertebral maturation and body height. Am J Orthod Dentofacial Orthop 2000;118:335–340
37. Chang HP, Liao CH, Yang YH, Chang HF, Chen KC. Correlation of cervical vertebra maturation with hand-wrist maturation in children. Kaohsiung J Med Sci 2001;17:29–35
38. Minars M, Burch J, Masella R, Meister M. Predicting skeletal maturation using cervical vertebrae. Today's FDA 2003;15:17–19
39. Grave K, Townsend G. Hand-wrist and cervical vertebral maturation indicators: how can these events be used to time Class II treatments? Aust Orthod J 2003;19:33–45
40. Kopecky GR, Fishman LS. Timing of cervical headgear treatment based on skeletal maturation. Am J Orthod Dentofacial Orthop 1993;104:162–169
41. Baccetti T, Franchi L, Cameron CG, McNamara JA Jr. Treatment timing for rapid maxillary expansion. Angle Orthod 2001;71:343–350
42. Van Erum R, Mulier M, Carels C, de Zegher F. Short stature of prenatal origin: craniofacial growth and dental maturation. Eur J Orthod 1998;20:417–425
43. Hedges C. Airport dentist crucial to INS gatekeeping. NY Times on the web, July 22, 2000
44. Friedrich RE, Ulbricht C, von Maydell LA. Dental caries and fillings in wisdom teeth as an aid in forensic dentistry for determining chronologic age over 18. Radiologic studies of orthopantomography images of children and adolescents. Arch Kriminol 2003;212:74–82
45. Flores-Mir C, Burgess CA, Champney M, Jensen RJ, Pitcher MR, Major PW. Correlation of skeletal maturation stages determined by cervical vertebrae and hand-wrist evaluations. Angle Orthod 2006;76:1–5
46. Baccetti T, Franchi L, McNamara JA Jr. An improved version of the cervical vertebral maturation (CVM) method for the assessment of mandibular growth. Angle Orthod 2002;72:316–323
47. Kjaer I, Hansen N, Becktor KB, Birkebaek N, Balslev T. Craniofacial morphology, dentition, and skeletal maturity in four siblings with Seckel syndrome. Cleft Palate Craniofac J 2001;38:645–651
48. Nadler GL. Earlier dental maturation: fact or fiction? Angle Orthod 1998;68:535–538
49. Anonymous. Aging horses by examining the teeth—a centuries old inexact science. Special report. J Vet Dent 1997;14:97–98

TEST: Assessing growth and development with panoramic radiographs and cephalometric attachments: a critical tool for dental diagnosis and treatment planning

1. Panoramic radiography provides a better assessment of growth potential of the jaws than does the lateral cephalogram.

   True ☐ **False** ☐

2. Panoramic radiography provides a better assessment of patient chronological age than does the lateral cephalogram.

   True ☐ **False** ☐

3. Failure to detect causes of impaction until after the normal eruption sequence of an affected tooth can complicate treatment planning and reduce the prognosis for successful intervention.

   True ☐ **False** ☐

4. Using the Classification of Hassel and Farman, the most significant growth potential is found in patients designated as being in the "Transition Stage"

   True ☐ **False** ☐

5. The adductor bone usually commences calcification at a younger age in girls than in boys.

   True ☐ **False** ☐

6. Second-hand smoke has been indicated as a possible cause of delayed dental development.

   True ☐ **False** ☐

7. Whereas individual variation can make accurate assessment of chronological age using radiographs somewhat problematic, the presence of filled third molars is a good predictor of the person concerned being 18 years or older.

   True ☐ **False** ☐

8. When assessing growth potential of the mandible, dental maturity is a better indicator than skeletal maturity using hand-wrist radiographs.

   True ☐ **False** ☐

9. Root completion for the first permanent molar occurs around 6 years of age.

   True ☐ **False** ☐

10. Excepting the third molars, by age 16 years all permanent teeth should be erupted and have completed root formation.

    True ☐ **False** ☐

Chapter

10

Panoramic Radiographic Appearance of the Mandibular Canal in Health and in Disease

Allan G. Farman
in association with Christoffel J. Nortjé

Learning Objectives

- Gain knowledge of the variations in normal anatomy of the mandibular canals and the effect of various pathological pathoses on the panoramic appearance of these anatomical landmarks
- Differentiate between lesions based upon location in relation to the canal and the effects on outline and position of the canal

The mandibular canal is of particular importance to the dentist and dental specialist as it carries both the dental division of the trigeminal nerve and the nerve supply for the lower lip. The trigeminal nerve ent Mandibular Foramen ers the inner surface of the mandibular ramus at the mandibular foramen, in the vicinity of a bony eminence, the lingula. This is a fact learned in study of anatomy and reinforced by the everyday necessity of locating an inferior dental block injection for local analgesia required in many dental procedures. What is not so well understood is that normal is a range and that variations do occur in which there may be more than one canal entry point, a factor that might account for failed anesthesia in at least a small percentage of patients. Such variations have been described both during studies of macerated mandibles from cadavers and also from the study of panoramic radiographs.

Panoramic radiographs may also help find the position of the mental foramen, through which the nerve supply to the lower lip passes. Failure to protect the mental foramen can lead to permanent loss of normal sensation in the lower lip. The panoramic radiographic positioning of the mental foramen and the mandibular canal also has been used as an indication of bone loss following dental extractions.

A comprehensive study of variations in the mandibular canal in patients who had not suffered mandibular pathoses or trauma found that the mandibular canals are usually, but not invariably, bilaterally symmetrical, and that the majority of hemimandibles contain only one major canal [1]. The position of the canal varies with respect to the apices of the tooth roots and the lower border of the mandible. They can be classified as high (Type I, close to the apices of the teeth), intermediate (Type II), or low (Type III, close to the lower cortex of the mandible) varieties [2]. The proportions of types varies with the investigation perhaps indicating a geographic or ethnic variability [1, 2]. Neither study showed a sex difference with respect to the positioning of the canal. There were almost equal numbers of high and low canals in a South African study with few intermediate canals [1]. In a Greek study there were few high canals and almost equal proportions of intermediate and low canals [2]. The Greek study also found asymmetry in canal positioning in almost one in five of those studied; whereas the South African study found this to occur in less than one in a hundred [1, 2]. It can be concluded that in a single panoramic radiograph the mandibular canal should not be used as a set reference point for assessment of bone loss following extractions. To make such an assessment requires sequential panoramic radiographs on a given patient.

Supplemental mandibular canals large enough to be seen on panoramic radiography are rare but are occasionally present, the most common being duplicate canals commencing from a single mandibular foramen, and the least common arising from two separate foramina (Figs. 10.1, 10.2) [1–3]. Such duplicate canals are found in only 0.5–1.0% of studied adult populations [1, 2, 4]. They are sometimes termed bifid canals [2, 4]. That such bifid canals are a reality rather than a projection artifact has been proven both by anatomical dissection [5] and also by computed tomography [6]. Whether the contents are neural, neurovascular or simply vascular is a contentious point. If nerves were present in the two canals, this might account for some failure to achieve local anesthesia when applying inferior dental anesthesia block injections.

On occasion, duplicated mental foramen are observed (Fig. 10.3). True duplication needs to be distinguished from the separate depictions of the mental canal at its origin from the mandibular canal central within bone, and at its exit from the facial cortex of the mandible.

It is possible that bifid canals represent a minor expression of structural twinning. Very rarely, the mandible may evidence augnathus, a variant of paragnathus

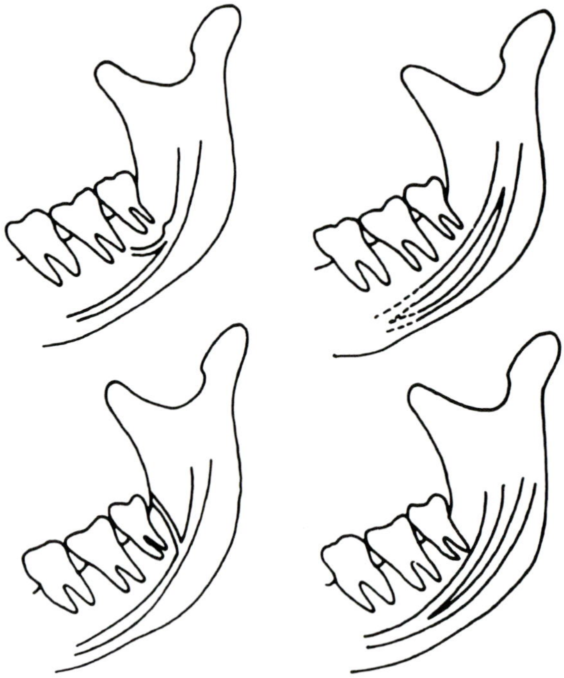

Fig. 10.1 Examples of bifid, or duplicate, mandibular canals. Such canals have been confirmed in various studies both using anatomical dissection and by computed tomography

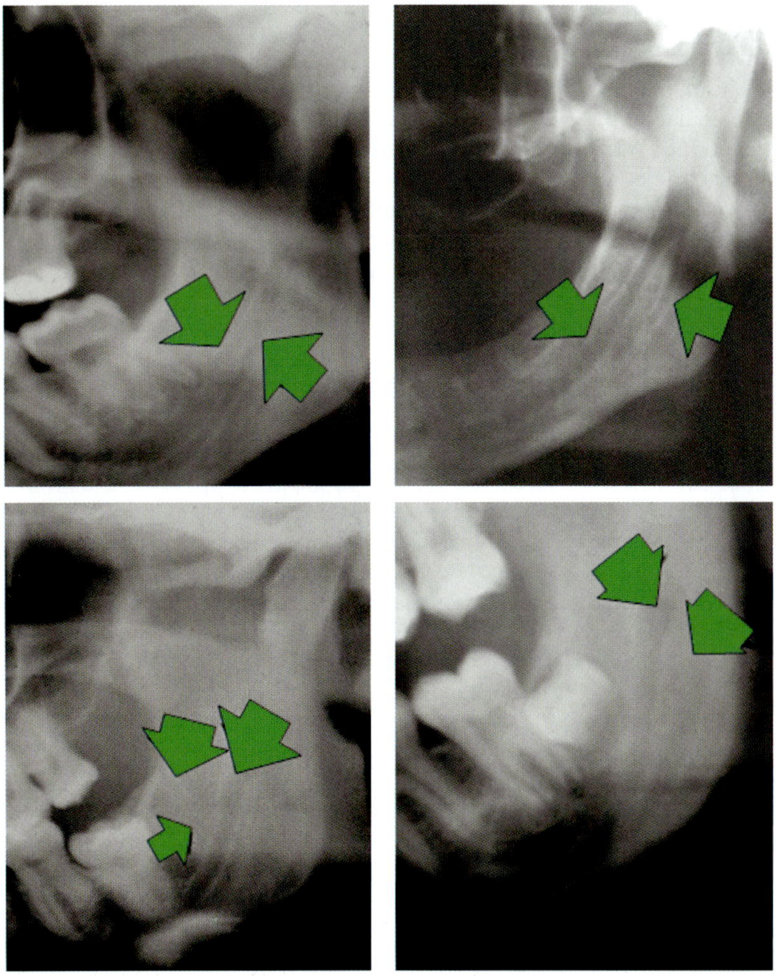

Fig. 10.2 Details from panoramic radiographs demonstrating various duplicate, or bifid, mandibular canals

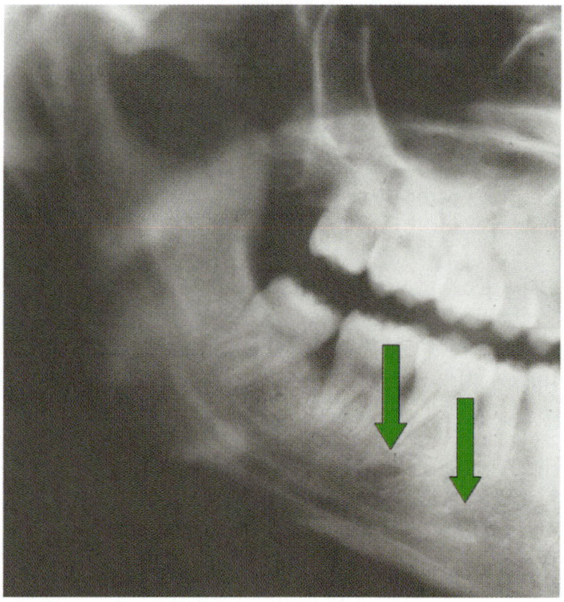

Fig. 10.3 Duplicated mental foramen (detail from panoramic radiograph)

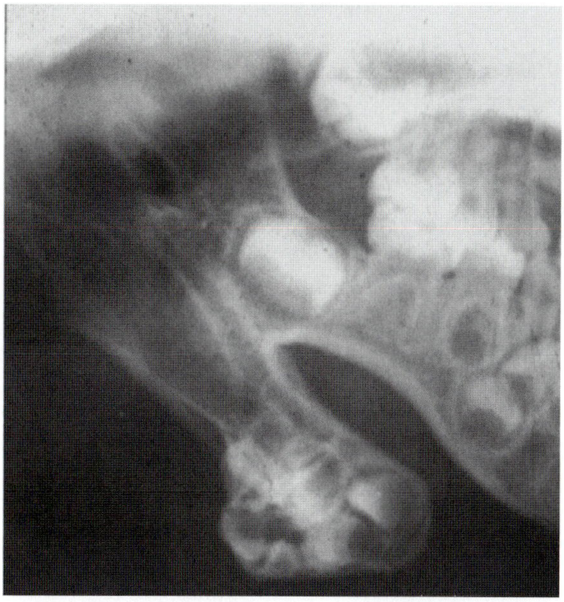

Fig. 10.4 Augnathus (a variant of paragnathus) demonstrating an extreme form of duplication of the mandibular canal. (Case treated by Professors D. Davis and M. Breytenbach, Cape Town, South Africa)

[7]. Such a case, subsequently treated successfully by surgeons Davis and Breytenbach in Cape Town, South Africa, is illustrated in Fig. 10.4. In this case, unilateral duplication of the mandible was accompanied by duplication of the mandibular canal and also of the dentition for that jaw quadrant.

Pathological Conditions of the Mandible

The effects of pathological conditions of the mandible on the panoramic appearance of the mandibular canal was first reported by the authors of this chapter several decades ago [8]. It was found that disease processes can affect the panoramic radiographic appearance of the mandibular canal in a variety of ways.

Localized loss of the canal cortex was found with chronic apical periodontitis, chronic pericoronitis, advanced chronic destructive periodontitis (in patients having a high mandibular canal), and rarely also with very large Stafne bone cavities. Generalized loss of the canal's cortex was usually indicative of severe infection or aggressive neoplasia, and was found in association with rarefying osteomyelitis, invasive squamous cell carcinoma, multiple myeloma, osteogenic sarcoma, and occasionally with ameloblastoma.

Displacement of the canal suggested a benign cystic or neoplastic process, and was found with large apical dental (radicular) cysts, residual dental cysts, dentigerous cysts, and the cementifying-ossifying fibroma among other benign conditions.

Primary lesions developing within the mandibular canal are frequently neural or vascular in origin.

Benign Lesions Within the Mandibular Canal

Primary lesions developing within the mandibular canal are frequently neural or vascular in origin. Benign neoplasm within the canal will tend to widen the canal and cause superior and inferior displacement of the canal as the lesion expands. Especially with slow growing lesions the cortical plate of the canal will remain intact. Figure 10.5 illustrates a case of neurilemmoma arising within the mandibular canal. This is a homogeneously radiolucent lesion that has caused widening of the canal in the site of the tumor. The normal canal blends with the lesion both mesially and distally with the cortical plate expanding to encompass the lesion. Certainly, not all neurilemmonas of the mandible are associated with widening of the mandibular canal, especially if they are situated in the premolar or anterior regions [10]. However, widening of the mandibular canal, when present, does suggest a lesion epicenter within the canal.

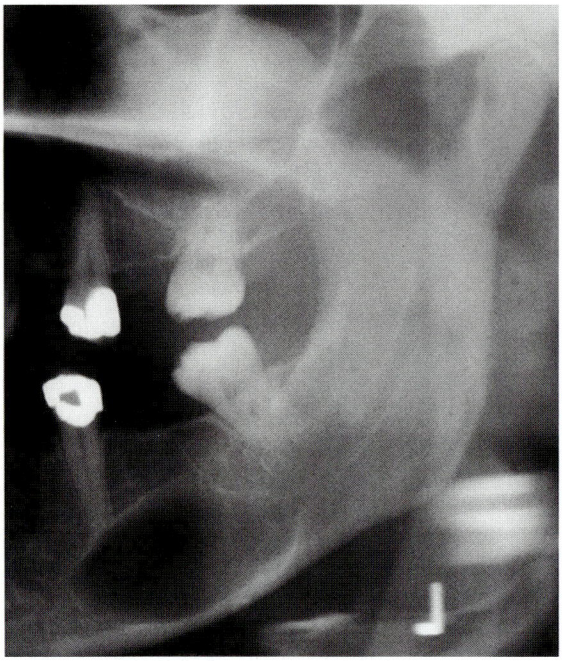

Fig. 10.5 Neurilemmoma within the mandibular canal. The canal is greatly expanded by this homogeneously radiolucent benign neoplasm

Shapiro et al. (1984) investigated the maxillofacial radiographic manifestations of neurofibromatosis (von Recklinghausen disease), a condition affecting 1 in 3,000 live births in which those affected are prone to develop benign neural tumors, neurofibromas [11]. They found that 72% of the 22 subjects studied had oral or maxillofacial radiological signs of the disease such as widened mandibular canals (six cases) or enlarged mandibular foramina (six cases including two who also had widened canals). Lee et al. (1996) found that 6 of 10 patients with neurofibromatosis showed enlargement of the mandibular foramen [12].

Malignant Lesions Within the Mandibular Canal

Primary malignancies arising within the mandibular canal are extremely rare [13]. When they do arise they will reflect a tissue of origin from the site concerned; i.e., neural, vascular, fibrous, or smooth muscle. Figure 10.6 illustrates a case of primary leiomyosarcoma arising in the left mandibular body and causing destruction of the canal outline. The young male patient evidenced paresthesia of the left side of the lower lip. No other site of disease was found so this is presumed a primary lesion.

Not all malignancies cause destruction of the canal outline. Extranodal non-Hodgkin lymphoma has been reported to cause enlargement of the canal not unlike that described for benign tumors [14, 15]. Metastases affecting the mandibular canal site are also rare, but certainly more common than primary malignancies.

Benign Lesions Peripheral to the Mandibular Canal

Slow growing benign cysts and tumors peripheral to the mandibular canal are likely to cause gradual displacement of the canal rather than resorption of the canal cortices.

Slow growing benign cysts and tumors peripheral to the mandibular canal are likely to cause gradual displacement of the canal rather than resorption of the canal cortices. Examples of such conditions are illustrated in Figs 10.7–10.11. When a homogeneous radiolucency is associated with expansion of the apical periodontal ligament space of a non-vital root canal, and the lesion is large enough to cause displacement of the mandibular canal, the most likely diagnosis is an apical dental (radicular) cyst (Fig. 10.7). If a homogeneous radiolucency surrounds the crown of an unerupted tooth and is attached to the tooth at the enamel-cemental junction. The most likely diagnosis is a dentigerous cyst. It should be cautioned that a variety of other conditions can envelope the crown of a tooth; hence, histopathological confirmation is required. Large dentigerous cysts can cause the displacement of the affected tooth and when aprproaching the mandibular canal are likely to displace this structure (Fig. 10.8). Benign tumors can also cause canal displacement. The most common benign odontogenic neoplasm is the ameloblastoma (Fig. 10.9) and this can either cause displacement or resorption of the canal, or can in some cases simply camouflage the canal by addition of septa and "soap bubble" trabecular patterns. Figure 10.10 is a detail from a panoramic radiograph of a patient having a calcifying epithelial odontogenic tumor. The lesion has displaced an adjacent tooth and there is widening of the follicle space resembling a dentigerous cyst. This is presumably due to invasion of the follicle space by tumor. This highlights the importance of histopathological evaluation of tissue from supposed dentigerous cysts. The displaced tooth has also resulted in displacement of the mandibular canal in this case.

Figure 10.11 illustrates a cementoblastoma that has displaced the mandibular canal toward the lower cortex of the mandible. This condition is entirely benign [16]. While this particular case was excised in its entirety, it is sometimes possible to endodontically treat an affected tooth and then simply surgically excise the lesion.

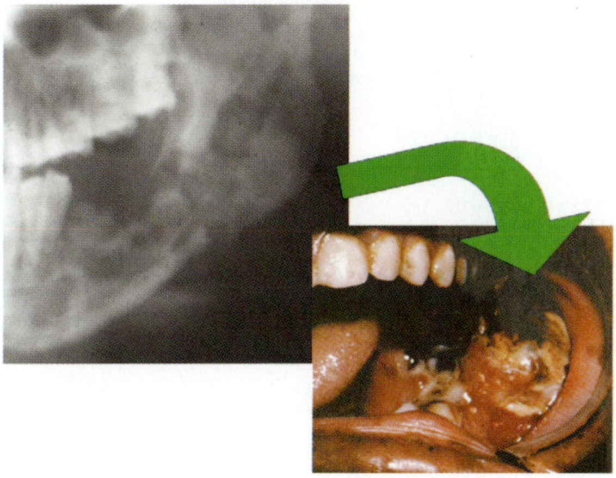

Fig. 10.6 Leiomyosarcoma (malignant neoplasm of smooth muscle), epicentered on the mandibular canal, with destruction of the canal's cortical outlines

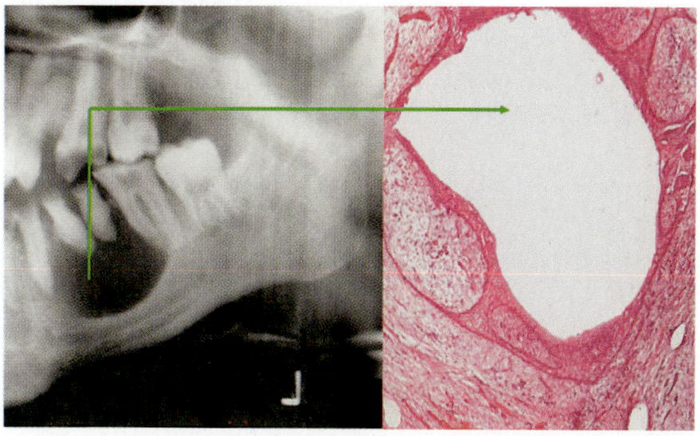

Fig. 10.7 Apical dental (radicular) cyst arising from the grossly decayed left mandibular first permanent molar tooth. Pressure developing within the cyst due to an osmotic gradient causes growth of the lesion and displacement of adjacent structures including the mandibular canal

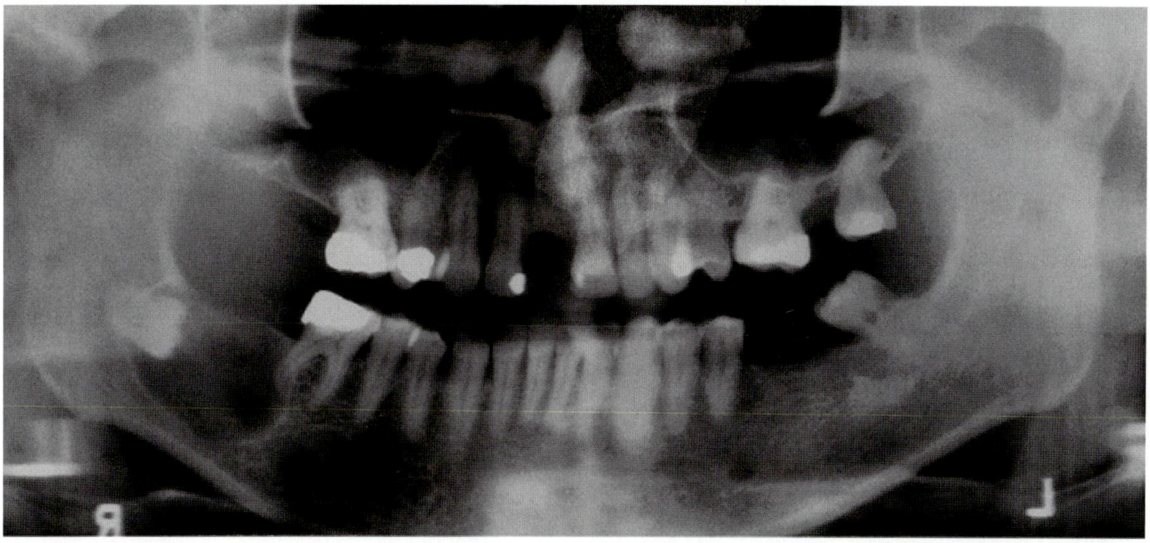

Fig. 10.8 Large dentigerous cyst associated with the crown of a horizontally positioned unerupted third molar tooth in the right side of the mandible. The right mandibular canal is displaced downward in comparison with the contralateral canal

Malignant Lesions Peripheral to the Mandibular Canal

A study of gingival carcinoma found no statistical difference between the diagnostic accuracy of panoramic radiographs and computed tomography for the determination of the superoinferior invasion of the mandible.

Both severe infections, such as suppurative osteomyelitis, and malignant neoplasms are not infrequently associated with an irregular erosion or lysis of the affected jaw. The mandibular canal is not spared in this process. The most common malignancy affecting the oral cavity is squamous cell carcinoma arising in the oral mucosa. The lesion can secondarily invade adjacent bone (Fig. 10.12). Lesions arising within bone generally have a "brandy glass" appearance when they erode outward.

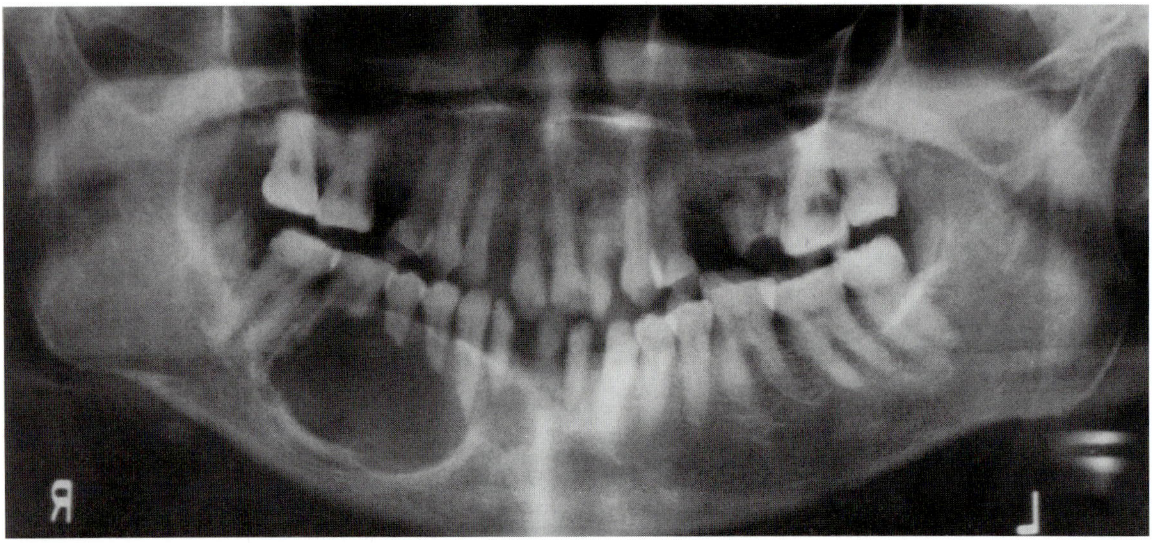

Fig. 10.9 Ameloblastoma in the right mandibular body. The lesion resulted in resorption of the apices of the superjacent teeth, but in downward displacement of the intact subjacent mandibular canal

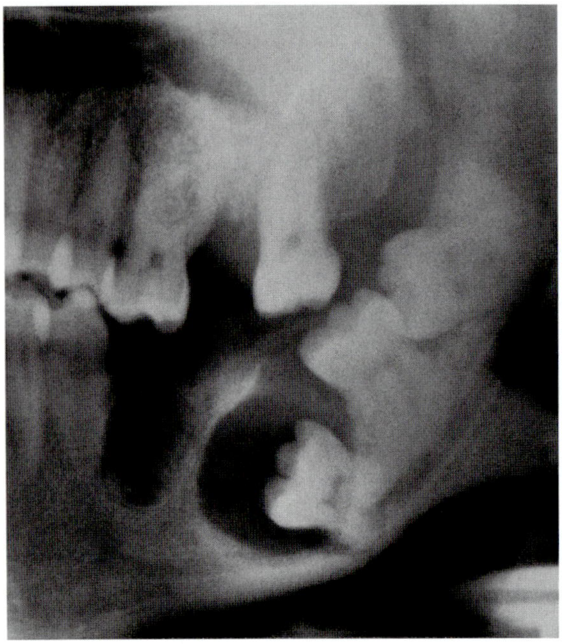

Fig. 10.10 Calcifying epithelial odontogenic tumor causing downward displacement of the mandibular first permanent molar which shows envelopment of the crown by a radiolucency resembling a dentigerous cyst. The mandibular canal is displaced toward the lower border of the mandible

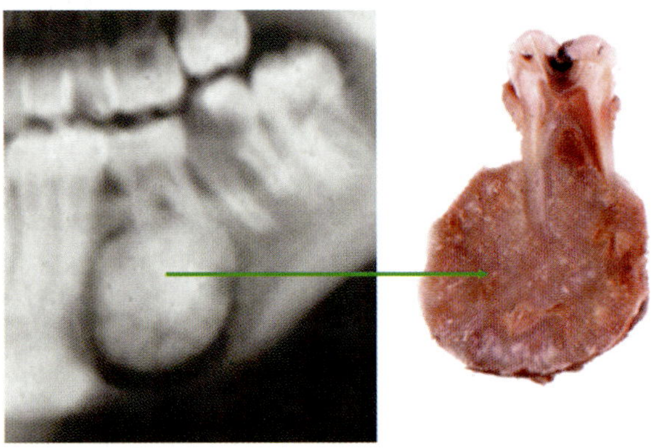

Fig. 10.11 Cementoblastoma of the mandibular first molar tooth displacing the roots of the second premolar and permanent second molar teeth. The mandibular canal has been displaced downward

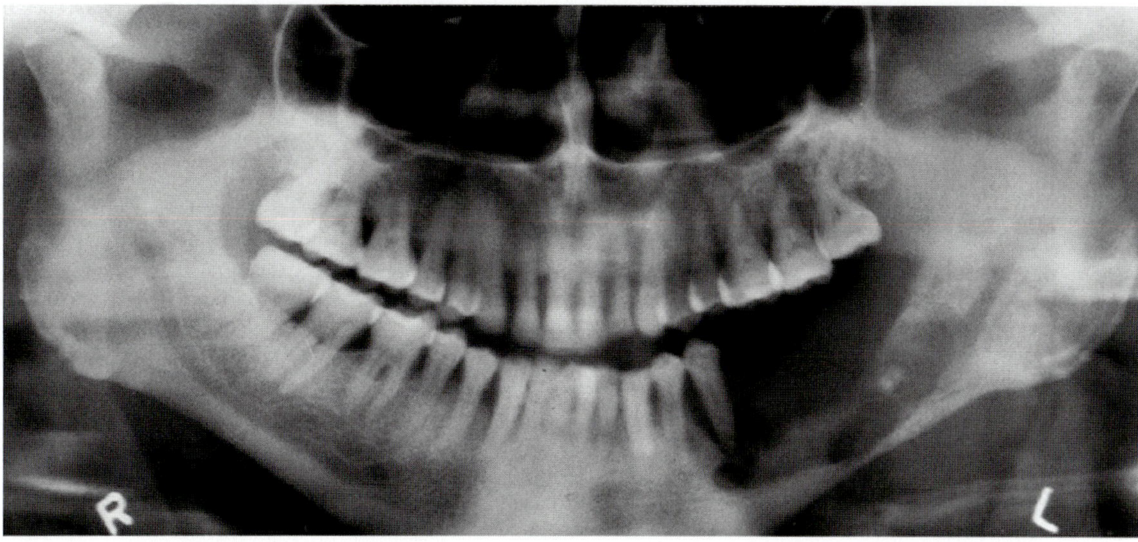

Fig. 10.12 Squamous cell carcinoma invading the left mandibular body and ramus and eroding the mandibular canal cortices. The lesion originated peripherally to bone and hence is "saucer-shaped" (saucerized)

In comparison, lesions arising peripherally, such as invading squamous cell carcinoma, produce a "saucerized" appearance. The mandibular canal might be thought of as a "highway for metastases" hence, erosion of this structure can be viewed as a negative factor regarding prognosis. A study of gingival carcinoma found no statistical difference between the diagnostic accuracy of panoramic radiographs and computed tomography for the determination of the superoinferior invasion of the mandible [17].

The most common malignancy of bone is myeloma. This condition tends to occur in late middle age and in the elderly with "punched out" radiolucencies often being found in many bones, but showing a particular predilection to the calvarium. An example of a lytic lesion forming centrally within the mandible is illustrated in Fig. 10.13. This particular lesion has not spared the mandibular canal and has resulted in a pathological fracture.

Less common malignancies of the jaws include the osteogenic sarcoma and the chondrosarcoma. Both of these conditions cause lysis of normal bone, including the cortices of the mandibular canal when the lower jaw is affected. Both can also demonstrate abnormal bone formation including floccules or "sunburst" appearances. A "sunburst" appearance is demonstrated in the osteogenic sarcoma illustrated in Fig. 10.14 where trabeculations of abnormal new bone are superimposed on the basic lytic lesion. This case also demonstrates a "floating tooth" where the bone supporting a left mandibular molar has been destroyed and growth of the lesion has elevated the tooth.

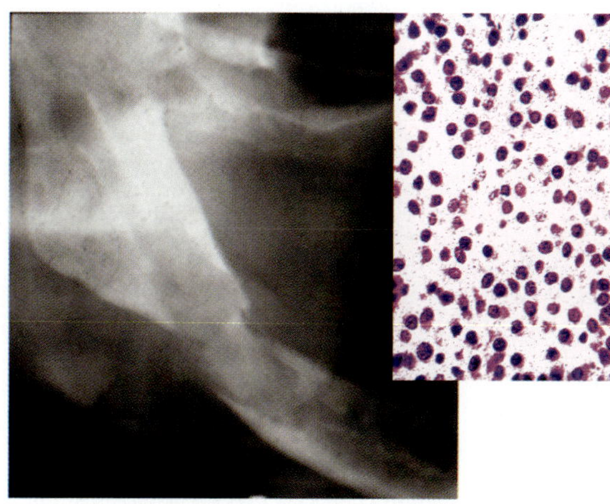

Fig. 10.13 Myeloma. The lesion has destroyed the cortices of the mandibular canal and also resulted in a pathological fracture of the jaw

Lesions Obscuring the Mandibular Canal

Some conditions can obscure the mandibular canal through producing a complex trabecular pattern that camouflages the canal. Conditions that cause this effect include such benign tumors as the odontogenic myxoma, and hamartomas including intraosseous hemangiomas and the familial fibro-osseous condition, cherubism (Fig. 10.15). Cherubism is a dominantly inherited condition that is usually bilateral and predominantly affects both sides of the mandible. Other

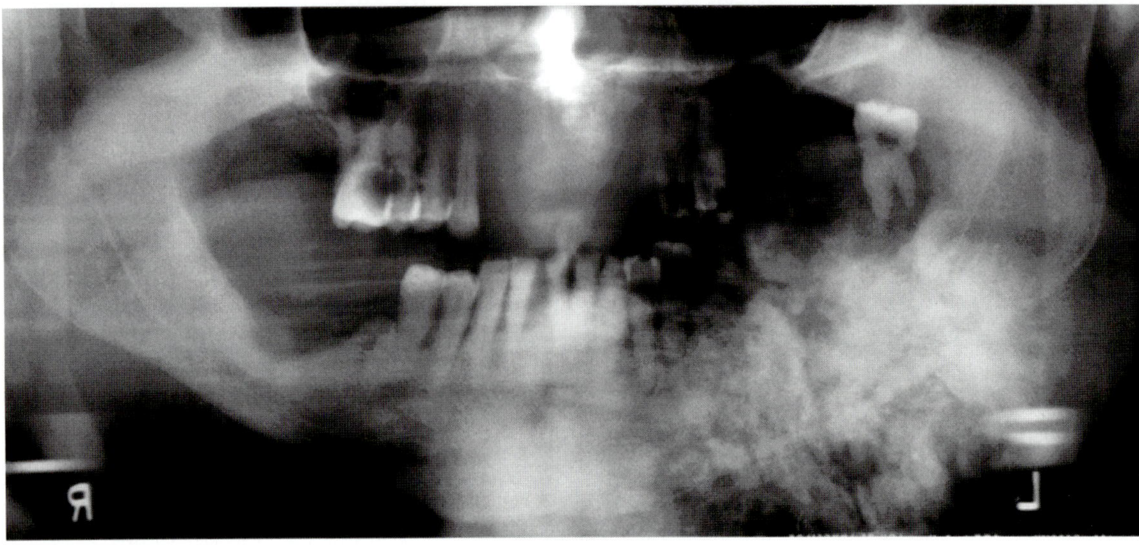

Fig. 10.14 Osteogenic sarcoma of the left mandible. The lytic phase of the lesion has destroyed the outline of the mandibular canal. Note the "sunburst" appearance of new bone formation that is considered a classic, but not invariable, feature of the condition

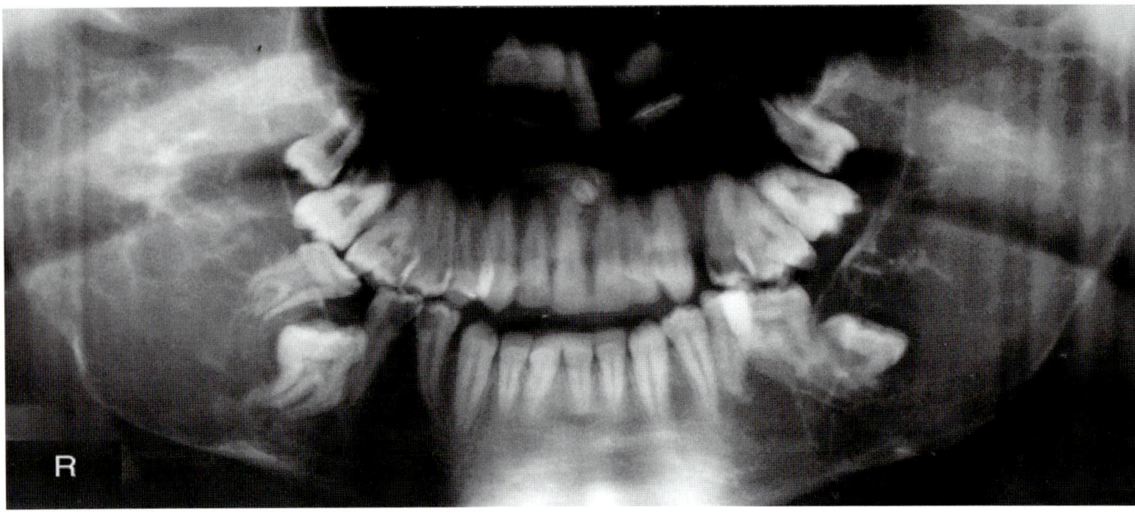

Fig. 10.15 Cherubism. The trabecular patterns within the bilateral lesions of the mandible obscure the outlines of the mandibular canals in the affected areas

conditions that can obscure the mandibular canal are those in which dense bone is deposited. Conditions that procedure dense bone include osteopetrosis, late stage fibrous dysplasia (Fig. 10.16) and florid osseous dysplasia (Fig. 10.17). Fibrous dysplasia arises in young individuals and causes expansion of the jaw unilaterally and typically does not cross the midline. Sclerosis occurs by early adulthood. Florid osseous dysplasia most frequently is found in middle age and older women of African extraction.

Concluding Remarks

It is sometimes believed that the special anatomical structures of the jaws, especially the teeth, make the radiologic interpretation of disease entities affecting the jaws particularly difficult as they hinder comparison with lesions of a similar nature found in bones elsewhere in the body [18]. The converse can be the case if the effects on these very structures are used as clues to discovering the nature of the condition. The mandibular

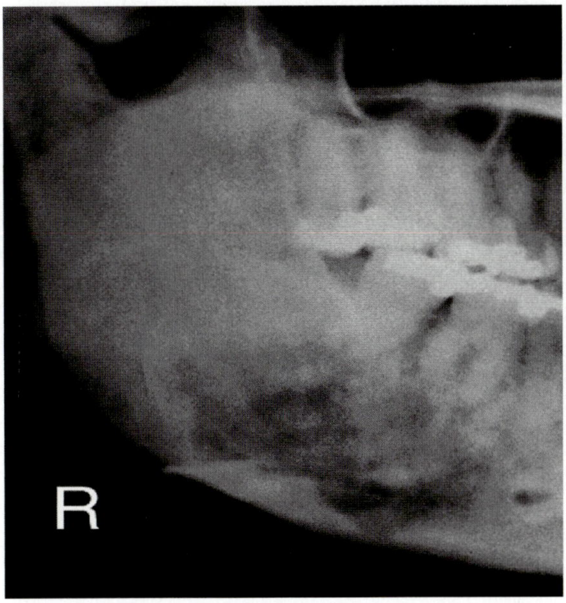

Fig. 10.16 Fibrous dysplasia (late phase): the frosted glass trabeculations that develop in the latter stages of fibrous dysplasia have reduced the clarity of the mandibular canal

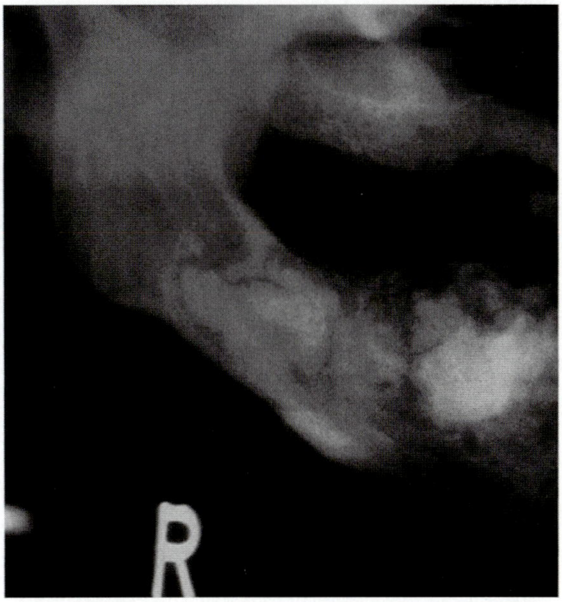

Fig. 10.17 While most lesions of florid osseous dysplasia occur above the mandibular canal, large lesions combined with factors of panoramic projection geometry conspire to obscure the mandibular canals

canal is usually clearly depicted in the panoramic dental radiograph. The dentist's familiarity with the normal range for its anatomy, and the ways in which it can be affected by various disease entities, should be an advantage in detection and interpretation of the normal versus disease. It should be kept in mind that while some disease entities produce consistent features that might help radiologic differentiation, others (e.g., ameloblastoma) show variable or non-specific changes. Nevertheless, in combination with the other well-described radiologic features of these lesions, interpretation of changes concerning the canal as shown on panoramic radiography may well assist in deriving a more accurate differential diagnosis list. In particular, canal displacement is almost invariably a feature of benign lesions, whereas extensive loss of the canal cortical plate is usually a feature of severe infection or aggressive neoplasia.

References

1. Nortjé CJ, Farman AG, Grotepass FW. Variations in the normal anatomy of the inferior dental (mandibular) canal: a retrospective study of panoramic radiographs from 3612 routine dental patients. Br J Oral Surg 1977;15:55–63
2. Zografos J, Kolokoudias M, Papadakis E. Types of the mandibular canal. Hell Period Stomat Gnathopathoprosopike Cheir 1990;5:17–20
3. Nortjé CJ, Farman AG, Joubert JJ de V. Radiographic appearance of the inferior dental canal: additional variation. Br J Oral Surg 1977;15:171–172
4. Langlais RP, Broadus R, Glass BJ. Bifid mandibular canals in panoramic radiographs. J Am Dent Assoc 1985;110:923–926
5. Carter RB, Keen EN. The intramandibular course of the inferior alveolar canal. J Anat 1971;108:433–440
6. Quattrone G. Furloni E, Bianciotti M. Bilateral bifid mandibular canal, presentation of a case. Minerva Stomatol 1989;38:1183–1185
7. Farman AG, Escobar V. Duplication of the oral and maxillofacial structures. Quintessence Int 1986;17:731–737
8. Farman AG, Nortjé CJ, Grotepass FW. Pathological conditions of the mandible: their effect on the radiographic appearance of the inferior dental (mandibular) canal. Br J Oral Surg 1977;15:64–74
9. Xie Q, Wolf J, Tilvis R, Ainamo A. Resorption of the mandibular canal wall in edentulous aged population. J Prosthet Dent 1997;77:596–600
10. Nakasato T, Katoh K, Ehara S, Tamakawa Y, Hoshino M, Izumizawa M, Sakamaki K, Fukuta Y, Kudoh K. Intraosseous neurilemmoma of the mandible. AJNR Am J Neuroradiol 2000;21:1945–1947
11. Shapiro SD, Abramovitch K, Van Dis ML, Skoczylas LJ, Langlais RP, Jorgenson RJ, Young RS, Riccardi VM. Neurofibromatosis: oral and radiographic manifestations. Oral Surg Oral Med Oral Pathol 1984;58:493–498
12. Lee L, Yan YH, Pharoah MJ. Radiographic features of the mandible in neurofibromatosis: a report of 10 cases and review of the literature. Oral Surg Oral Med Oral Pathol Oral Radiol Endod 1996;81:361–367

13. Farman AG, Kay S. Leiomyosarcoma of the oral cavity. Oral Surg Oral Med Oral Pathol 1977;43:402–409
14. Yamada T, Kitagawa Y, Ogasawara T, Yamamoto S, Ishii Y, Urasaki Y. Enlargement of mandibular canal without hypesthesia caused by extranodal non-Hodgkin's lymphoma. Oral Surg Oral Med Oral Pathol Oral Radiol Endod 2000;89:388–392
15. Bertolotto M, Cecchini G, Martinoli C, Perrone R, Garlaschi G. Primary lymphoma of the mandible with diffuse widening of the mandibular canal. Eur Radiol 1996;6: 637–639
16. Farman AG, Köhler WW, Nortjé CJ, van Wyk CW. Cementoblastoma. J Oral Surg 1979;37:198–203
17. Nakayama E, Yoshiura K, Yuasa K, Tabata O, Araki K, Kanda S, Ozeki S, Shinohara M. Detection of bone invasion by gingival carcinoma of the mandible: a comparison of intra-oral and panoramic radiography and computed tomography. Dentomaxillofac Radiol 1999;28:351–356

TEST: Panoramic radiographic appearance of the mandibular canal in health and in disease

1. The relative position of the mandibular canal as demonstrated on a single panoramic radiograph of an edentulous patient can be used to accurately measure the amount of bone loss subsequent to exodontia.

   True ☐ **False** ☐

2. Bifid mandibular canals are found in what proportion of the general adult population?
   (a) 25–50%
   (b) 5–10%
   (c) 0.5–1%
   (d) None of the above

3. Neurofibromatosis is most frequently associated with which of the following alterations in the mandibular canal?
   (a) Localized erosion of the cortices
   (b) Downward displacement
   (c) Obscuring the canal cortices
   (d) Widening of the canal

4. The most common malignancy affecting the oral cavity is:
   (a) Squamous cell carcinoma
   (b) Myeloma
   (c) Osteogenic sarcoma
   (d) Chondrosarcoma

5. Displacement of the mandibular canal that leaves the cortices intact is a common feature of suppurative osteomyelitis.

   True ☐ **False** ☐

6. Panoramic radiographs have been proven equal to computed tomographs for the evaluation of the superoinferior extension of gingival carcinoma of the mandible.

   True ☐ **False** ☐

7. The complex trabecular pattern of the odontogenic myxoma may “camouflage” the cortical outlines of the mandibular canal.

   True ☐ **False** ☐

8. Lesions found enveloping the crown of unerupted teeth are invariably dentigerous cysts and therefore do not require histopathological verification.

   True ☐ **False** ☐

9. "Punched-out" radiolucencies are most typical of:
   (a) Osteogenic sarcoma
   (b) Multiple myeloma
   (c) Cementoblastoma
   (d) Ameloblastoma

10. Extranodal non-Hodgkin's lymphoma has been reported to cause widening of the mandibular canal.

    True ☐ **False** ☐

Chapter

Pathological Conditions affecting the Maxillary Sinus

11

Allan G. Farman
in association with Christoffel J. Nortjé

Learning Objectives

- Gain knowledge of the range of effects of pathoses in the dental arches on the adjacent maxillary sinuses
- Understand that lesions from the upper jaw can extend into the sinus and be larger in reality that they appear clinically
- Realize that the maxillary sinuses extend beyond the focal layer of the panoramic radiograph; hence, that pathoses within the sinuses may not always be clearly demonstrated by this imaging modality

Overview of alternative imaging modalities

Radiography of the maxillary sinuses is often undertaken using computed tomography, magnetic resonance imaging, or the occipitomental plain radiographic projection (Waters projection). However the panoramic radiograph has been found useful for detection of "cyst-like densities" and can clearly demonstrates lesions arising from the maxillary dental arch [1]. Waters projection demonstrates the superior, inferior, and lateral margins of the maxillary sinuses while reflecting the shadows of the petrous temporal bones downward below the inferior margin of the maxillary sinuses [2]. It demonstrates well any soft tissue or fluid contents of the maxillary sinus [1]; however, this method does not display the cortices of the anterior and posterior wall of the maxillary sinus. Neither does the panoramic radiograph; hence computed tomography and magnetic resonance imaging are the methods of choice for imaging the maxillary and other paranasal sinuses.

While computed tomography and magnetic resonance imaging are well suited to demonstrate the maxillary sinuses, it should be remembered that these methods are only employed if there are signs and symptoms of disease, by which time the patients prognosis when afflicted by such insidious disease as squamous cell carcinoma can be poor [3]. Extensive lesions occupying the maxillary sinus can result in surprisingly few clinical signs and symptoms [4]. For this reason, the panoramic radiograph made for dental inspection can sometimes be the primary indicator of maxillary sinus disease. Nevertheless, while panoramic radiography can sometimes detect maxillary sinus disease, it should never be used to entirely exclude sinus pathology. Only the portions of the sinus that are within the image layer will be demonstrated. As the panoramic image layer most closely reflects the dental arch, sinus disease can well arise within the sinuses outside the panoramic image layer.

Maxillary sinus disease frequencies

Diseases of the maxillary sinus are comparatively frequent even in apparently young individuals with rates in excess of one in five individuals examined using the Waters projection (mucosal thickening 12.3%; cysts or polyps 7.2%; opacified sinus 3.3%) [5]. For this reason, it is incumbent upon the practitioner to understand the panoramic radiological features of disease and normal variations within the paranasal sinuses as represented by standard dental radiographic projections. Certainly the patient should not be referred to an ear, nose, and throat specialist for every instance of antral mucosal thickening or mucous retention phenomenon (Figs. 11.1, 11.2), but neither should the practitioner ignore features that could reflect an early malignancy. The reputation of a practitioner is greatly enhanced given appropriate referrals that can make the difference between life and death. Failure to diagnose obvious changes within standard dental radiographic projections can result in liability and unwanted notoriety.

Inflammatory conditions

Inflammatory conditions of non-odontogenic origin are usually clearly demonstrated on panoramic radiography if they involve mucosal thickenings arising from the floor of the maxillary sinus. The most frequent such a process is the mucous retention phenomenon. This is

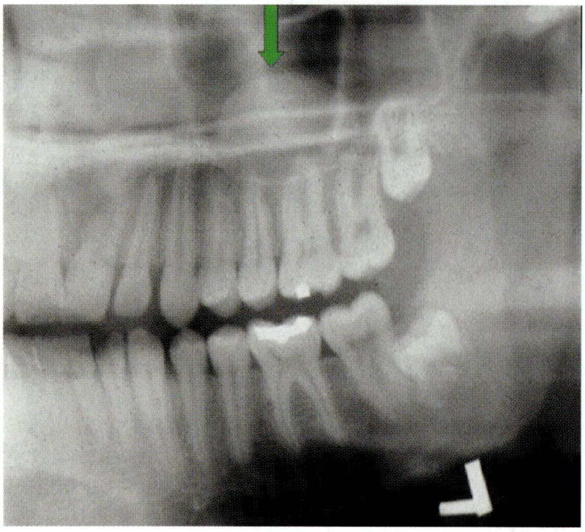

Fig. 11.1 Mucous retention phenomenon: detail from panoramic radiograph shows a smooth-outlined dome-shaped soft tissue density in left maxillary sinus (*arrow*)

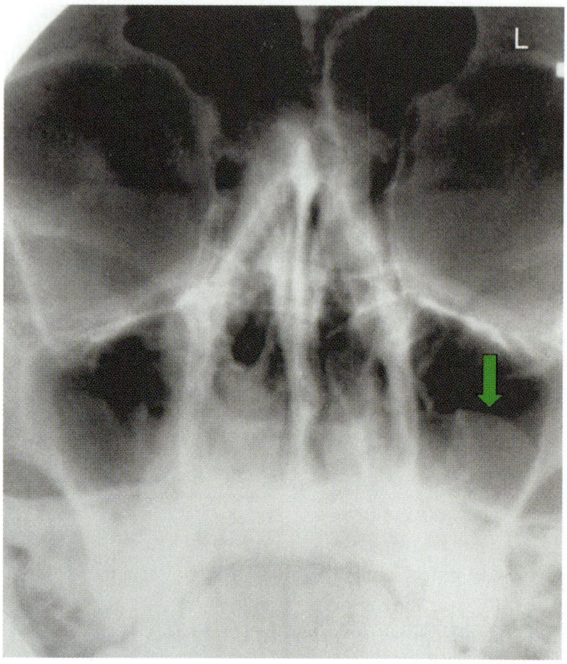

Fig. 11.2 Mucous retention phenomenon of maxillary sinus (*arrow*) shown using the occipitomental projection (Waters projection). This projection can be made using the cephalometric attachment available for use with panoramic systems

commonly seen on panoramic radiographs as a smooth dome-shape swelling of the mucosa with homogeneous radiodensity. The sinus floor is not displaced or eroded. A mucous retention phenomenon is rarely symptomatic; it requires no treatment. Antral polyps are only clearly demonstrated when situated in the panoramic image layer. This is rarely the case; hence, other radiographic views are preferred. Opacified sinuses or fluid levels may be found with acute sinusitis, which accompanies the common cold in 0.5–5% of cases [5, 6]. Fluid levels are not as well demonstrated in panoramic radiographs as they are using the Waters method or computed tomography.

Mucous retention (extravasation) phenomenom

Nortjé et al. [3] comprehensively studied the appearance on panoramic dental radiographs of pathological conditions affecting the maxillary sinuses, comparing inflammatory conditions of dental origin, iatrogenic disease, foreign bodies, non-odontogenic inflammatory conditions, cysts, benign neoplasms, malignant neoplasms, and dysplasias affecting the maxilla.

One should always remember that prevalence of mucous retention phenomenon in the maxillary sinus averages around 5%, but varies considerably from report to report, perhaps as a function of population, geography and season; hence most lesions found on panoramic radiography are likely to be of little importance [15–18]. The prevalence is approximately twice as high in men as in women. The detection and correct interpretation of the retention phenomenon is important for preventing unnecessary diagnostic procedures or surgical intervention [19]. It has been demonstrated that the retention phenomenon, unlike the antral mucocele, has no relationship to sinus obstruction [20]. Antral mucoceles are associated with osteal closure and complete sinus opacification, pain, jaw expansion, and erosion of the antral outline [21, 22]. True mucoceles of the sinuses are comparatively rare in occurrence, but are a serious matter when encountered. Evidence of irregular erosion of the maxillary sinus outline indicates the need to refer the patient to an ear, nose, and throat specialist or oncologist for a second opinion.

Adjacent dental pathoses

Chronic dental abscesses can result in a loss of the continuity of the outline of the lower border of the sinus where it abuts the associated tooth apices, and a related thickening of the sinus mucosa is occasionally evident. Panoramic radiographs are ideal to demonstrate this change as they are specifically designed to illustrate the structures within the dental arches.

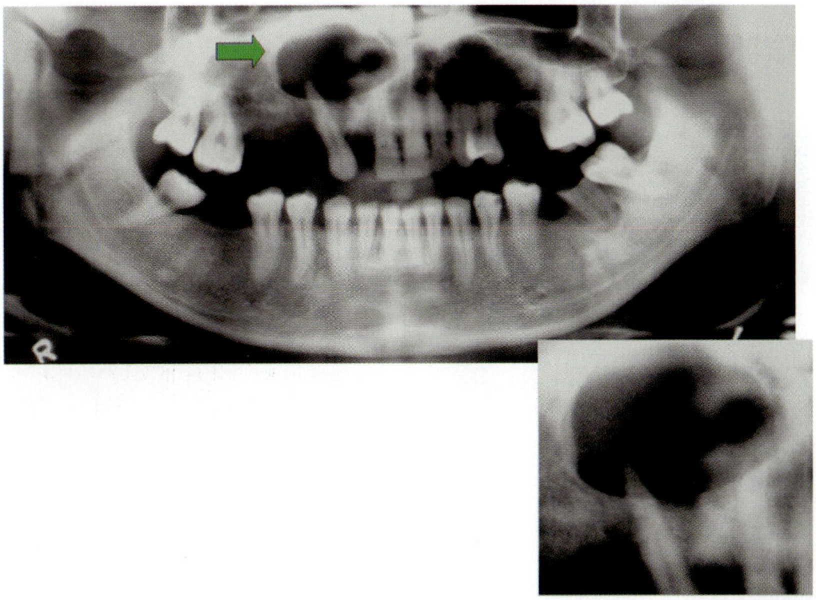

Fig. 11.3 Apical dental cyst (*arrow*) on carious right maxillary lateral incisor. The lesion is a well-delineated unilocular homogeneous radiolucency. It has grown so large that it has caused a displacement of the ipsilateral anterior wall and floor of the maxillary sinus

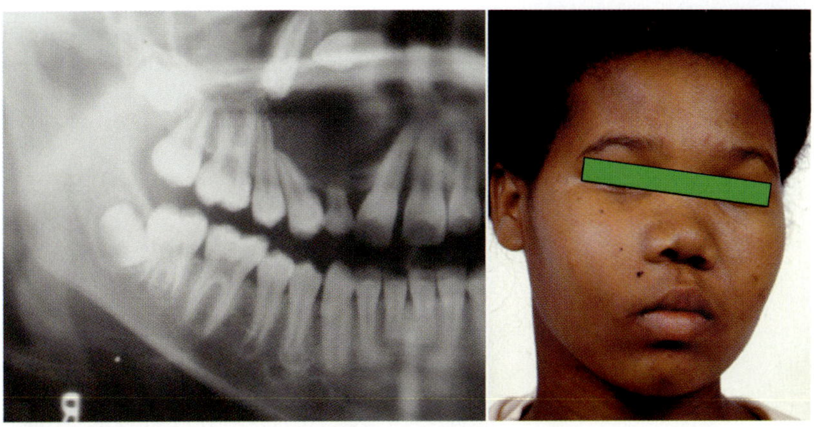

Fig. 11.4 Solitary keratocystic odontogenic tumor displacing the floor of the right maxillary sinus in a 15-year-old female. The permanent lateral incisor and canine teeth are displaced superiorly while displacing the roots of ipsilateral central incisor and first premolar teeth mesially and distally, respectively. The retained primary canine shows normal physiological resorption of the root

Benign cysts and neoplasms

Benign cysts and neoplasms arising in maxillary bone tend to displace the floor or wall of the sinus and can expand to a large size within the maxillary sinus with little in the way of clinically obvious jaw expansion. For example, apical dental cysts (generally associated with the root apex of a carious or fractured tooth) and residual cysts cause an upward displacement of the floor of the sinus, but the cortical outline usually remains intact. Apical dental cysts can extend into the sinus away from the original epicenter in the alveolar ridge (Fig. 11.3). Even a very large cyst arising in the maxilla can result in surprisingly little in the way of clinically noticeable jaw expansion. Dentigerous cysts have a similar effect on the floor of the maxillary sinus to that observed for apical dental cysts, however, the dentigerous cyst envelopes the crown of an unerupted tooth. As the tooth is displaced there is sometimes the appearance of a tooth "suspended" within the sinus.

Other benign radio-opacity

Concerning benign neoplasms, the keratocystic odontogenic tumor (previously termed the odontogenic keratocyst) results in a homogeneous radiolucency that might be unilocular, crenulated, or multilocular in outline, and occasionally can envelope unerupted teeth (Figs. 11.4, 11.5). These also tend to displace the sinus floor and to extend into the sinus while producing little in the way of jaw expansion. In fact, benign tumors in general displaced the sinus floor and expanded into the maxillary sinus rather than outward (Figs. 11.6–11.9). Trabeculation within multilocular tumors such as the myxoma and the ameloblastoma can sometimes be

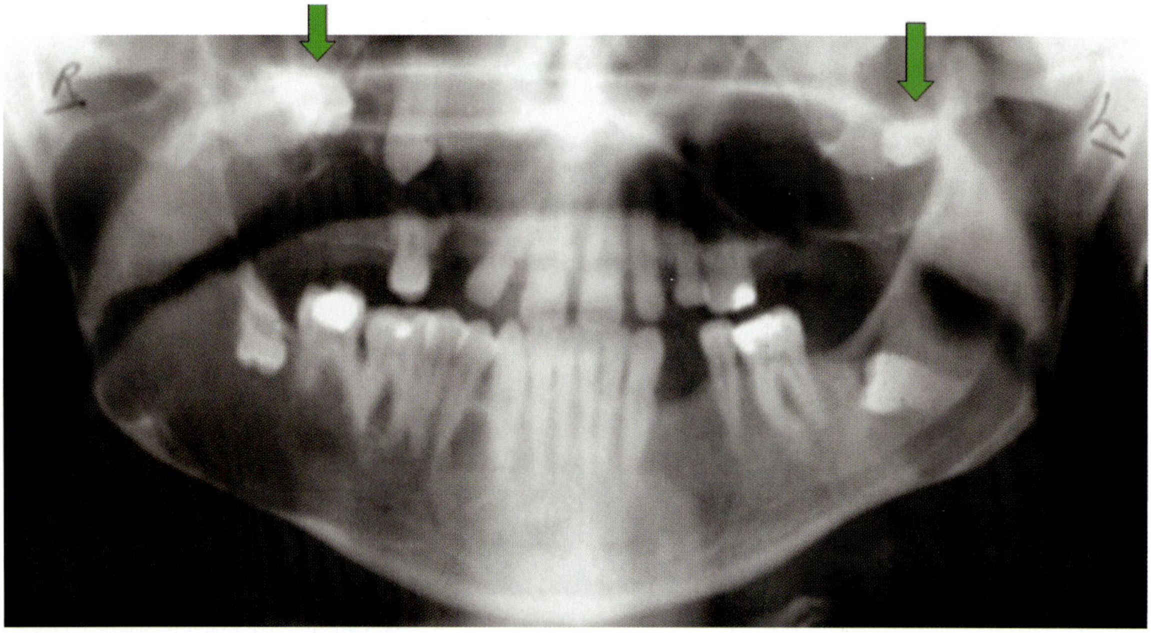

Fig. 11.5 Keratocystic odontogenic tumor: multiple lesions in both jaws in nevoid basal cell carcinoma syndrome. The maxillary lesions are unilocular while the mandibular lesions are crenulated and multilocular. There is displacement of "enveloped" teeth, some of which apparently "float" in the maxillary sinuses (e.g., *arrows*)

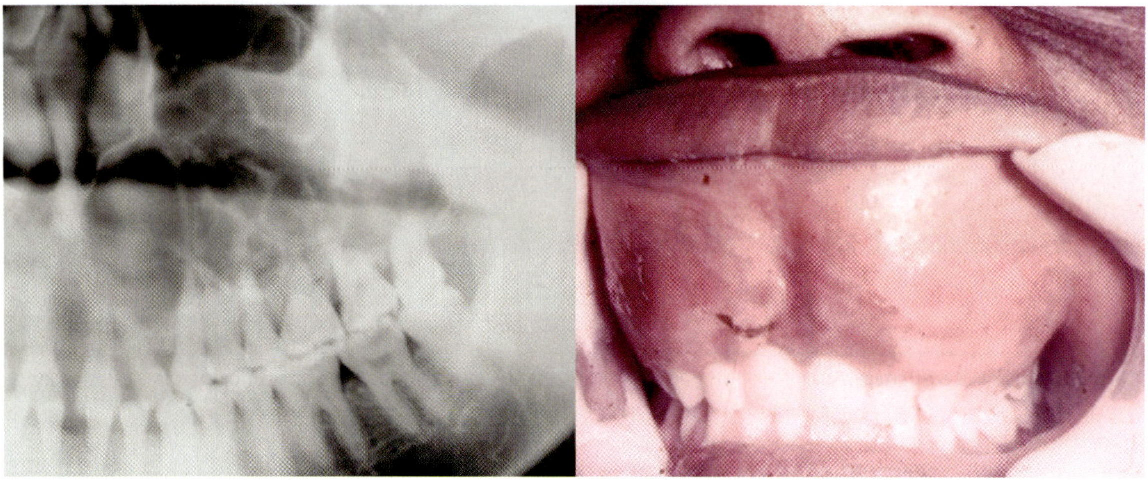

Fig. 11.6 Large maxillary ameloblastoma crossing the midline. *Left* Panoramic detail of the left maxillary sinus. The lesion is a well-delineated multilocular homogeneous radiolucency that occupies the whole maxillary sinus space. *Right* Jaw expansion is evident

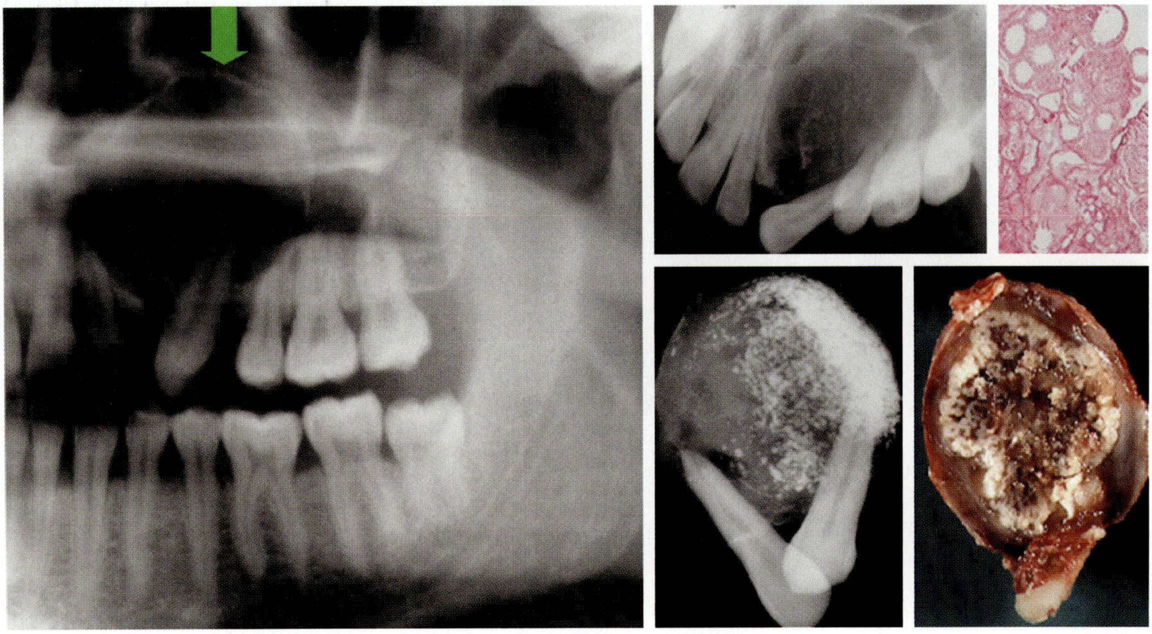

Fig. 11.7 Benign neoplasm, adenomatoid odontogenic tumor: unilocular lesion in the left maxilla subjacent to the canine tooth (cropped panoramic, occlusal, and specimen radiographs). Note displacement of maxillary sinus floor (*arrow*)

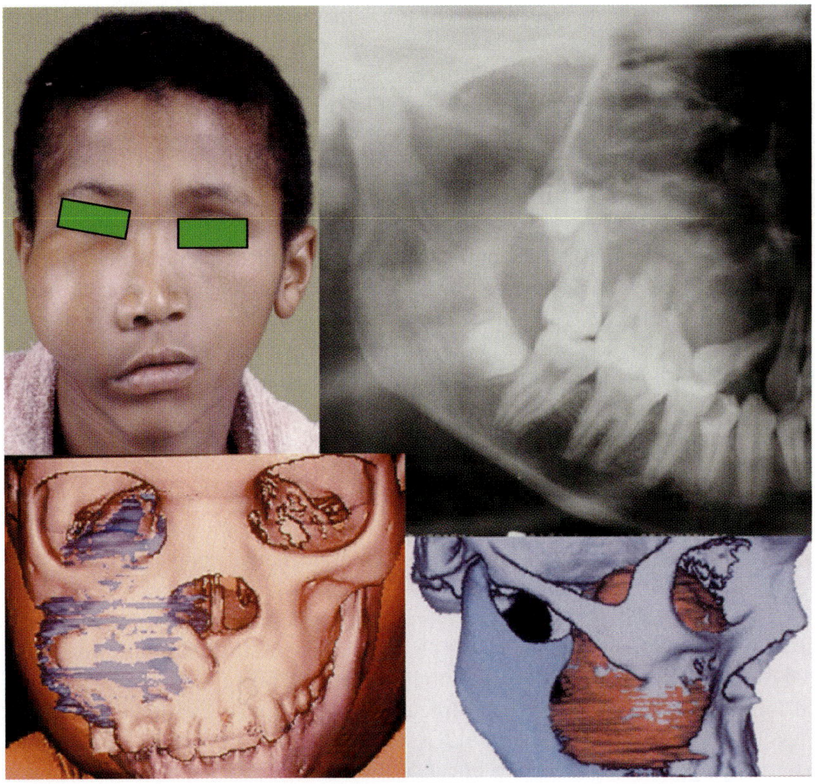

Fig. 11.8 Cementifying-ossifying fibroma displacing and occupying the whole maxillary sinus space on the right side. *Lower images* represent reformatted computed tomography reconstruction of this benign neoplasm

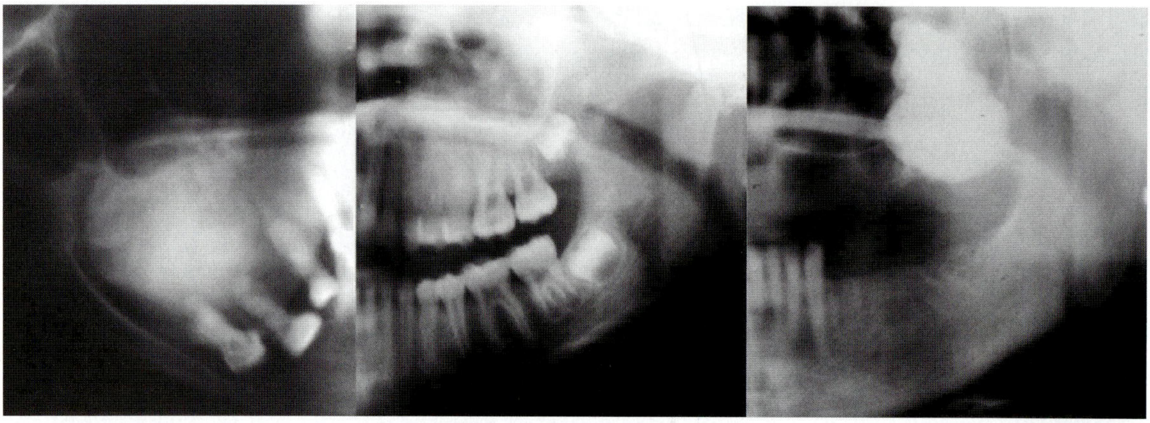

Fig. 11.9 Comparisons of three benign radio-opaque lesions involving the maxillary sinus. *Left* Mature cementifying-ossifying fibroma following mineralization. Note the radiolucent "capsule" at the periphery signifying this to be a benign neoplasm. *Center* Mature instance of fibrous dysplasia. This lesion melds imperceptibly with normal surrounding bone and is not "encapsulated." *Right* Complex odontoma and is more intensely radio-opaque than the other conditions in its mature phase

mistaken for septa within the sinus in the absence of noticeable jaw expansion. Care should be taken to inspect for such features suggesting disease as tooth displacement and tooth root external resorption in the case of the ameloblastoma.

Owing to their radio-opacity, roots or whole teeth displaced into the sinus are readily apparent even when not centered within the image layer. These need to be differentiated from sinus bone nodules and antroliths (calcified "stones" arising in the antral lining) both of which entities could be mistaken for teeth or displaced roots [6]. Foreign bodies, such as bullets, are clearly demonstrated; however, care needs to be made to differentiate between clearly demarcated real images, and blurred magnified ghost images of foreign bodies or jewelry more distally and lower placed in or on the contralateral side of the face. Oroantral fistulas following dental extraction are only noticeable on panoramic radiography when large and within the panoramic image layer.

Dysplastic conditions affecting the maxillary sinuses

The maxilla can also be the site of a variety of dysplastic and fibro-osseous conditions. Fibrous dysplasia can cause the partial or complete occlusion of the sinus on the affected side of the maxilla (Figs. 11.9, 11.10). This may arise in young children and is usually apparent by adolescence. It is generally unilateral. By way of comparison, Paget disease of bone can also cause occlusion of the sinus, but can affect both sides of the maxilla and is found in an aging population (Fig. 11.11).

Detection of maxillary sinus malignant neoplasia

The early detection of insidious maxillary sinus disease can be very important for the patient' prognosis, especially in the case of malignant neoplasia.

In comparison with benign neoplasms, malignant tumors affecting the portion of the sinus screened by the plane of the panoramic radiograph tend to result in erosion of bone. Primary malignancies most commonly arising in the maxillary sinus are squamous cell carcinoma, adenoid cystic carcinoma, and adenocarcinoma [7]. The maxillary sinus may also be affected secondarily by extension malignancies of the oral soft tissues or jaw, and also, although rare, is the site of metastases from distant sites [8].

The early detection of insidious maxillary sinus disease can be very important for the patient's prognosis, especially in the case of malignant neoplasia. By the time of overt signs of squamous cell carcinoma of the maxillary antrum (e.g., neck node metastasis or palatal fistula, Figs. 11.12–11.15), the 5-year survival is only one in six [7]. Substantial progress is being made with multimodality treatment of cancer; hence, the dentist may well make a difference in patient longevity by the early detection of cancer from astute reading of the panoramic radiograph [9]. Early detection can result in an 80%, or better, treatment success rate as determined by 5-year

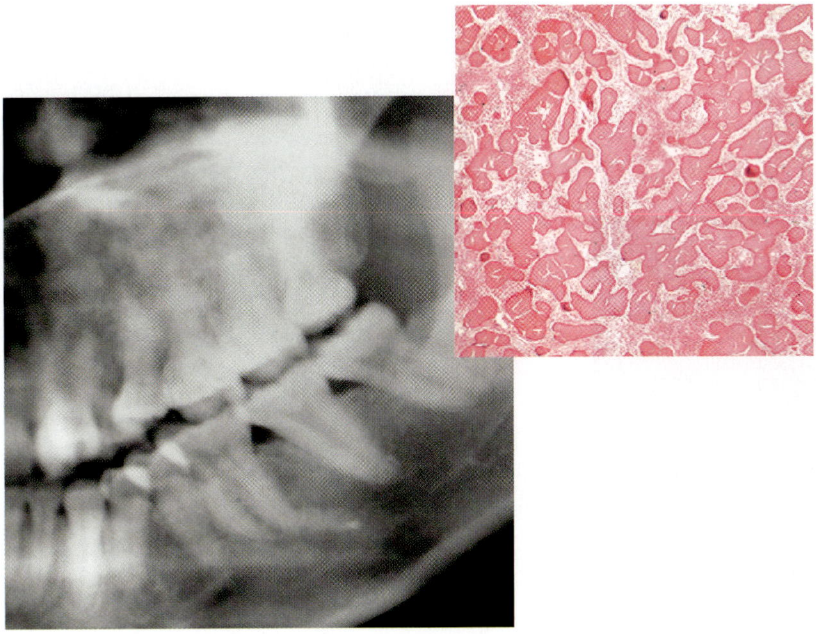

Fig. 11.10 Fibrous dysplasia: cropped panoramic radiograph showing mature (late) lesion of the left maxilla, obscuring the sinus. The lesion is radio-opaque with some radiolucent mottling. It has a ground (frosted) glass appearance. The lesion melds with the normal surrounding bone

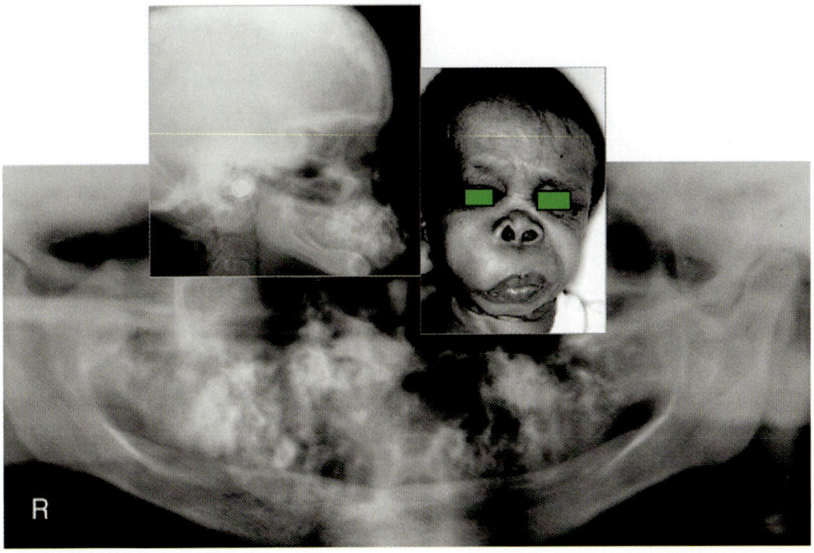

Fig. 11.11 Paget disease of bone. Note cotton-ball radio-opaque sclerotic deposits. There is maxillary cortical expansion. The lesion is bilateral, crossing the midline (panoramic and lateral skull radiographs)

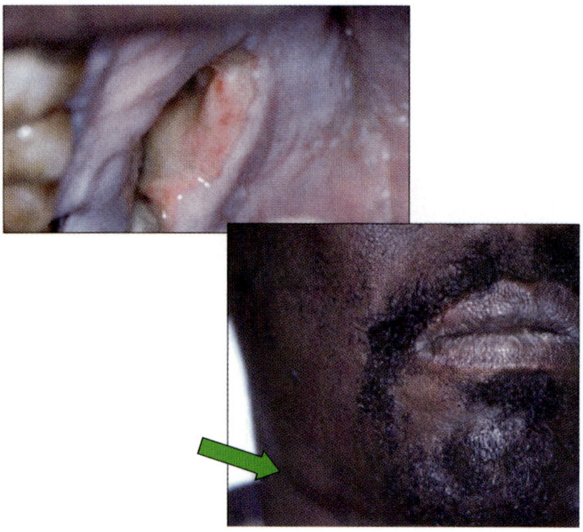

Fig. 11.12 Late stage maxillary sinus squamous cell carcinoma eroding through the palate. Prognosis is poor. This patient has fixed cervical lymph nodes due to metastasis (*arrow*)

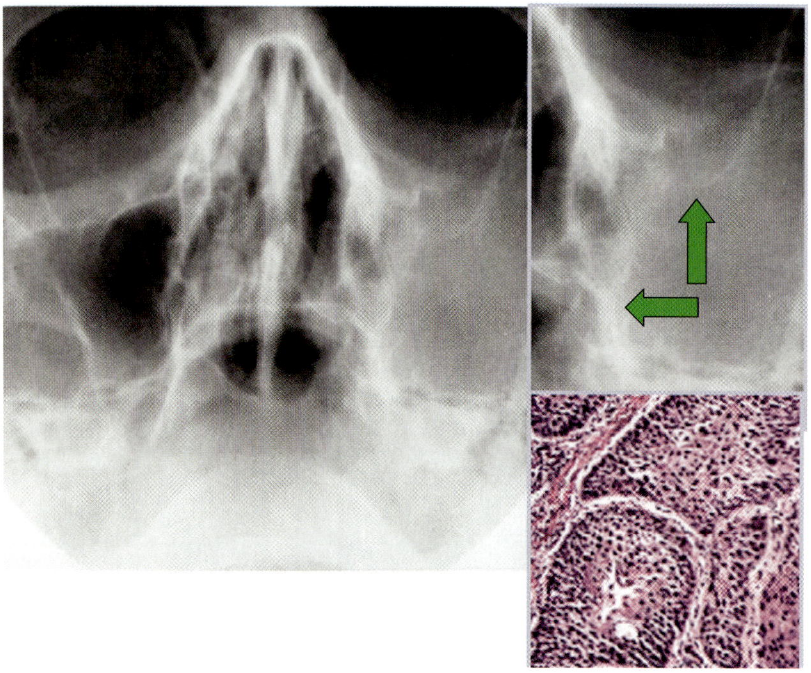

Fig. 11.13 Squamous cell carcinoma. Waters view showing opacification of left maxillary antrum (sinus) with destruction of nasal and orbital walls (*arrows*)

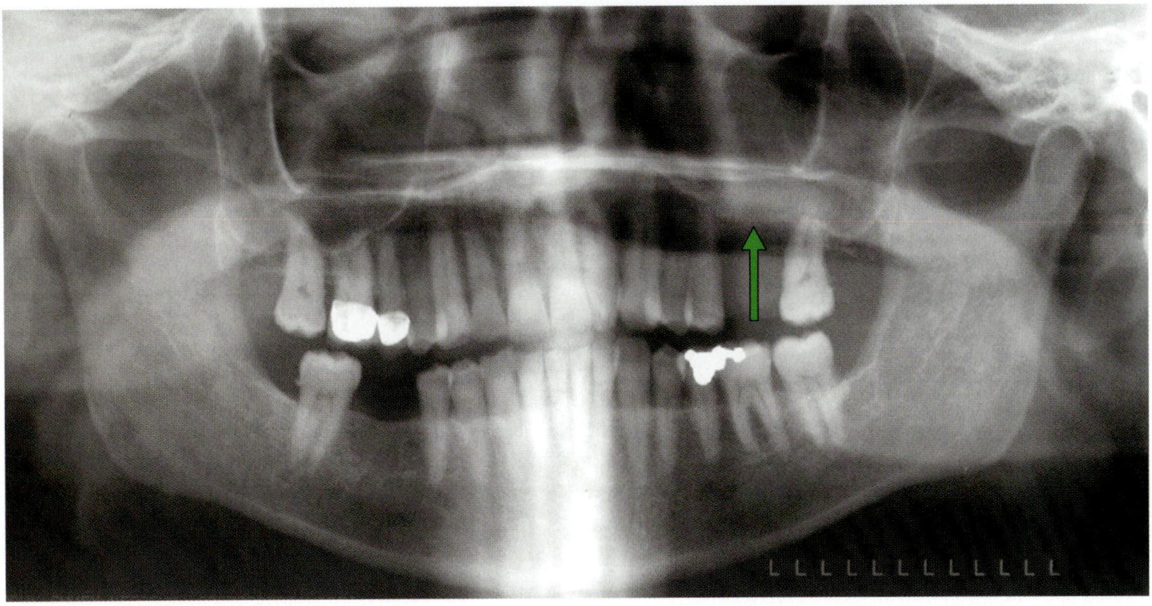

Fig. 11.14 Panoramic radiograph of maxillary squamous cell carcinoma. There is a loss of the lower cortex of the sinus (*arrow*); however the feature is relatively subtle in this view

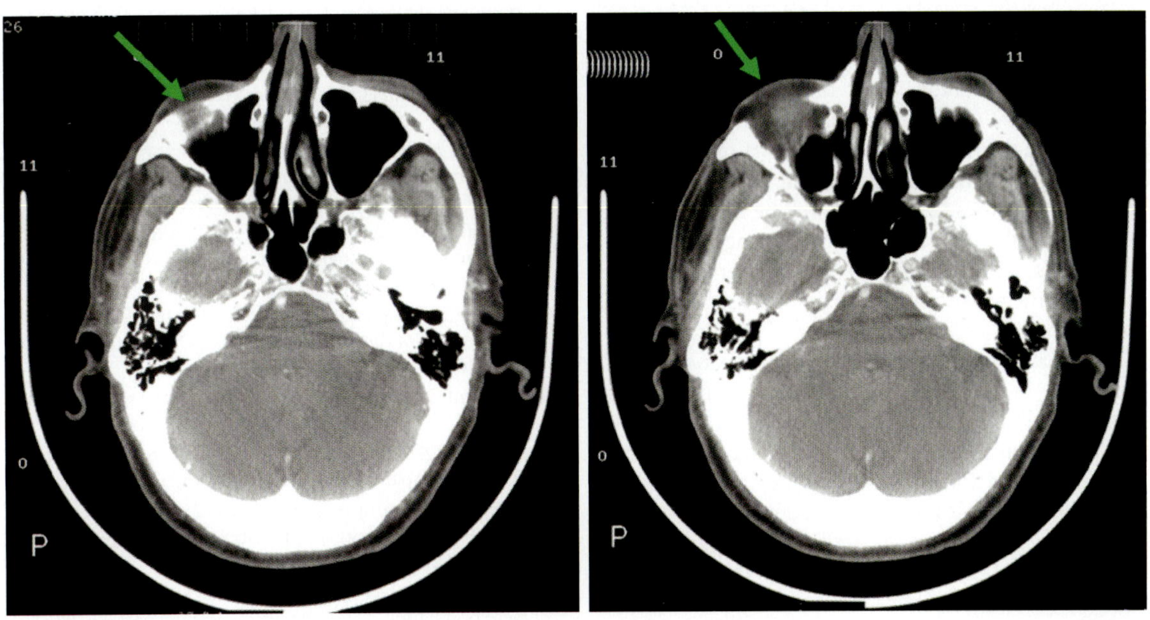

Fig. 11.15 Axial multislice computed tomographic view of same case as that shown in Fig. 11.14. The carcinoma has caused erosion of the anterior sinus wall and soft tissue proliferation is now apparent. The panoramic radiograph was the initial examination; however, computed tomography was needed to better define the lesion and represents the appropriate next step in imaging in this case

survival [10, 11]. It has been found that panoramic radiography can demonstrate antral malignancy at the time of diagnosis in 90% of cases [12]. However, occasional individual case reports do show that, dependent on the lesion's precise site, even large squamous cell carcinomas might be missed when relying on panoramic radiographs alone [13, 14].

...the dentist may well make a difference in patient longevity by the early detection of cancer from astute reading of the panoramic radiograph.

Summary

In summary, the growth of tumors within the maxilla is not concentric; hence, the site of origin is not necessarily the epicenter of the lesion. The maxillary sinus, or antra, constituted the path of least resistance for the growth of such maxillary lesions as cysts and benign neoplasms. Even very large benign tumors and cysts might be present without resulting in clinically noticeable jaw expansion. Hence, the panoramic radiograph is of value in detection of unsuspected disease.

Antral malignancies are usually insidious and produce clinical signs and symptoms relatively late, when the prognosis is often quite poor. Panoramic radiographs have been found of utility in detection of antral carcinoma, particularly that affecting the posterior wall of the sinus [23]. Caution should be used in that the panoramic radiograph is not the technique of choice for viewing the maxillary sinuses; however, it is incumbent on the dentist to evaluate the portion of the maxillary sinus shown in the panoramic radiograph made for other purposes. This might well be the first sign of disease and the only reason for pursuing further diagnostic tests. Early detection of such sinister occurrences improves the prognosis for the unfortunate afflicted patient.

There are limitations to the use of panoramic radiography in the detection of maxillary sinus disease; namely, only the areas within the selected image layer will be in focus. Experimental studies have shown that axial computed tomography provides a better evaluation of osteolytic lesions in the laterosuperior or middle of the posterior sinus wall than will panoramic radiograph [24, 25]. Lesions affecting the floor of the maxillary sinus are better identified and localized with panoramic radiographs than with the Waters projection [26]. When dentists are reading the radiographs, panoramic radiographs have been found equal to Waters projection for determination of sinusitis [27]. These two techniques, and computed tomography, should be considered complementary rather than alternatives [1].

References

1. Ohba T, Katayama H. Comparison of panoramic and Waters projection in the diagnosis of maxillary sinus disease. Oral Surg Oral Med Oral Pathol 1976;42:534–538
2. Waters CA, Waldron CW. Roentgenology of the accessory nasal sinuses describing a modification of the occipitofrontal position. Am J Roentgenol (Detroit) 1915;2:633
3. Nortjé CJ, Farman AG, de V Joubert JJ. Pathological conditions involving the maxillary sinus: their appearances on panoramic dental radiographs. Br J Oral Surg 1979;17:27–32
4. Farman AG, Nortjé CJ, Grotepass FW, Farman FJ, van Zyl JA. Myxofibroma of the jaws. Br J Oral Surg 1977;15:3–18
5. Savolainen S, Eskelin M, Jousimies-Somer H, Ylikoski J. Radiological findings in the maxillary sinuses of symptomless young men. Acta Otolaryngol Suppl 1997;529:153–157
6. Jain RK, Frommer HH. Incidental finding of antroliths in panoramic radiography. N Y State Dent J 1982;48:530–531
7. Lee RJ, O'Dwyer TP, Sleeman D, Walsh M. Dental disease, acute sinusitis and the orthopantomogram. J Laryngol Otol 1988;102:222–223
8. Kim GE, Chung EJ, Lim JJ, Keum KC, Lee SW, Cho JH, Lee CG, Choi EC. Clinical significance of neck node metastasis in squamous cell carcinoma of the maxillary antrum. Am J Otolaryngol 1999;20:383–390
9. Koscielny S. The paranasal sinuses as metastatic site of renal cell carcinoma. Laryngorhinootologie 1999;78:441–444
10. Hayashi T, Nonaka S, Bandoh N, Kobayashi Y, Imada M, Harabuchi Y. Treatment outcome of maxillary sinus squamous cell carcinoma. Cancer 2001;15:1495–1503
11. Tiwari R, Hardillo JA, Mehta D, Slotman B, Tobi H, Croonenburg E, van der Waal I, Snow GB. Squamous cell carcinoma of maxillary sinus. Head Neck 2000;22:164–169
12. Epstein JB, Waisglass M, Bhimji S, Le N, Stevenson-Moore P. A comparison of computed tomography and panoramic radiography in assessing malignancy of the maxillary antrum. Eur J Cancer B Oral Oncol 1996;32B:191–201
13. Lilienthal B, Punnia-Moorthy A. Limitations of rotational panoramic radiographs in the diagnosis of maxillaryn lesions. Case report. Aust Dent J 1991;36:269–272
14. Haidar Z. Diagnostic limitations of orthopantomography with lesions of the antrum. Oral Surg Oral Med Oral Pathol 1978;46:449–453
15. Halstead CL. Mucosal cysts of the maxillary sinus: report of 75 cases. J Am Dent Assoc 1973;87:1435–1441
16. Myall RW, Eastep PB, Silver JG. Mucous retention cysts of the maxillary antrum. J Am Dent Assoc 1974;89:1338–1342
17. Ruprecht A, Batniji S, el-Neweihi E. Mucous retention cyst of the maxillary sinus. Oral Surg Oral Med Oral Pathol 1986;62:728–731
18. MacDonald-Jankowski DS. Mucosal antral cysts in a Chinese population. Dentomaxillofac Radiol 1993;22:208–210
19. Bohay RN, Gordon SC. The maxillary mucous retention cyst: a common incidental panoramic finding. Oral Health 1997;87:7–10
20. Tufano RP, Mokadam NA, Montone KT, Weinstein GS, Chalian AA, Wolf PF, Weber RS. Malignant tumors of the nose and paranasal sinuses: hospital of the University of Pennsylvania experience 1990–1997. Am J Rhinol 1999;13:117–123

21. Bhattacharyya N. Do maxillary sinus retention cysts reflect obstructive sinus phenomena? Arch Otolaryngol Head Neck Surg 2000;126:1369–1371
22. Barsley RE, Thunthy KH, Weir JC. Maxillary sinus mucocele. Report of an unusual case. Oral Surg Oral Med Oral Pathol 1984;58:499–505
23. Greenbaum EI, Rappaport I, Gunn W. The use of panoramic radiography in detection of posterior wall invasion by maxillary antrum carcinoma. Laryngoscope 1969;79:256–263
24. Perez CA, Farman AG. Diagnostic radiology of maxillary sinus defects. Oral Surg Oral Med Oral Pathol 1988;66:507–512
25. Ohba T, Ogawa Y., Shinohara Y, Hiromatsu T, Uchida A, Toyoda Y. Limitations of panoramic radiography in the detection of bone defects in the posterior wall of the maxillary sinus. Dentomaxillofac Radiol 1994;23:149–153
26. Duker J, Fabinger A. Evaluation of the basal parts of the maxillary sinus by means of panoramic tomography. Dtsch Zahnarztl Z 1978;33:823–826
27. Lyon HE. Reliability of panoramic radiography in the diagnosis of maxillary sinus pathosis. Oral Surg Oral Med Oral Pathol 1973;35:124–128

TEST: Pathological conditions of the maxillary sinus

1. The Waters method uses an occipital-mental projection to demonstrate the maxillary sinuses.

   True ☐ **False** ☐

2. The sex ratio for the prevalence of mucosal retention phenomenon in the maxillary sinus is?
   (a) 1M:1F
   (b) 1M:2F
   (c) 2M:1F
   (d) None of the above

3. With early detection the prognosis for 5-year survival of maxillary sinus squamous cell carcinoma is improved to approximately?
   (a) 100%
   (b) 80%
   (c) 60%
   (d) 40%

4. Which of the following lesion outlines occurs with the keratocystic odontogenic tumor?
   (a) Unilocular
   (b) Crenulated
   (c) Multilocular
   (d) Any of the above

5. Opacified maxillary sinuses from acute sinusitis is associated with the common cold with which of the following frequencies?
   (a) 0.5–5%
   (b) 10–15%
   (c) 25–40%
   (d) >50%

6. Fibrous dysplasia is generally unilateral and tends to be detected during childhood or adolescence.

   True ☐ **False** ☐

7. Jaw swelling is a frequent first sign of early changes due to benign neoplasms affecting the maxillary sinuses.

   True ☐ **False** ☐

8. Trabeculation within multilocular tumors such as the myxoma and the ameloblastoma frequently obscured the maxillary sinus outline.

   True ☐ **False** ☐

9. Panoramic radiographs of the maxillary sinus clearly demonstrate the position of metallic foreign bodies and are not subject to confusing ghosting artifact.

True ☐ **False** ☐

10. The image layer for panoramic radiography rarely if ever covers the entire maxillary sinus.

True ☐ **False** ☐

Chapter

Panoramic Radiology: Endodontic Considerations

12

Allan G. Farman
in association with Stephen J. Clark

Learning Objectives

After reading this article, the reader should be able to:

- Understand how a panoramic radiograph provides a comprehensive overview that can be important in detection of additional teeth requiring endodontic treatment
- Determine where a panoramic radiograph is vital to properly image and interpret a periapical lesion extending beyond the margins of a periapical radiograph
- Explain the dynamic interrelationships between the various periapical pathoses of inflammatory origin

Panoramic imaging can serve as an important endodontic diagnostic tool as well as an effective method to evaluate the success of endodontic therapy. This article provides a number of clinical examples that illustrate the effectiveness of utilizing panoramic imaging as a valuable adjunct to endodontic treatment planning.

Periapical Pathoses

Endodontics is concerned with the morphology, physiology, and pathology of the human dental pulp and periradicular tissues. Radiology is especially important for diagnosis in the detection of periapical lesions, and to assess treatment success including post-treatment healing [1].

The pathoses of the pulp and dentally associated periapical lesions can be considered as a continuum of conditions rather than isolated entities (Fig. 12.1). Following irreversible pulpitis, the pulp will inevitable undergo necrosis. Early in the inflammatory process there may be no radiographic evidence of irreversible pulpitis. With the spread of the pulpal inflammation to the periapical tissues, the patient's pain will often become more localized with the development of percussion sensitivity. Radiographically, a widened periodontal ligament space may develop. During the acute phase of periapical periodontitis simply not enough time has passed for cell types necessary to effect resorption of bone to be present. Acuteness has nothing to do with severity. It is simply a reflection of a relatively short passage of time from the onset of the condition. If the irritant is sufficiently strong for tissue destruction, then pus will form. The patient then has an abscess. When the lesion has existed long enough for chronic inflammatory cells to be present, there is an attempt to seal off irritation through the generation of granulation tissue, and this is usually associated with development of a periapical radiolucency.

Different portions of the lesion can demonstrate different cellular activities. There may still be tissue breakdown and pus formation, in which case there is a chronic abscess, walled by granulation tissue. Within the granuloma, epithelial remnants of the root sheath of Hertwig (the rests of Malassez) can be stimulated to proliferate (Fig. 12.2). As the central cells within the proliferating epithelial islands are distanced from their blood supply, there may be breakdown and micro-cyst formation. Growth occurs due to osmotic pressures within the cyst cavity. Periapical radiolucencies that appear to be larger than 1 cm in diameter on radiograph most likely contain a cystic component (Figs. 12.3–12.5), although smaller lesions can also be cystic. Early radiolucencies, not involving the cortex of the affected jaw can be difficult to detect regardless of the radiographic method. Lesions large enough to be seen on periapical radiographs are usually clearly demonstrated by panoramic radiographs. The panoramic radiograph has the advantage of demonstrating the full extent of larger lesions that can extend beyond the margins of a periapical radiograph.

Given reduced host resistance, or increased virulence of infectious agents, there can be tissue destruction and a cyst may convert to a chronic abscess following the loss of the epithelial lining. Given drainage of pus, increased host resistance, or antibiotics, such lesions can deteriorate (Fig. 12.1). At a distance beyond the radiolucency there can be bony sclerosis (Fig. 12.6). Such increased mineralization inflammatory origin is termed condensing osteitis.

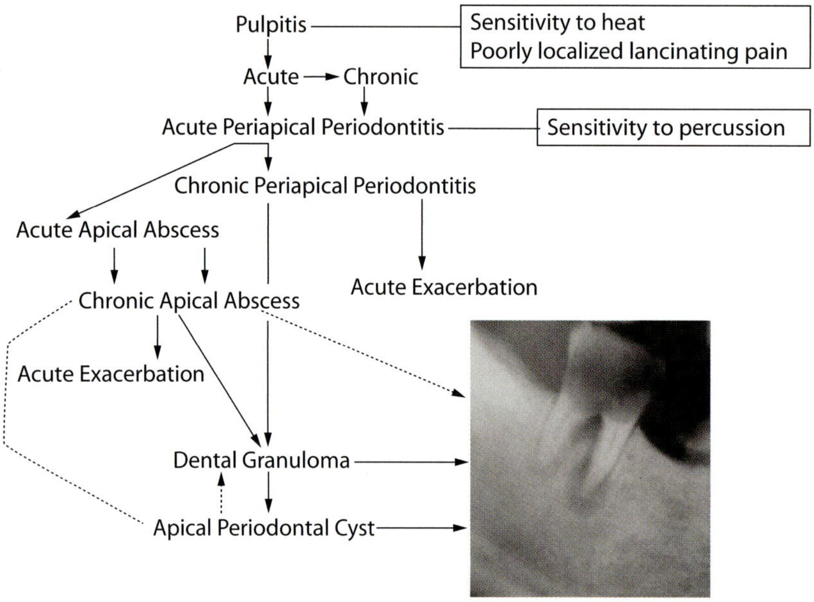

Fig. 12.1 Dynamics of pulpal and inflammatory periapical pathoses

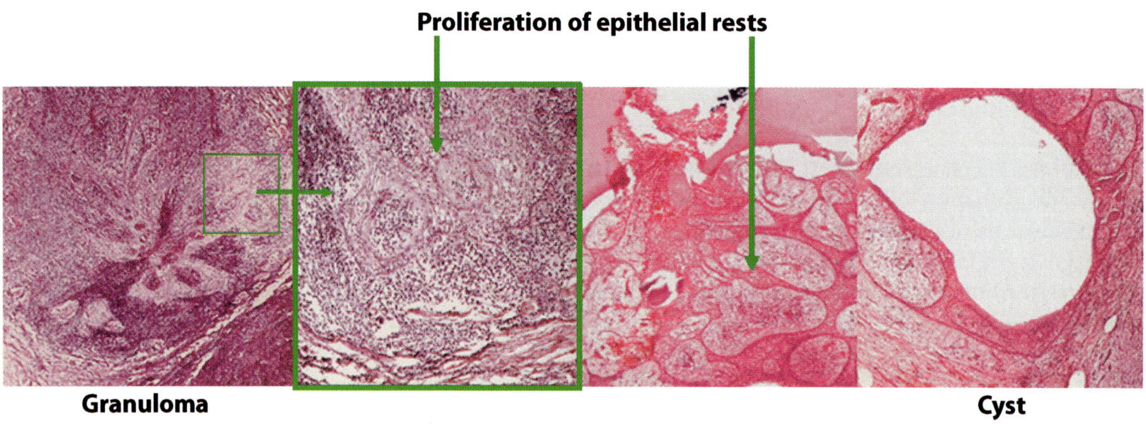

Fig. 12.2 Histological progression from dental granuloma (*left*) to apical periodontal (*radicular*) cyst (*right*). *Vertical arrows* indicate proliferation of epithelial rests

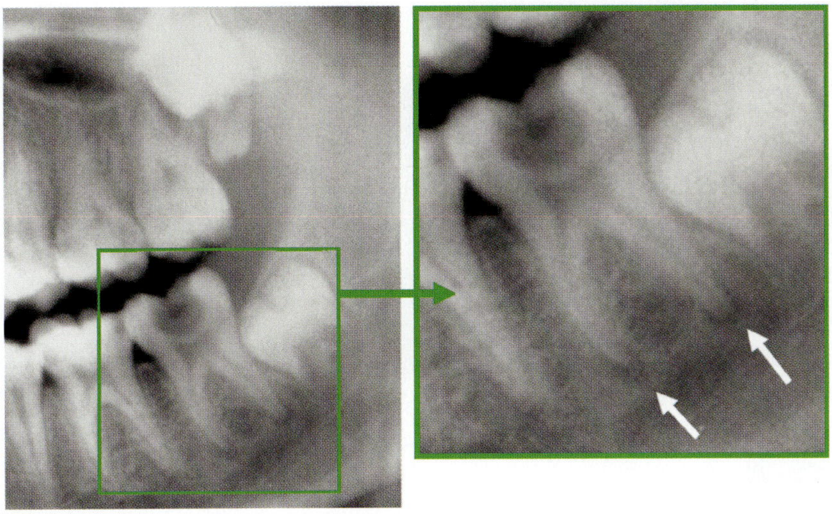

Fig. 12.3 Details of a panoramic radiograph demonstrating development of periapical radiolucencies (*arrows*) at the root apices of a mandibular permanent molar tooth having extensive occlusal dental caries involving the pulp

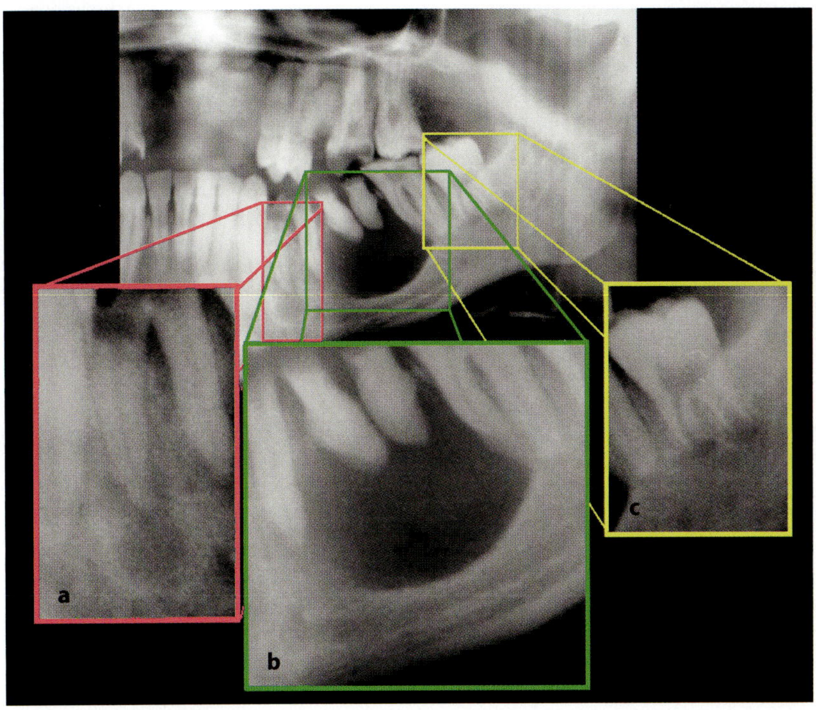

Fig. 12.4 Details of panoramic radiograph showing moderate (**a**) and large (**b**) periapical radiolucencies, and normal tooth development (**c**) where the root apices have not fully formed

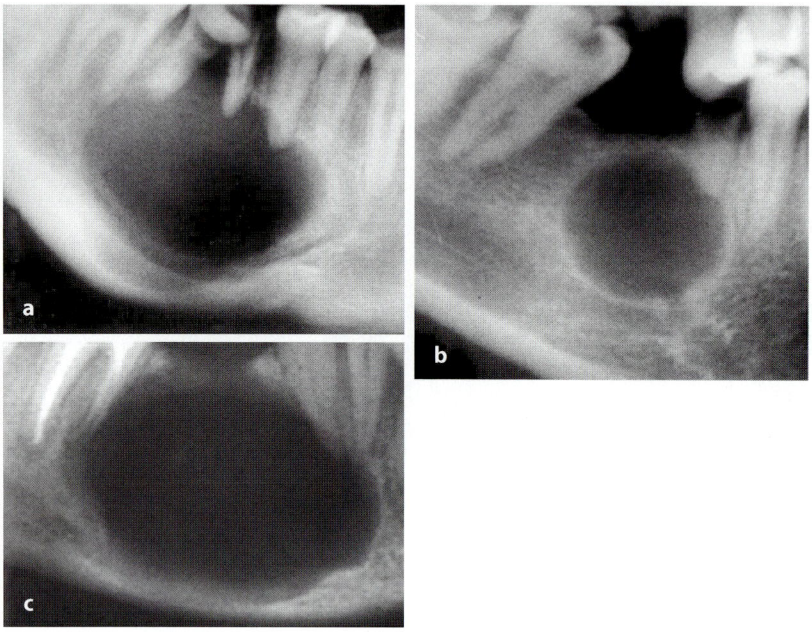

Fig. 12.5 Large apical periodontal cyst on a mandibular first molar (**a**) and premolar (**b**); and residual radicular (apical periodontal) cyst (**c**) following removal of the "causative" tooth. Note the small periapical radiolucency associated with the overfilled distal root of the adjacent molar tooth in (**c**)

Occasionally, infections of dental origin do not remain localized, especially in patients with reduced host resistance due to immunosuppression. Highly destructive suppurative osteomyelitis may ensue (Fig. 12.7a). The panoramic radiograph is a useful method to explore the boundaries of such lesions. Spread of infection in the form of periostitis ossificans is also possible, but is more frequent in young individuals who exhibit a high resistance to infection (Fig. 12.7b, c).

Providing a Comprehensive Radiographic Overview

If patients are referred to the endodontist to have root canal therapy performed to treat pulpal and periradicular diseases, the only radiograph to accompany the patient is often the periapical radiograph. Boodle et al. (2003) notes that such individual periapical radiographs are inadequate for the detection of asymptomatic pathoses present in other areas of the maxilla and mandible [2].

Frequently, the referring dentist has made a panoramic radiograph, but does not see a need to provide anything other than the selected periapical view. In the case of the US armed forces, the military's readiness mission requires that a panoramic radiograph be part of the patient's dental record. In addition to its use for personal identification purposes, the panoramic radiograph is an excellent diagnostic tool that can give the clinician an overall view of the dentoalveolar structures.

A retrospective study at Fort Gordon, Georgia by Bodley et al. evaluated randomly selected panoramic radiographs from US military personnel and recorded the presence of radiolucent and radio-opaque areas that would not be evident on a referral periapical radiograph [2]. The results of this study found a 4.2% occurrence of undiagnosed pathoses that would otherwise have gone undetected, and that could well impact on military readiness at a critical juncture. Ahlqwist et al. (1986), in conjunction with an epidemiological study of oral health in women investigated the diagnostic yield of the panoramic radiograph in comparison with the intraoral full mouth survey including posterior bitewing radiographs [3]. Full mouth surveys and panoramic radiographs of 75 women were compared for gross characteristics such as distribution of teeth, missing teeth, restorations, and endodontic treatment as well as for osteolytic lesions at the root, marginal bone loss and carious lesions. Nearly a 100% correlation was found both for gross characteristics and also for osteolytic lesions associated with teeth. Furthermore the coefficient of correlation was 0.96 for individual mean marginal bone scores. Poor agreement was found only for carious lesions with only 36% of those carious lesions extending well into the dentin being found both in the intraoral radiographs and in the panoramic radiographs. It was concluded that, except

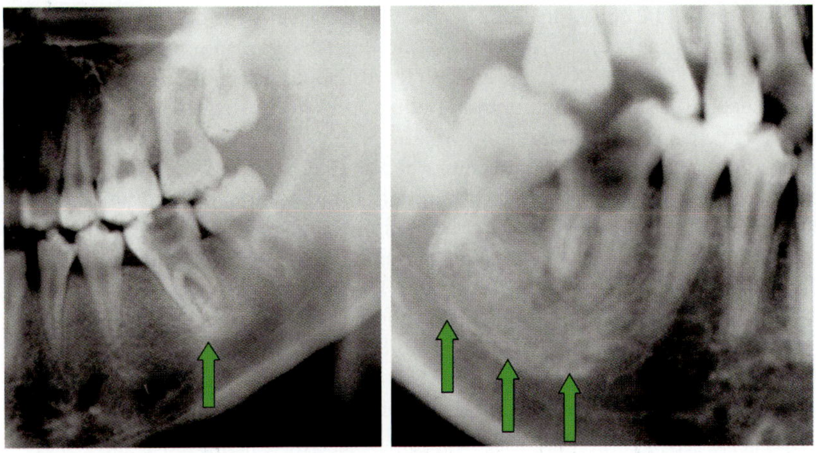

Fig. 12.6 Details from panoramic radiographs demonstrating examples of focal sclerosing osteomyelitis (condensing osteitis). In both instances, bony sclerosis is seen beyond the apical rarefactions subjacent to the carious first molar tooth (*arrows*)

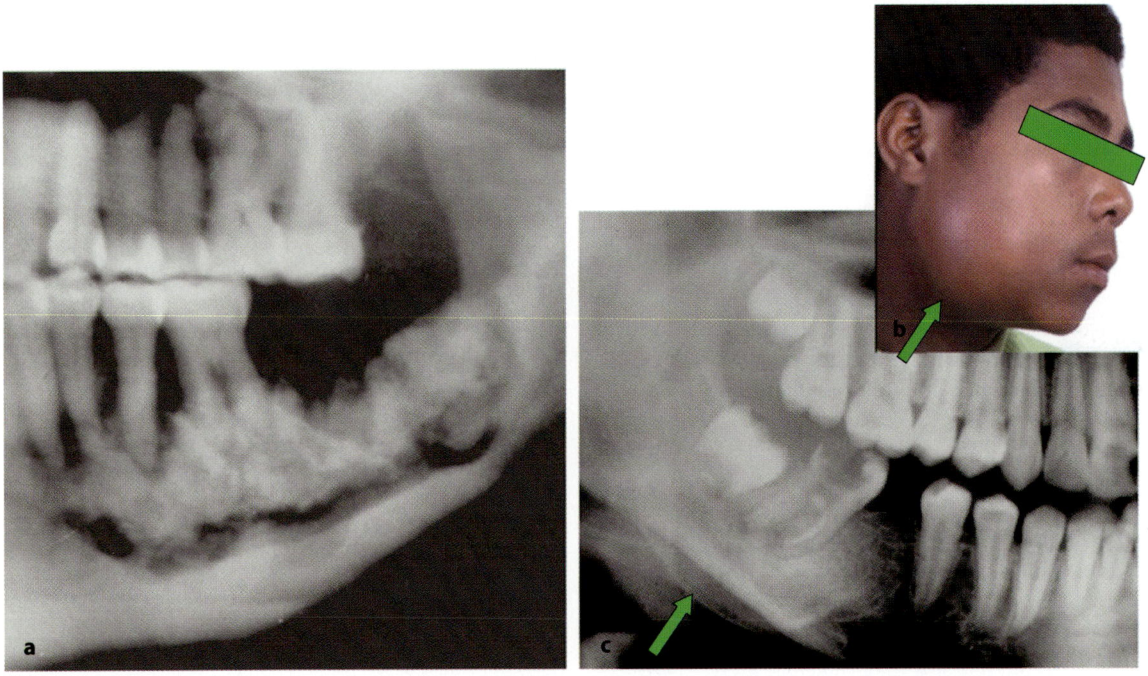

Fig. 12.7 **a** Suppurative osteomyelitis. Note irregular radiolucency and sequestration of dead bone. **b** Clinical photograph of patient illustrated in **c**. Note swelling of right cheek with "onion peel" proliferation of the lower mandibular cortex (*arrows*). This is proliferative periostitis and represents chronic irritation from the carious first molar tooth that has a periapical pathosis

for dental caries, the panoramic radiograph can be considered as adequate as the intraoral radiographic survey for studies of oral health.

Using panoramic radiographs, De Cleen et al. (1993) determined the periapical status of all teeth and the prevalence of endodontic treatment in a group of 184 Dutch adults [4]. For this population, 5.2% of all non-endodontically treated teeth showed signs of periapical pathoses and 2.3% of the teeth were root-filled. Around the apices of 39.2% of the endodontically treated teeth in this survey, radiologic signs of periapical pathology were observed. Using the level of the root canal filling as a criterion for evaluating the quality of the root canal treatment, 50.6% of the endodontic treatments were assessed to be inadequate. There was a significant correlation between the presence of periapical pathology and underfilling of the root canal(s). Nearly half of the patient sample (44.6%) had at least one tooth with radiographic signs of periapical pathosis, indicating a substantial future need for endodontic treatment [4].

A similar study was conducted in Gottingen by Hulsmann et al. (1991) to determine the incidence, distribution, and quality of endodontic treatment using panoramic radiographs of 200 periodontal patients [5]. While only 3.2% of all teeth had root-canal fillings, 87% of all root-canal fillings ended more than 2 mm from the apex and more than 60% exhibited insufficient obturation. Periapical lesions were clearly depicted in panoramic radiographs for 60% of all teeth having root-canal fillings [5].

Follow Up Evaluation

Lupi-Pegurier et al. (2002) conducted a study to determine the periapical status and the quality of root-canal treatment amongst an adult population attending the dental school in Nice, France [6]. The survey involved 344 patients: 180 women and 164 men. Panoramic radiographs, made by a trained radiology assistant, were used. The periapical areas of all teeth (with the exception of third molars) were examined. Technical quality of root fillings was evaluated for both apical extension and density. Statistical analyses were conducted using ANOVA, Chi^2, Fisher's PLSD, and Cohen's Kappa tests. Men had significantly fewer natural remaining teeth than women ($p < 0.03$) so it is perhaps not surprising that the average number of root-filled teeth was lower for men than for women ($p < 0.01$). The majority of root fillings were considered of poor technical quality. While non-root-filled teeth ($n = 6{,}126$) had significantly fewer signs of periapical pathology than root-filled teeth ($n = 1{,}429$) (1.7% versus 31.5%, $p < 0.0001$). There was a significant correlation between the presence of periapical pathology and inadequate root-canal fillings ($p < 0.001$). The results of the study indicated that many endodontic treatments were technically unsatisfactory in terms of quality and treatment outcome. There was a need for comprehensive evaluation of the need for endodontic retreatment in the population examined. Panoramic radiography proved effective for this evaluation [6].

Hulsmann et al. (1991) of the University of Gottingen used panoramic radiographs to determine the incidence, distribution, and quality of endodontic treatment in 200 patients [5]. Root-canal fillings were found in 3.2% of teeth. Eighty-seven percent of all root-canal fillings ended more than 2 mm from the apex and more than 60% exhibited insufficient obturation. Periapical lesions were detected in 60% of all teeth with root canal fillings. Panoramic radiographs were made of 392 Estonian schoolchildren (33% boys and 67% girls) aged 14–17 years, 197 in Tartu and 195 in Tallinn [7]. The mean number of permanent teeth was 31.5 with 14% of the children having one to four teeth (excluding wisdom teeth). Endodontic treatment had been given to 13% of the subjects in Tartu and to 46% in Tallinn, the success rates being only 47% and 44%, respectively. Furthermore, eight odontogenic cysts, one nasopalatine duct cyst, and one solitary bone cavity were found by analyzing the diagnostic panoramic in addition to two odontomas, two cementifying-ossifying lesions, and one osteoma.

Ainamo et al. (1994) evaluated 169 dentate persons, aged 76, 81, and 86 years, living at home in Helsinki, Finland by means of panoramic radiography supplemented by intraoral radiographs [8]. The older the age group, the fewer teeth remained. The proportion of endodontically treated teeth was 19% in the 76-year-olds and rose to 26% in the 86-year-olds.Of these subjects, 41% had periapical periodontitis, which was more common in endodontically treated teeth (18%) than in teeth without root fillings (4%). Periapical lesions were more common in men than women. The relatively high frequency of periapical lesions could be interpreted as radiographic evaluation of the dentate elderly being a relatively high-yield procedure.

Maxillary Sinus Disease Related to Endodontic Therapy

Endo-antral syndrome

Selden first reported the "endo-antral syndrome" as an endodontic complication in 1989 [9]. This "syndrome" results from the spread of pulpal disease beyond the periapex into the maxillary sinus [9–11]. Selden described this syndrome as being characterized by the following: (a) occurrence in a tooth with pulpal disease whose apices approximate the floor of the maxillary sinus, (b) presence of a periapical radiolucency with the involved tooth, (c) radiographic loss of the lamina dura at the inferior border of the maxillary sinus over the involved tooth, (d) a radio-opaque mass that approximates the sinus above the apex of the involved tooth (representing localized swelling and thickening of the sinus mucosa), and (e) radio-opacity of differing degrees in the sinus space (Fig. 12.8). Selden felt that all five features were not necessarily to be found in all cases and that most cases of this syndrome responded well to non-surgical endodontic therapy. He concluded that it would be of "strategic clinical value" for the endodontic diagnostic evaluation to include the status of the adjacent maxillary sinus at the beginning of root canal therapy if only to establish a baseline for follow up.

Aspergillosis

Aspergillosis of the maxillary sinus is a relatively rare disease in nonimmunocompromised patients. Khongkhunthian and Reichart (2001) report that in recent years a number of cases of aspergillosis of the maxillary sinus have been reported in association with overextension of root canal fillings with certain root canal cements [12]. It has been suggested that zinc oxide-based root canal cements might promote the infection with the Aspergillus species. In particular *Aspergillus fumigatus* has been found to be associated with the maxillary sinus infection. Radiographically the unique appearance of a dense opacity foreign body reaction in the maxillary sinus is considered a characteristic finding in maxillary sinus aspergillosis (Fig. 12.9). Two cases where root canal overfilling was associated with aspergillosis of the maxillary sinus in young healthy female patients were reported from Chiang Mai University, Thailand [12]. In both patients the first maxillary molar was involved. Patients were asymptomatic and the diagnosis was made incidentally; however surgical inspection confirmed both patients to have aspergillomas, microscopically showing characteristic branching hyphae and conidiophores typical of Aspergillus.

Giardino et al. reported a case with overextension of root canal sealer (a 9-mm radio-opaque mass) into the maxillary sinus [13]. Surgical biopsy revealed aspergillosis. They also noted that zinc oxide–eugenol-based filling materials might be a stimulant to growth of Aspergillus.

Horre et al. (2002) also reported that fungal infections of the maxillary sinus can be associated with overfilling of dental root canals, when zinc-containing filling materials are used [14]. They reported a maxillary sinus aspergilloma patient caused by *Aspergillus emericella*

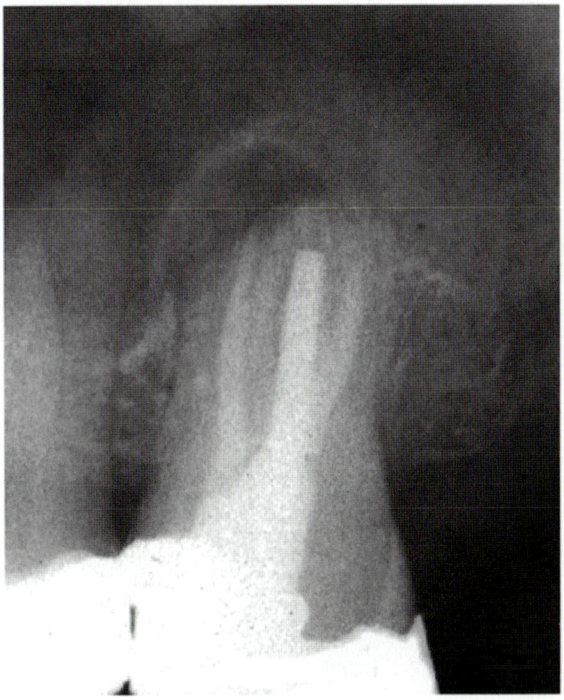

Fig. 12.8 Endo-antral syndrome. Radicular cyst causing displacement of maxillary sinus floor and reaction in sinus lining mucosa. This lesion actually had areas of cyst, granuloma, and abscess when examined histologically (see Fig. 12.2.—this is the same case)

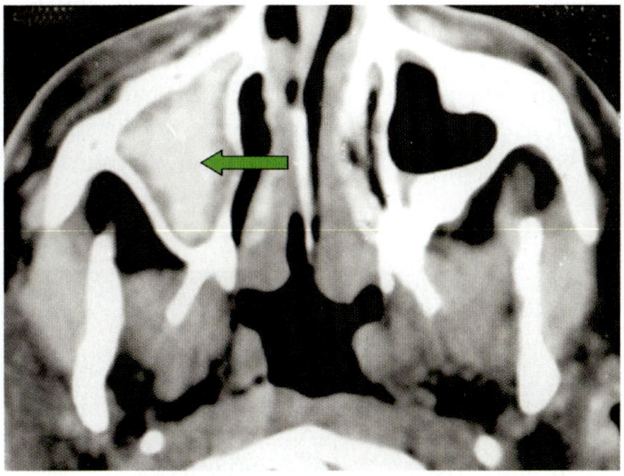

Fig. 12.9 Cropped axial CT scan showing Aspergillus sinusitis (*arrow*)

(rather than *A. fumigatus*) in a young immunocompetent female.

Conditions that May Simulate Dental Periapical Pathoses

There are a number of landmarks and conditions that need to be differentiated from periapical pathoses of dental cause. The most important radiologic consideration is whether the apical periodontal ligament space is intact. Acute apical periodontitis will leave the lamina dura intact, but the tooth may be elevated in the socket due to accumulation of pus and/or inflammatory exudates. This is easy to differentiate from the normal circumstance in view of being associated with pain, particularly on dental occlusion or tapping the tooth. With chronic periapical pathoses there is generally a remodeling of the apical periodontal space with an apical radiolucency having walls that merge with the lamina dura. By way of comparison, normal anatomic landmarks are superimposed on the undisturbed periodontal ligament space. Such anatomical structures include the mental foramen, incisive fossa, and maxillary sinus.

Periapical cementifying-osseous dysplasia is a fairly common condition, particularly in middle-aged women of African ancestry. The condition is found particularly in association with the apices of mandibular anterior teeth. The initial lesions are homogeneous radiolucencies. These later calcify over time. With care it is possible to demonstrate that periodontal space remains intact, as this condition actually arises in the supporting bone rather than in cementum. In any event, vitality testing of the pulp is key. In periapical cemental dysplasia the teeth remain vital.

Stafne was the first to report the presence of "bone cavities" or depressions in the angle of 35 mandibles [15]. Such cavities generally appear below the mandibular canal toward the lower border between the mandibular first molar and the mandibular angle, and are not considered rare. However, Stafne bone cavity is relatively rare in the anterior mandible. As a result, diagnosis in the anterior mandible may be missed. Treatment modalities such as endodontic treatment, bone trephining, and bone exploration may be conducted. In the absence of a non-vital tooth or other obvious etiology, computed tomography is a suitable noninvasive diagnostic and follow up modality for this bony configuration on panoramic or intraoral radiographs of the anterior mandible [15]. While this is considered a developmental anomaly, it may not become apparent until the patient is in their late teens or early twenties.

Various cysts and neoplasms can also be superimposed over the apices of teeth, and can, on occasion, result in resorption of the lamina dura and tooth roots (Fig. 12.10). Panoramic radiology can sometimes provide the wider view needed to reveal the actual extent of such lesions and thereby help develop a more accurate differential diagnosis. In many instances the teeth concerned remain vital to pulp testing.

The systemic condition, secondary hyperparathyroidism, common in end-stage renal disease may cause brown tumors resulting in loss of lamina dura simulating a periapical lesion of dental origin, but again the involved tooth or teeth are vital (Fig. 12.10). A panoramic radiograph can be heplful in screening for additional

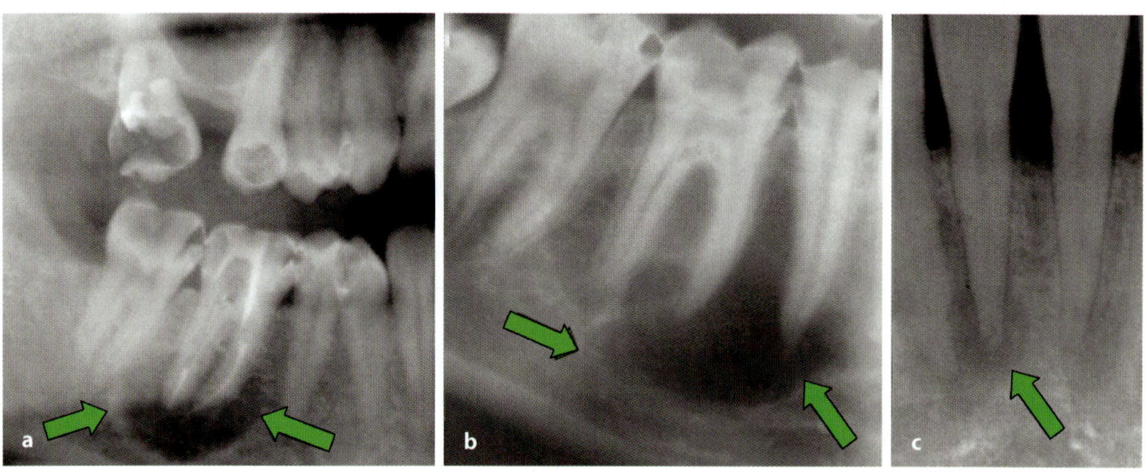

Fig. 12.10 **a** Cementifying-ossifying fibroma seen as a circumscribed unilocular radiolucency incidentally associated with first molar roots (detail from panoramic radiograph). **b** Keratocystic odontogenic tumor detail from panoramic radiograph. Note the homogeneous radiolucency that surrounds the roots of the right premolar and molar teeth. The definitive diagnosis awaits histopathology in such cases (*inset*). **c** Brown tumor in secondary hyperparathyroidism superimposed over root of left mandibular central incisor tooth

radiolucent lesions if secondary hyperparathyroidism is suspected (see Chapter 15).

Conclusion

When performing both basic and advanced endodontic procedures, it is important to have a comprehensive overview of the dentition as a whole, and to use an imaging technique that provides full coverage of any detected periapical pathosis. While individual periapical radiographs are essential for evaluation of root canal morphology, a panoramic radiograph provides the desired comprehensive overview and also is valuable in correctly assessing and interpreting large periapical lesions. The panoramic radiograph can be considered more than just a useful adjunct in comprehensive endodontic evaluation.

References

1. Brynolf I. Radiography of the periapical region as a diagnostic aid. II. Diagnosis of pulp-related changes. Dent Radiogr Photogr 1979;52:25–47
2. Bodey TE, Loushine RJ, West LA. A retrospective study evaluating the use of the panoramic radiograph in endodontics. Mil Med 2003;168:528–529
3. Ahlqwist M, Halling A, Hollender L. Rotational panoramic radiography in epidemiological studies of dental health. Comparison between panoramic radiographs and intraoral full mouth surveys. Swed Dent J 1986;10:73–84
4. De Cleen MJ, Schuurs AH, Wesselink PR, Wu MK. Periapical status and prevalence of endodontic treatment in an adult Dutch population. Int Endod J 1993;26:112–119
5. Hulsmann M, Lorch V, Franz B. Studies on the incidence and quality of root fillings. Evaluation by orthopantomograms. Dtsch Zahnarztl Z 1991;46:296–299
6. Lupi-Pegurier L, Bertrand MF, Muller-Bolla M, Rocca JP, Bolla M. Periapical status, prevalence and quality of endodontic treatment in an adult French population. Int Endod J 2002;35:690–697
7. Peltola JS, Wolf J, Mannik A, Russak S, Seedre T, Sirkel M, Vink M. Radiographic findings in the teeth and jaws of 14- to 17-year-old Estonian schoolchildren in Tartu and Tallinn. Acta Odontol Scand 1997;55:31–35
8. Ainamo A, Soikkonen K, Wolf J, Siukosaari P, Erkinjuntti T, Tilvis R, Valvanne J. Dental radiographic findings in the elderly in Helsinki, Finland. Acta Odontol Scand 1994;52:243–249
9. Selden HS. The endo-antral syndrome: an endodontic complication. J Am Dent Assoc 1989;119:397–398, 401–402
10. Selden HS. Diagnostic radiographic findings and symptom-free teeth. J Endod 1994;20:100–102
11. Selden HS. Endo-antral syndrome and various endodontic complications. J Endod 1999;25:389–393
12. Khongkhunthian P, Reichart PA. Aspergillosis of the maxillary sinus as a complication of overfilling root canal material into the sinus: report of two cases. J Endod 2001;27:476–478
13. Giardino L, Pontieri F, Savoldi E, Tallarigo F. Aspergillus mycetoma of the maxillary sinus secondary to overfilling a root canal. J Endod 2006;32:692–694
14. Horre R, Schumacher G, Marklein G, Kromer B, Wardelmann E, Gilges S, De Hoog GS, Wahl G, Schaal KP. Case report. Maxillary sinus infection due to Emericella nidulans. Mycoses 2002;45:402–405
15. Katz J, Chaushu G, Rotstein I. Stafne's bone cavity in the anterior mandible: a possible diagnostic challenge. J Endod 2001;27:304–307

TEST: Panoramic radiology: endodontic considerations

1. When there is a periapical pathosis caused by spread of infection from a necrotic dental pulp, the lamina dura surrounding the periodontal ligament space is generally unaffected.

   True ☐ **False** ☐

2. An acute periapical abscess is usually very easy to detect using standard radiographs.

   True ☐ **False** ☐

3. The Stafne bone cavity is most frequently located beneath the mandibular canal toward the angle of the mandible.

   True ☐ **False** ☐

4. Aspergillus infections have been found in association with endodontic filling overextension in the maxilla.

   True ☐ **False** ☐

5. The endo-antral syndrome can be associated with thickening of the mucosa in the maxillary sinus.

   True ☐ **False** ☐

6. Radiographically, it is always a simple matter to differentiate between periapical cysts, granulomas, and abscesses.

   True ☐ **False** ☐

7. Periapical cemental dysplasia has a predilection to occur in middle-aged women of African ancestry.

   True ☐ **False** ☐

8. Using panoramic radiographs, De Cleen et al. (1993) found more than 5% of all nonendodontically treated teeth showed signs of periapical pathoses.

   True ☐ **False** ☐

9. A study of elderly patients in Finland found that more than 40% has periapical periodontitis affecting one or more tooth.

   True ☐ **False** ☐

10. Both the keratocystic odontogenic tumor and the ossifying fibroma may at times simulate apical periodontal pathoses.

    True ☐ **False** ☐

Chapter

Panoramic Radiology of Pericoronal Pathoses

13

Allan G. Farman in association with Christoffel J. Nortjé and Robert E. Wood

Learning Objectives

After studying this chapter, the reader should be able to:

- Define the role of panoramic radiology in the detection of pericoronal pathoses
- List differential possibilities for pericoronal radiolucencies and mixed radiolucency–radio-opacities
- Understand the subtle radiographic signs that can help more closely determine the nature of pericoronal lesions
- Understand the importance of histopathological analysis in developing a definitive diagnosis

Panoramic radiography has a role in supporting the detection and delineation of pathological conditions in the jaws. This chapter concentrates on the detection and differential interpretation of conditions arising in association with the crown of a tooth or teeth.

The crowns of unerupted teeth are normally surrounded by the dental follicle, a remnant of the enamel forming organ that is lined by reduced enamel epithelium. The enamel follicle is necessary for tooth eruption. The follicle appears as a homogeneous radiolucent halo surrounding the crown of the tooth, arising in the region of the enamel-cemental junction [1]. This "halo" has a thin outer radio-opaque border that is continuous with the lamina dura surrounding the periodontal ligament space. The follicle space can vary considerably under normal conditions and tends to enlarge during tooth eruption. Guidelines to differentiate between a normal and an abnormal dental follicle space include: pericoronal space exceeding 2.5 mm for teeth other than maxillary canines on periapical radiographs or 3 mm in panoramic radiographs [2], or follicular radiolucency exceeding 2.5 cm. It is recommended that in the absence of clinical symptoms, equivocally enlarged or enlarging follicles be followed radiographically for up to 6 months—or until it is apparent that tooth eruption is being delayed, the tooth is being displaced or the tooth erupts [1]. This can be accomplished by use of panoramic radiography. Professional clinical judgment is always needed as it is impossible to distinguish radiographically or histopathologically between a small dentigerous cyst and an enlarged dental follicle.

Follicular Cysts

Cysts forming within the dental follicle, and lined by a thin layer of "flattened" epithelial cells resembling the reduced enamel epithelium, are termed follicular cysts [1]. When they envelope the tooth crown and originate within bone, they are termed "dentigerous." When the cyst is entirely within soft tissue, the term "eruption cyst" is employed. If the cyst is displaced distally or buccally, the term "paradental" cyst has been applied.

Dentigerous cysts occur most often in sites where dental impaction is most common, namely, surrounding the crown of an unerupted mandibular third molar or maxillary canine tooth followed by mandibular premolars and maxillary third molars. They are most frequently detected in individuals in the second or third decade of life. Between 2% and 3% of individuals with delayed tooth eruption have been found to have dentigerous cysts and about 0.8% of impacted third molars have been so associated [1].

Clinically, the dentigerous cyst is usually asymptomatic, except for delay in eruption of the involved tooth and possible local jaw expansion. Aspiration of the cyst contents yields straw-colored fluid that may contain cholesterol crystals. There is no sex predilection. Radiologically (Fig. 13.1), there is a well delineated unilocular homogeneous radiolucency enveloping the crown of an unerupted tooth. The radiolucency starts at the junction of the enamel and cementum at the neck of the tooth and usually has a thin radio-opaque outline that is continuous with the lamina dura of the periodontal ligament space. Marked displacement of the affected tooth is not uncommon. The dentigerous cyst may also displace adjacent teeth and frequently results in root resorption of such neighboring teeth [3, 4]. Resorption of the roots of adjacent teeth has been reported to occur in 55% of cases [1].

Manganaro (1998) from the Brooke Army Medical Center, San Antonio, Texas investigated the likelihood of finding occult histopathology on routine third

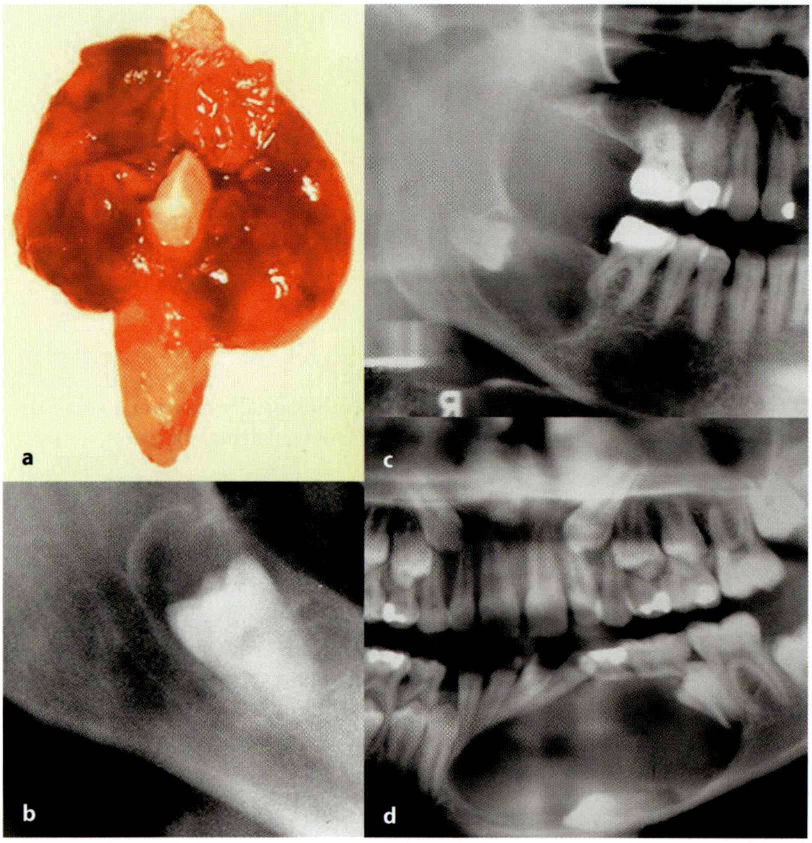

Fig. 13.1 The dentigerous cyst develops within the dental follicle space resulting in a soft tissue sac surrounding the crown of the affected tooth and attached at the enamel-cemental junction. **a** Photograph of extracted tooth with attached dentigerous cyst. **b** Small dentigerous cyst surrounding a distoangular third molar impaction. **c** Horizontally impacted third molar tooth with medium-sized dentigerous cyst. **d** Panoramic detail of large dentigerous cyst from an impacted left mandibular canine. The affected canine has been displaced to the lower border of the mandible. There is displacement of adjacent teeth and marked resorption of the roots of the primary molar teeth adjacent to this lesion

molar extractions [5]. The study involved 42 patients with 101 bony or soft tissue impacted teeth. The most fequent microscopic histopathology observed was dentigerous cyst. Of the 101 teeth evaluated, 46 (45.5%) were concluded to have dentigerous cyst. The male to female ratio was 1:1, and the average age was 23.3 years. Frequently, a pericoronal radiolucent width of 2.0 mm on the panoramic radiograph was associated with the interpretation of dentigerous cyst histopathology. The range of widths of the radiolucency associated with the dentigerous cysts was 0.1–3.0 mm. Other histopathological entities were not identified [5].

Shibata et al. (2004) examined radiographically the relationship between the primary tooth and the dentigerous cyst of the permanent successor during the transitional dentition [6].

From a retrospective review, 70 patients under 16 years of age had histologically confirmed dentigerous cysts that had developed from the central incisor to the second premolar. These were identified and investigated using panoramic and periapical radiographs. In most cases (54; 77%) the cyst was in the premolar region. Of the 54 premolars with dentigerous cysts, the overlying primary tooth had already been previously extracted in seven cases. Of the 47 remaining premolars with an associated primary tooth, 35 (75%) had bone resorption of the periapical or bifurcation region, or irregular resorption of the associated primary tooth. Of the remaining 12 primary teeth with no periapical lesions, nine had been treated with root canal therapy. Thus, 44 of these 47 cases (94%) had the possibility of inflammation at the primary tooth associated with the dentigerous cyst. It was concluded that inflammatory change at the apex of the primary tooth may bring on a dentigerous cyst of the permanent successor [6]. This finding needs to be kept in perspective: dentigerous cysts do occur on the crowns of permanent molars and such teeth have no primary predecessors.

Table 13.1 Pericoronal lesions

Homogeneous radiolucency		Other pericoronal radiolucencies (uncommon)	Mixed radiolucency and radio-opacity [14]
Unilocular	Multilocular		
• Dilated dental follicle	• Cherubism	• Langerhans' cell disease [13]	• Adenomatoid odontogenic tumor (late stage)
• Dentigerous cyst	• Ameloblastoma	• Ewing's sarcoma	• Ameloblastic fibro-odontoma (late stage)
• Envelopmental keratocystic odontogenic tumor	• Ameloblastic fibroma	• Leukemia	• Calcifying odontogenic cyst (late stage)
• Unicystic (mural) ameloblastoma	• Ameloblastic fibro-odontoma (early stage)	• Squamous odontogenic tumor	• Regional odontodysplasia
• Adenomatoid odontogenic tumor (early stage)	• Odontogenic myxoma	• Odontogenic carcinoma	• Calcifying epithelial odontogenic tumor
• Calcifying odontogenic cyst (early stage)		• Pseudotumor of hemophilia	

Management of the dentigerous cyst usually is accomplished by enucleation; however in very large cases marsupialization can be used to reduce the cyst size prior to excision [7, 8]. As a variety of other pathoses can grow into the follicle space and resemble clinically and radiologically the dentigerous cyst, it is important to have all tissues removed from the lesion examined histologically [9].

Adams and Walton (1996) did report a case of spontaneous regression of a radiolucency associated with an impacted mandibular third molar with spontaneous regression in a patient who failed to attend for surgical enucleation [10]. Hence a period of expert observation might be appropriate if there is uncertainly of whether the case is a dilated follicle versus a dentigerous cyst.

Scheifele et al. (2005) investigated the occurrence of epithelium in the soft tissues associated with routine surgical removal of 150 mandibular third molars [11]. Histological examination was made on soft tissues removed with 150 consecutive surgical third molar extractions. The diagnostic criteria were defined as a pericoronal translucency >2.5 mm for dentigerous cysts and a distal translucency >2.5 mm and inflammation for inflammatory paradental cysts. Pericoronal translucencies were found for only four third molars, and paradental cysts were found in 47.The prevalence was 2% for dentigerous cyst and 10% for inflammatory paradental cyst in the Danish population examined.

By way of comparison, Rakprasitkul (2001) investigated whether the incidence of pathological conditions affecting the pericoronal tissue of unerupted third molars justifies the "routine" removal of such teeth [12]. The pericoronal tissue associated with completely unerupted third molars in a Thai population was submitted for histological examination after surgical tooth removal was performed in 37 males and 55 females, aged 13–63 years. The 104 unerupted third molars comprised 68 mandibular third molars (65%) and 36 maxillary third molars (35%). The incidence of normal tissue of a dental follicle was 41%, and the incidence of pathological tissue was 59% (dentigerous cyst, 51%; chronic nonspecific inflammatory tissue, 5%; keratocystic odontogenic tumor, 2%; ameloblastoma, 1%). The incidence of pathological conditions was higher than that of normal conditions in all third molar positions. In younger patients, normal tissue was more commonly found, but in patients older than 20 years, the incidence of pathological tissue was higher than the incidence of normal tissue. It was concluded that unerupted third molars should be removed before pathological changes can occur in their pericoronal tissues and was used as a justification for the removal of unerupted third molars from patients older than 20 years of age [12].

Conditions to consider in the differential interpretation of pericoronal radiolucencies are listed in Table 13.1. Representative examples of such conditions are described in this chapter.

Envelopmental Keratocystic Odontogenic Tumor

The pathogenesis of the keratocystic odontogenic tumor (formerly known as odontogenic keratocyst) is believed to be proliferation of dental lamina. The lesion is a unilocular or multilocular homogeneous radiolucency that can envelope the crown of an unerupted tooth (Fig. 13.2) [15]. Jaw expansion is a late finding. It may be sporadic or part of the nevoid basal cell carcinoma syndrome. Lam and Chan (2000) evaluated keratocystic odontogenic tumors [16]. The clinical records and pathological features of keratocystic odontogenic tumors from 69 ethnic Hong Kong Chinese (40 male

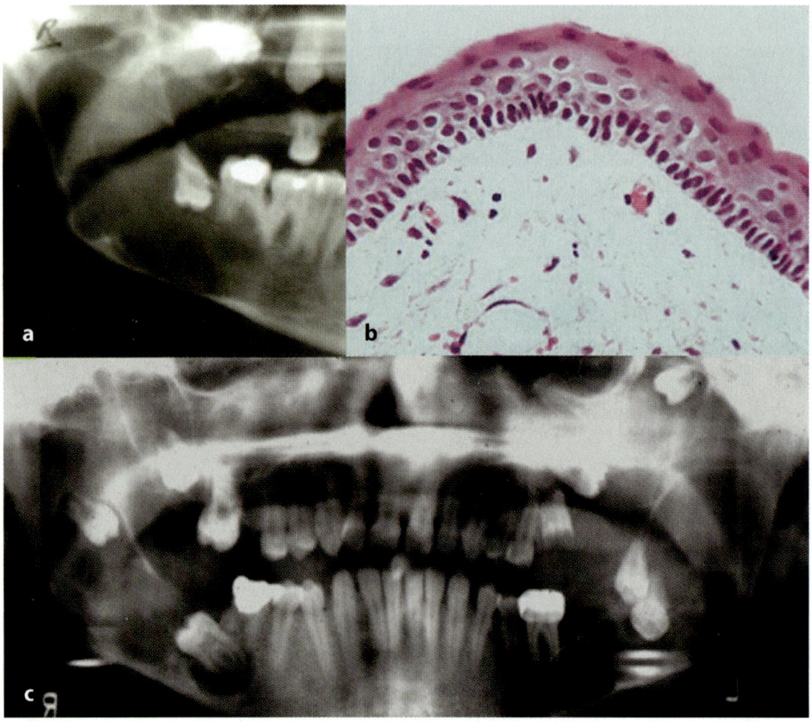

Fig. 13.2 **a** Crenulated lesion of solitary keratocystic odontogenic tumor incidentally involving inverted impaction of mandibular third molar tooth. **b** Histological analysis reveals parakeratinized epithelium with cuboidal basal cells and no rete and few or no inflammatory cells in the absence of secondary inflammatory stimulus. Hematoxylin and eosin, high magnification. **c** Multiple keratocystic odontogenic tumors in all four quadrants, many enveloping unerupted teeth, in a case of multiple basal cell carcinoma syndrome

and 29 female patients) were reviewed. The male-to-female ratio was 1.4:1; patient age ranged from 6 to 69 years with a modal peak in the third decade (mean age 28 years; median age 23 years).The preoperative diagnosis was correct in 78% of the cases and the most common misdiagnosis was dentigerous cyst. Sixty-two percent of the cysts were found in the mandible, and 38% in the maxilla. It was concluded that pathological examination of keratocysts is important, because keratocysts have different clinicopathological features and carry a risk for clinical misdiagnosis.

Ameloblastoma

The ameloblastoma is the most common odontogenic neoplasm. It is usually central. With more than 80% of cases occuring in the mandible, especially at the angle. The unicystic variety represents approximately 5% of all ameloblastomas and can develop as a mural change within a dentigerous cyst or secondary invasion of the dental follicle space [1]. Unicystic ameloblastoma can occur in locations not necessarily contacting teeth. The unicystic ameloblastoma tends to occur in a younger age group than other types of ameloblastoma, those affected being diagnosed on average at 22 years of age, an age group where the dentigerous cyst is also fairly common. Ameloblastomas are homogeneous radiolucencies (Fig. 13.3). Cortical expansion is a frequent finding. Lesions tend to displace tooth crowns and resorb adjacent tooth roots.

Adenomatoid Odontogenic Tumor

The adenomatoid odontogenic tumor is most frequently found in children or adolescents [14, 17, 18]. This lesion frequently, but not invariably, envelopes the crown of an unerupted tooth—especially a maxillary canine (Fig. 13.4) [19, 20]. It is most frequently unilocular, but can be loculated. Adenomatoid odontogenic tumors generally have a well delineated margin. The radiologic content is a homogeneous radiolucency initially but later develops calcified “floccules” as internal structure.

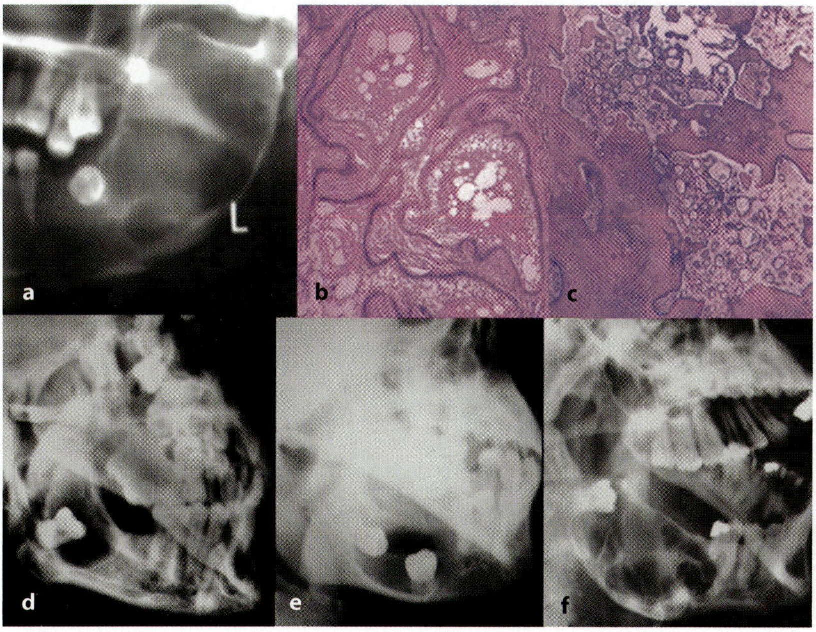

Fig. 13.3 a Ameloblastoma seen as expansile crenulated radiolucency in the mandibular ramus, incidentally associated with a displaced third molar tooth. **b** Follicular ameloblastoma. The histology is comprised of follicles with columnar basal cells surrounding tissue reminiscent of the stellate reticulum of the developing tooth. Hematoxylin and eosin, intermediate magnification. **c** The ameloblastoma is a relatively aggressive benign neoplasm. Histology showing infiltration of a bone. Hematoxylin and eosin, low magnification. **d** Case of unicystic ameloblastoma with slight crenulations (superiorly) and extension beyond the enamel-cemental junction (lateral-oblique radiograph). **e** Unicystic ameloblastoma enveloping the crowns of two molar teeth (lateral-oblique radiograph). **f** Lateral-oblique radiograph showing expansile multilocular homogeneous radiolucency enveloping and displacing a mandibular third molar. (Note: The lateral-oblique radiograph can be made using the cephalometric attachment to a panoramic machine.)

Cortical expansion may occur. Adenomatoid odontogenic tumor tends to displace rather than cause resorption of adjacent teeth.

Ameloblastic Fibroma and Fibro-odontoma

The ameloblastic fibroma and ameloblastic fibro-odontoma are most frequently found in children and adolescents [1, 21]. Both are quite uncommon. They can be unilocular, crenulated, or multilocular (Fig. 13.5). Their outline is usually well-delineated and corticated. The ameloblastic fibroma is a homogeneous radiolucency, whereas the ameloblastic fibro-odontoma can contain "salt and pepper" calcifications. Cortical expansion is a late finding. They cause displacement of teeth. They are usually less aggressive locally than nonunicystic ameloblastomas.

Ameloblastic fibro-odontoma is a benign odontogenic tumor with similar features to ameloblastic fibroma, but with the addition of calcifications that can produce a "milky way" lumen appearance on radiography. This lesion is also mostly found in children and adolescents.

Odontogenic Myxoma

The odontogenic myxoma (myxofibroma) is another homogeneously radiolucent odontogenic tumor that has on occasion been found above an unerupted tooth or teeth [1, 21, 22]. This condition usually has fine angular trabeculations and tends not to cause cortical expansion or erosion. Resorption of adjacent teeth is also uncommon.

Calcifying Odontogenic Cyst

The calcifying odontogenic cyst is an epithelially lined cavity that may be found over a wide age range but usually detected in individuals under 40 years of age [22, 23]. More than 70% occur in the maxilla. They may be unilocular or multilocular and frequently are found to

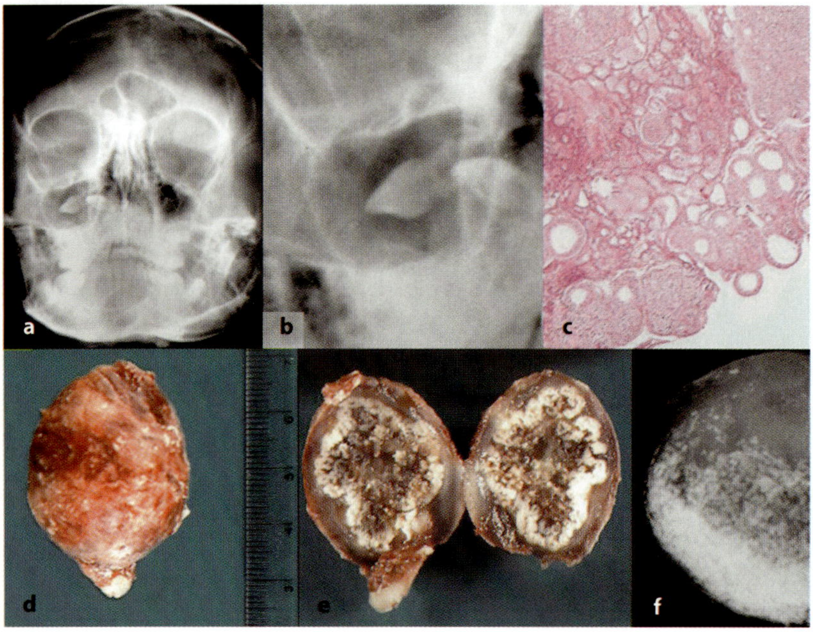

Fig. 13.4 **a** Waters protection made using a "ceph" attachment reveals a unilocular, well-delineated radiolucency enveloping the crown of a developing maxillary canine tooth and causing displacement of the tooth. This proved to be an adenomatoid odontogenic tumor. **b** Detail of same case of adenomatoid odontogenic tumor. **c** Histological examination showing the typical "adenomatoid" appearance. The apparent ducts actually have the basement membrane centrally located and represent folds in the neoplastic epithelial sheets rather than actual ducts. Hematoxylin and eosin, low magnification. **d** Gross specimen of adenomatoid odontogenic tumor in maxillary canine region. **e** Sectioned gross specimen. **f** Radiograph of gross specimen showing floccules of calcification. Such floccules are common to late adenomatoid odontogenic tumor lesions. Initially the lesions appear to be a homogeneous radiolucency and can be misdiagnosed as dentigerous cyst on radiologic study

envelope crown of an unerupted tooth or less frequently odontoma. The radiologic content of the lesion can be either a homogeneous radiolucency or "salt and pepper" calcifications.

Calcifying Epithelial Odontogenic Tumor

Calcifying epithelial odontogenic tumor is most frequently found in adults [1, 22]. It is very rare. Lesions can be unilocular, crenulated, or multilocular and the outline can be well or poorly delineated (Fig. 13.6a). It is a homogeneous radiolucency initially but later develops calcified "floccules." Cortical expansion may occur. Calcifying epithelial odontogenic tumor can cause displacement or resorption of tooth roots.

Malignancies Associated with Envelopmental Radiolucencies

Acute leukemia is sometimes associated with collections of leukemia cells in the jaws. These collections of malignant cells can on occasion envelope a developing tooth or teeth (Fig. 13.6b). More rarely, carcinoma is reported arising in a dental follicle or dentigerous cyst [24–26].

Regional Odontodysplasia

Regional odontodysplasia is a localized failure of permanent teeth (and less commonly primary teeth) to develop normally [27]. It is of unknown etiology. Unerupted "ghost teeth" form in a segment of the dentition while the rest of the teeth develop normally (Fig. 13.7). Widened "follicle spaces" with fine calcifications are found on occasion.

Cherubism

Cherubism is a hereditary condition with progressive bilateral swelling at the mandibular angles during childhood [22]. It is familial being autosomal dominant with varying expressivity. Radiologically there are usually bilateral multilocular radiolucencies at the angles of mandible and sometimes in the posterior maxilla (Fig. 13.8). Unilateral cases have been reported rarely.

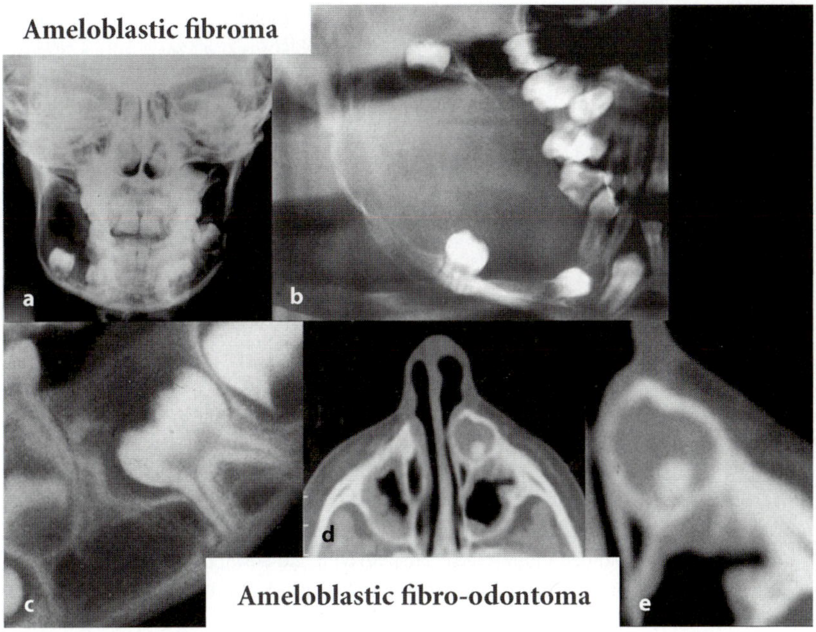

Fig. 13.5 Ameloblastic fibroma is a homogeneously radiolucent lesion found in children and adolescents that can incidentally involve developing adjacent teeth causing their displacement. **a** Posterior-anterior projection of ameloblastic fibroma. **b** Similar case using panoramic radiography. This particular lesion is expansile and has displaced developing premolars and first and second permanent molar teeth. **c** Small ameloblastic fibro-odontoma with calcification evident. This lesion overlies a developing mandibular first molar tooth (panoramic detail). **d** Axial CT of ameloblastic fibro-odontoma of the maxilla enveloping a canine tooth. The radiographic technique was of too low a resolution to demonstrate fine calcifications. **e** Detail of axial CT scan shown in (**d**)

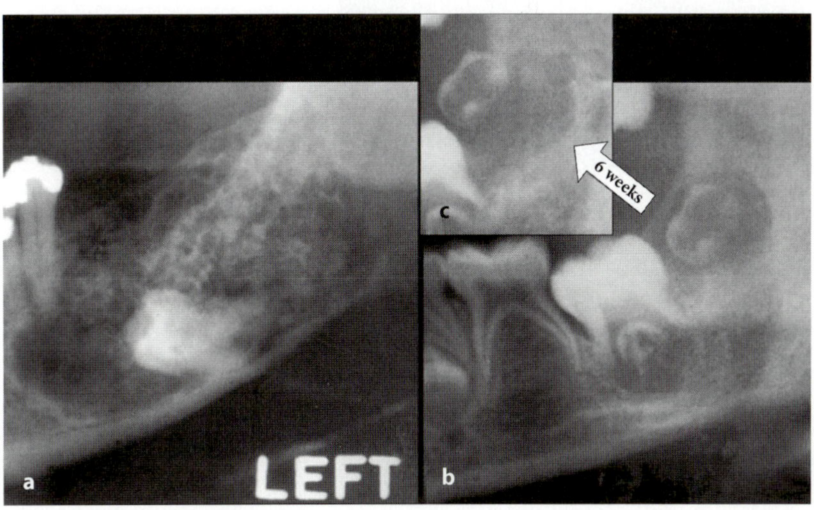

Fig. 13.6 **a** Calcifying epithelial odontogenic tumor. This is a relatively aggressive benign odontogenic tumor generally found in an older age group. The lesion envelopes a fully formed unerupted molar tooth in this instance. **b** Acute leukemia cell deposit completely surrounding a developing molar tooth. Not all pericoronal lesions are benign. **c** Six weeks later the lesion has displaced the tooth into premature eruption with expansion of the deposit now largely below the tooth

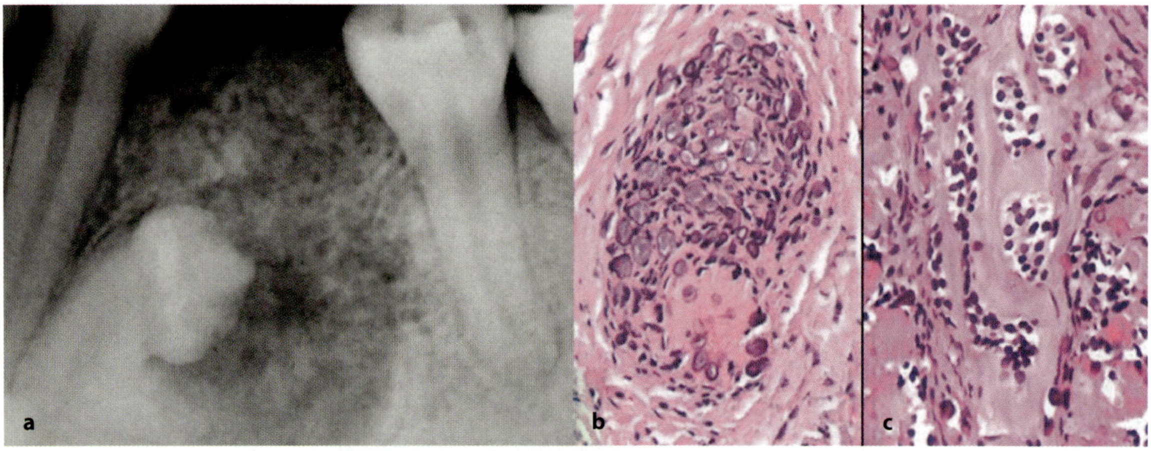

Fig. 13.7 **a** Radiologic appearance of pericoronal tissues in regional odontodysplasia. The "ghost" premolar tooth affected by the condition is unerupted and displaced; however, the pericoronal tissues are not entirely radiolucent. **b** Islands of cells with calcifications ("osteodentin") in area of regional odontodysplasia expanded tooth follicle. Hematoxylin and eosin, intermediate magnification. **c** Strands of cells with calcification ("osteodentin") in area of regional odontodysplasia expanded tooth follicle. Hematoxylin and eosin, intermediate magnification

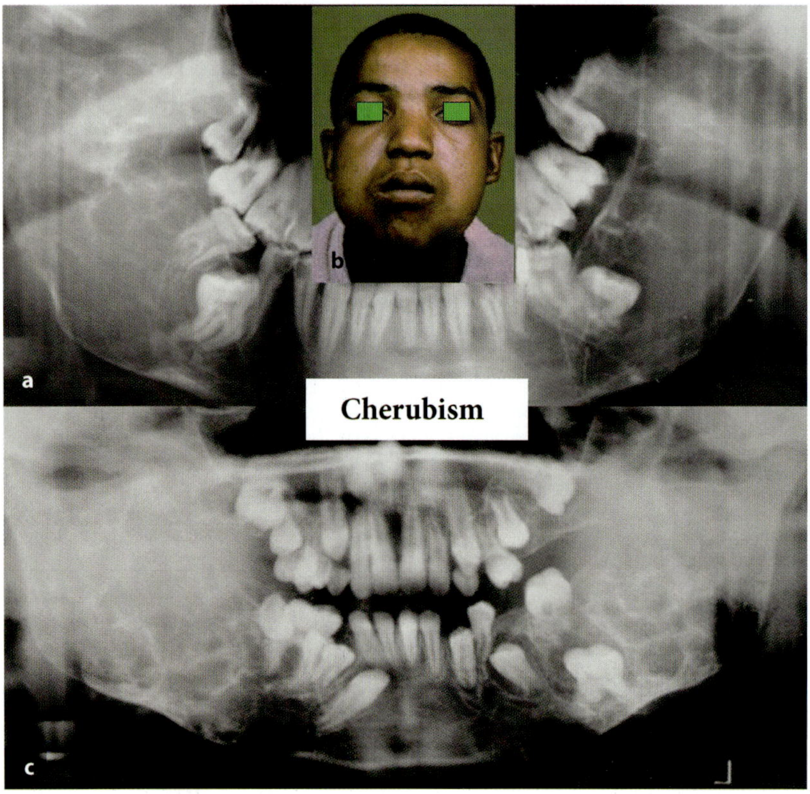

Fig. 13.8 Cherubism. **a** Panoramic radiograph showing bilateral expansile mandibular multilocular radiolucencies with displacement of enveloped developing molar teeth. **b** Clinical appearance of patient in (**a**). **c** A different case of cherubism. This patient also evidences displaced developing teeth

Displacement of teeth and toothbuds is common. The lesions spare the mandibular condyles. Opacification occurs during maturation [22].

Cyst Boundaries in Radiologic Differentiation

Ikeshima and Tamura (2002) tried to find a simple method to radiologically differentiate between the dentigerous cyst and benign tumors enveloping an unerupted tooth crown [28]. They conducted a study employing the radiographs of patients who visited Nihon University Dental Hospital at Matsudo and were pathologically defined as having a cyst or tumor. Using radiographs of these patients, they investigated the attachment point to the embedded tooth, and expressed the results as the proportion of the attachment point to the embedded tooth root length. The study was carried out in 100 patients with cysts (87 dentigerous cysts and 13 keratocystic odontogenic tumors), and 27 patients with benign tumors (24 ameloblastomas and 3 adenomatoid odontogenic tumors). The results showed that the discriminated boundary value (from the cementifying-enamel junction) was 0.38 for the embedded tooth root length. The cases showing a boundary value of less than 0.38 for the cementifying-enamel junction were judged to be cysts, and those showing a value of 0.38 or more were judged to be benign tumors. Using this assumption, the rate of misjudgment was 28% in the cyst group and 33% in the benign tumor group [28].

Concluding Remarks

Panoramic radiography plays valuable roles in detection, monitoring and post-operative follow up of pericoronal radiolucencies. Nevertheless, it should always be remembered that a variety of different lesions can appear pericoronally; hence, it is important that all removed tissues be submitted for careful appraisal histologically preferably by an oral pathologist or, where that is not feasible, by a general pathologist versed in diseases of the maxillofacial region.

References

1. Wood NK, Kuc IM. Pericoronal radiolucencies. In: Wood NK, Goaz PW (eds) Differential Diagnosis of Oral and Maxillofacial Lesions, edn 5, 1991; pp 279–295
2. Farah CS, Savage NW. Pericoronal radiolucencies and the significance of early detection. Aust Dent J 2002;47:262–265
3. Tumer C, Eset AE, Atabek A. Ectopic impacted mandibular third molar in the subcondylar region associated with a dentigerous cyst: a case report. Quintessence Int 2002;33:231–233
4. Counts AL, Kochis LA, Buschman J, Savant TD. An aggressive dentigerous cyst in a seven-year-old child. ASDC J Dent Child 2001;68:268–271
5. Manganaro AM. The likelihood of finding occult histopathology in routine third molar extractions. Gen Dent 1998;46:200–202
6. Shibata Y, Asaumi J, Yanagi Y, Kawai N, Hisatomi M, Matsuzaki H, Konouchi H, Nagatsuka H, Kishi K. Radiographic examination of dentigerous cysts in the transitional dentition. Dentomaxillofac Radiol 2004;33:17–20
7. Zhao YF, Liu B, Jiang ZQ. Marsupialization or decompression of the cystic lesions of the jaws. Shanghai Kou Qiang Yi Xue 2005;14:325–329
8. Jones TA, Perry RJ, Wake MJ. Marsupialization of a large unilateral mandibular dentigerous cyst in a 6-year-old boy: a case report. Dent Update 2003;30:557–561
9. Sadeghi EM, Sewall SR, Dohse A, Novak TS. Odontogenic tumors that mimic a dentigerous cyst. Compend Contin Educ Dent 1995;16:500–504
10. Adams AM, Walton AG. Case report. Spontaneous regression of a radiolucency associated with an ectopic mandibular third molar. Dentomaxillofac Radiol 1996;25:162–164
11. Scheifele C, Philipsen HP, Reichart PA. Occurrence of epithelium in the soft tissues associated with routine surgical removal of 150 mandibular third molars. Mund Kiefer Gesichtschir 2005;9:36–42
12. Rakprasitkul S. Pathologic changes in the pericoronal tissues of unerupted third molars. Quintessence Int 2001;32:633–638
13. Piattelli A, Rubini C, Iezzi G, Fioroni M. CD1a-positive cells in odontogenic cysts. J Endod 2002;28:267–268
14 Thunthy KH. Differential diagnosis of pericoronal radiolucencies with and without radiopacities. Gen Dent 1999;47:182–186
15. Tamashiro-Higa T, Mosqueda-Taylor A. Keratocystic odontogenic tumor in dentigerous position. A clinical case. Cir Cir 2005;73:127–131
16. Lam KY, Chan AC. Keratocystic odontogenic tumors: a clinicopathological study in Hong Kong Chinese. Laryngoscope 2000;110:1328–1332
17. Handschel JG, Depprich RA, Zimmermann AC, Braunstein S, Kubler NR. Adenomatoid odontogenic tumor of the mandible: review of the literature and report of a rare case. Head Face Med 2005;24;1–3
18. Olgac V, Koseoglu BG, Kasapoglu C. Adenomatoid odontogenic tumor: a report of an unusual maxillary lesion. Quintessence Int 2003;34:686–688
19. Walker LM, Wood AJ, McDonald A, Carpenter W. Unerupted mandibular second primary molar with an unusual histopathological finding: a case report. J Dent Child (Chic) 2004;71:77–79
20. Bravo M, White D, Miles L, Cotton R. Adenomatoid odontogenic tumor mimicking a dentigerous cyst. Int J Pediatr Otorhinolaryngol 2005;69:1685–1688
21. Yura Y, Yoshida H, Yanagawa T, Urata M, Nitta T, Sato M, Uemura S, Koike M, Komori A. An odontogenic myxofibroma related to an embedded third molar of the mandible. Report of a case. Int J Oral Surg 1982;11:265–269
22. Farman AG, Nortjé CJ, Wood R. Oral & Maxillofacial Diagnostic Imaging. 1993; Mosby: St Louis
23. Altini M, Farman AG. Calcifying odontogenic cyst. Oral Surg Oral Med Oral Pathol 1975;40:751–759

24. Gulbranson SH, Wolfrey JD, Raines JM, McNally BP. Squamous cell carcinoma arising in a dentigerous cyst in a 16-month-old girl. Otolaryngol Head Neck Surg 2002;127:463–464
25. Shimoyama T, Ide F, Horie N, Kato T, Nasu D, Kaneko T, Kusama K. Primary intraosseous carcinoma associated with impacted third molar of the mandible: review of the literature and report of a new case. J Oral Sci 2001;43:287–292
26. Olson JW, Miller RL, Kushner GM, Vest TM. Odontogenic carcinoma occurring in a dentigerous cyst: case report and clinical management. J Periodontol 2000;71:1365–1370
27. Gould AR, Farman AG, Marks ID. Pericoronal features of regional odontodysplasia. J Oral Med 1984;39:236–242
28. Ikeshima A, Tamura Y. Differential diagnosis between dentigerous cyst and benign tumor with an embedded tooth. J Oral Sci 2002;44:13–17

TEST: Panoramic radiology of pericoronal pathoses

1. Radiologic analysis is usually definitive in diagnosing pericoronal radiolucencies.

   True ☐ **False** ☐

2. For teeth other than the maxillary canines a pericoronal radiolucency exceeding 2.5 mm is usually construed as a sign of pathosis.

   True ☐ **False** ☐

3. Cherubism is a cause of radiolucencies that extend around the crowns of maxillary canine teeth.

   True ☐ **False** ☐

4. Regional widening of the pericoronal tissues surrounding unerupted teeth can be found in cases of odontodysplasia.

   True ☐ **False** ☐

5. Adenomatoid odontogenic tumor, when it does occur, is frequently found in adolescents.

   True ☐ **False** ☐

6. The calcifying odontogenic cyst is more frequently encountered in the maxilla than in the mandible.

   True ☐ **False** ☐

7. The unicystic ameloblastoma tends to occur in younger individuals than do other forms of ameloblastoma.

   True ☐ **False** ☐

8. The pathogenesis of the keratocystic odontogenic tumor is believed to involve a proliferation of the dental lamina.

   True ☐ **False** ☐

9. Lesions typically appearing as a mixed radiolucency/radio-opacity include dentigerous cyst, keratocystic odontogenic tumor and ameloblastoma.

   True ☐ **False** ☐

10. The dentigerous cyst is almost invariably symptomatic.

    True ☐ **False** ☐

Panoramic Radiology in Maxillofacial Trauma

14

Allan G. Farman
in association with George M. Kushner

Learning Objectives
After studying this chapter, the reader should be able to:
- Define the role of panoramic radiology in the detection of mandibular fractures
- Describe the areas where fractures of the maxillofacial structures are not well illustrated by panoramic radiographs
- Understand the value panoramic radiography has over traditional computed tomography in the detection of fractures involving teeth and alveolar bone

Panoramic radiography has a role in support of maxillofacial surgery in the evaluation of suspected jaw fractures involving teeth, and in assessment of fractures of the mandibular body and angle. Panoramic radiographs, however, should not be relied upon for detecting subtle changes in the temporomandibular joint and condylar head consequent to trauma. To evaluate maxillary trauma, the panoramic radiograph should be considered merely adjunctive to computed tomography. While panoramic radiography is especially useful in demonstrating changes involving teeth and alveolar bone, modern computed tomography better defines the bony structures of the maxilla.

The panoramic radiograph is, without a doubt, one of the most frequently selected and utilized diagnostic images for the initial workup of maxillofacial surgery patients. It also is especially relevant when teeth are in close proximity to pathoses or intricately involved in bone fractures following facial trauma. However, this does not mean that the panoramic radiograph is always sufficient in itself. Quite often, clinical and panoramic radiographic findings will lead to selection of additional advanced imaging, including computed tomography with three-dimensional reconstruction. For maxillofacial surgery, panoramic radiography is helpful in evaluation of: (1) dental impactions; (2) mandibular and dental fractures; (3) maxillofacial cysts and tumors; and (4) other jaw pathoses. This chapter will focus mainly on the use of panoramic radiography in detection of fractures of the jaws, and conditions predisposing to such fractures consequent to maxillofacial trauma. Suspected maxillary bone fractures are better detected using computed tomography than with plain radiographs or panoramic images; however, panoramic radiography is still valuable for evaluation of dental fractures and fractures limited to the alveolar bone.

Fractures of Teeth and Alveolar Bone

Traumatic injuries can be localized to the dentition (Fig. 14.1a, b) and are usually demonstrated on either panoramic or periapical radiographs. While periapical radiographs have higher spatial resolution, their field of view is restrictive. Further, if such high resolution is needed to find a fracture line, it is quite likely that contrast considerations and beam geometry will obscure the fracture. Periapical radiographs also need to be placed in the mouth, and that might not be a pleasant experience for the patient with a bruised or lacerated lip. When the alveolar bone is also fractured, the extent of the injury can be difficult to assess simply by periapical radiography (Fig. 14.1c–e). Cardinal radiologic signs of traumatic injuries to teeth are listed in Table 14.1.

Fractures of the Body and Angle of the Mandible

At times, an alveolar fracture with dental subluxation is the obvious consequence of facial trauma; however, a panoramic radiograph still can be useful in detecting additional unsuspected fractures (Fig. 14.2a). In this case, alveolar fracture in the anterior mandible was accompanied by a hairline fracture through the mandibular body, extending from the roots of the one standing periodontally involved right molar tooth (Fig. 14.2a detail). It should be remembered that even a negative finding is of value in determining the correct treatment plan. The value of the panoramic view to clinical management should not be second guessed retrospectively away from the clinical situation that evoked radiograph selection. A more readily detected mandibular body/

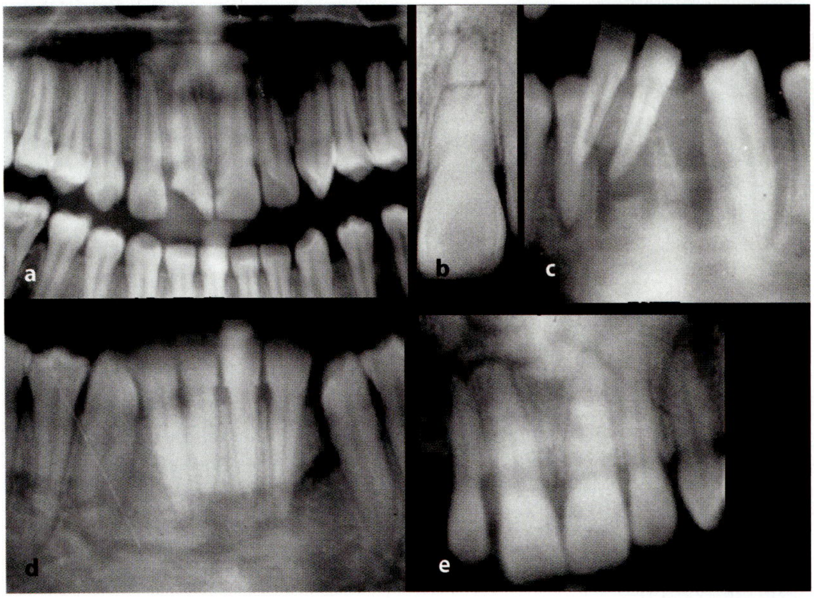

Fig. 14.1 Traumatic dental injuries. **a** Detail of panoramic radiograph showing fracture of crown of right maxillary central incisor tooth. **b** Periapical radiograph demonstrating root fracture to left maxillary central incisor tooth. **c** Panoramic detail of luxation of mandibular anterior teeth. **d** Panoramic detail of mandibular alveolar fracture. **e** Panoramic detail of maxillary alveolar fracture

Table 14.1 Radiologic signs of traumatic injuries to teeth

Recent tooth fracture
• Thin radiolucent line(s) extending through any portion of tooth
• "Step defect"
• Well-defined yet soft radiolucent band (where central X-ray beam cuts fracture line obliquely)
• For crown, transillumination and/or disclosing solutions often useful
Tooth displacement
• Concussion—no radiologic sign or periodontal ligament (pdl) space widening, most frequently apically
• Subluxation—often tooth mobility with no radiologic sign or pdl space widening
• Luxation—widened pdl (unless intrusive); minor alveolar fracture(s); step in dental occlusion
Later changes following luxation
• Pulp necrosis—widened pulp due to absence of continued secondary dentin formation
• Apical periodontal pathosis
• External root resorption and possible ankylosis
• Pulpal obliteration

angle fracture—also associated with the periodontal space of a molar tooth—is illustrated in Fig. 14.2a, b detail. Case 14.2b is more readily detected than Case 14.2a due to slight displacement of the bony fragments, obvious loss of continuity of the mandibular cortex, and the radiographic beam geometry being perfectly tangential to the fracture line. In Case 14.2a, there is little or no displacement of the bony fragments in the fracture of the mandibular body. The fracture line is "double" indicating that the beam geometry was not tangential to the fracture. Additional cases where teeth were associated with mandibular fracture are illustrated in Fig. 14.3. This leads to the question of the role of teeth in predisposition to jaw fracture.

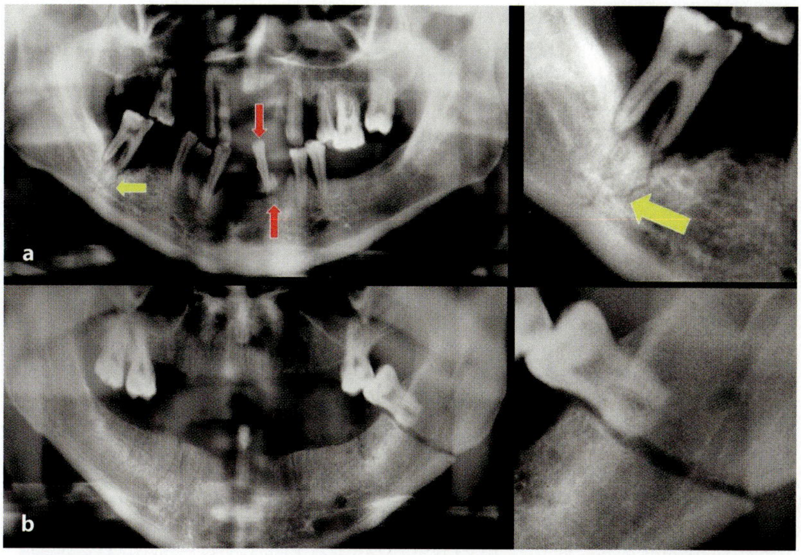

Fig. 14.2 **a** Alveolar fracture in anterior mandible (*red arrows*). There is also a fracture in the right molar region of the same jaw (*yellow arrow* and *detail*). **b** Tooth-associated fracture of left mandibular angle

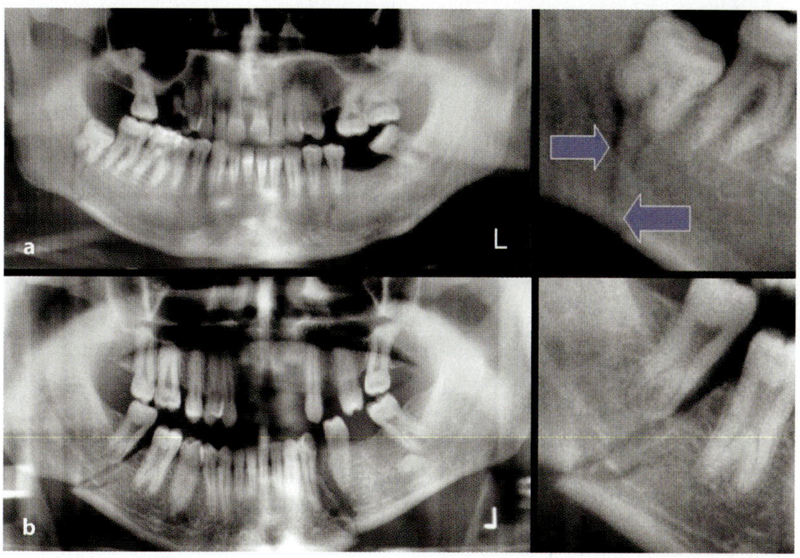

Fig. 14.3 **a** Mandibular fracture in right third molar region (*blue arrows*). **b** Mandibular fractures in right molar and left premolar regions (incidentally, molars are taurodonts)

Dental Impactions as Predisposing Factors to Mandibular Fracture

The question of whether the mandibular third molar is a risk factor for mandibular angle fracture was posed by several researchers [1–3]. Ma'aita and Alwrikat (Ammam, Jordan) in 2000 examined the medical records and panoramic radiographs of 615 patients who had suffered mandibular fractures [1]. The presence or absence and degree of impaction of the mandibular third molar teeth were assessed for each patient and related to the occurrence of fracture at the mandibular angle. Other information collected included patient age, sex, mechanism of injury, and specific location(s) of mandibular fracture(s). Chi^2 and Student t-tests were used to statistically evaluate the data, and the incidence of mandibular angle fracture was found to be significantly greater when an unerupted mandibular third molar was present ($p < 0.05$). Of the 426 maxillofacial trauma patients with an impacted mandibular third molar, 127 (29.8%) had angle fractures. Of the 189 patients without an impacted mandibular third molar, 25 (13.2%) had angle fractures. Hence, the mandibular angle that contains an impacted mandibular third molar is more susceptible to fracture when exposed to trauma than is the mandibular angle where the impacted mandibular third molar is absent.

Meisami et al. further assessed the influence of the presence, position, and severity of impaction of the mandibular third molar on the incidence of mandibular angle fractures [2]. A retrospective cohort study was designed for patients presenting to the Division of Oral and Maxillofacial Surgery, Toronto General Hospital for treatment of mandibular fractures from January 1995 to June 2000. The study sample comprised 413 mandibular fractures in 214 patients. The independent variables in this study were the presence, position, and severity of impaction of mandibular third molar teeth. The outcome variable was the incidence of mandibular angle fractures. Hospital charts and panoramic radiographs were used to determine and classify these variables. Demographic data collected included age, sex, mechanism of injury, and number of mandibular fractures. The incidence of angle fractures was found to be significantly higher in males than in females and was most commonly seen in the third decade of life. Assault was the most frequent etiological factor. Patients with impacted mandibular third molar had three times the risk of angle fractures when compared to patients without these teeth ($p < 0.001$). Impaction of one or more mandibular third molar significantly increased the incidence of angle fractures ($p < 0.001$); however, the severity and angulation of mandibular third molar impactions were not proven to be significantly associated with the incidence of fractures. This study provides evidence that patients with retained impacted mandibular third molars are significantly more susceptible to mandibular angle fracture than those without. The risk for angle fracture, however, was not proven to be influenced by the severity of tooth impaction.

Iida and co-workers (2005) from Heidelberg, Germany also investigated the risk of mandibular angle fractures in relation to the status of the incompletely erupted mandibular third molar [3]. They used panoramic radiographs to review 436 mandibular halves in 218 patients between the ages of 15 and 40 years old with mandibular fractures. The incidence of angle fractures in the mandibular halves with incompletely erupted mandibular third molar teeth was 30.8% and this was statistically significantly higher than that in controls ($p < 0.0001$). Moreover, the deeply located impacted mandibular third molar was associated with a higher incidence of mandibular angle fracture when compared with the adjacent second molar ($p < 0.0001$). This differs from the finding of Meisami et al. [2]. Iida and co-workers concluded that the incompletely erupted mandibular third molar close to the inferior border of the mandible significantly increases the risk of mandibular angle fractures in individuals subject to maxillofacial trauma [3].

Panoramic Radiographs in Third Molar Assessment for Relationship to the Inferior Dental Canal

If impacted teeth can predispose to certain mandibular fractures, perhaps they should be extracted in patients who are subject to facial trauma, such as persons involved in the martial arts or boxing. If this is to be considered, then the potential hazards of third molar removal need also to be considered. Blaeser et al. (Boston, MA) studied panoramic radiographic risk factors for inferior alveolar nerve injury after third molar extraction [4]. A case-control study design was used; the sample consisted of patients who underwent removal of impacted mandibular third molars. Cases were defined as patients with confirmed inferior alveolar nerve injury after mandibular third molar extraction, whereas controls were defined as patients without nerve injury. Five surgeons, who were blinded to injury status, independently assessed the preoperative panoramic radiographs for the presence of high-risk radiographic signs. Panoramic signs studied included diversion of the inferior alveolar canal, darkening of the third molar root, and interruption of the cortical white line of the canal. Bivariate analyses were completed to assess the relationship between radiographic findings and nerve injury. The sensitivity, specificity, and positive and negative predictive values were computed for each radiographic sign.

The sample comprised eight cases and 17 controls. Positive radiographic signs were statistically associated with an inferior alveolar nerve injury ($p < 0.0001$). The presence of panoramic radiographic sign(s) had positive predictive values that ranged from 1.4% to 2.7%, representing a 40% or greater increase over the baseline likelihood of injury (1%) for the individual patient. Absence of these radiographic findings had a strong negative (>99%) predictive value. This study confirms previous analyses showing that panoramic findings of diversion of the inferior alveolar canal, darkening of the third molar root, and interruption of the cortical white line are statistically associated with inferior alveolar nerve injury through impacted mandibular third molar removal. Based on the estimated predictive values, the absence of positive radiographic findings was associated with a minimal risk of nerve injury, whereas, the presence of one or more of the findings was associated with an increased risk for nerve injury during the surgical removal of mandibular third molar teeth.

Sedaghatfar et al. (2005), also from Boston, MA, evaluated panoramic radiographic findings as predictors of inferior alveolar nerve exposure following impacted mandibular third molar extraction [5]. The aim of their study was to estimate the sensitivity and specificity of panoramic radiographic findings in relation to inferior alveolar nerve exposure after impacted mandibular third molar extraction. The study used a retrospective cohort model. The primary predictor variable was the presence or absence of panoramic radiographic sign associated with an increased risk for nerve injury. The secondary predictor variable was surgeon assessment of inferior alveolar nerve exposure risk. The outcome variable was inferior alveolar nerve exposure, defined as direct visualization of the nerve at the time of impacted mandibular third molar extraction. The sample comprised 230 patients having 423 mandibular impacted third molar teeth evaluated and removed. Following impacted mandibular third molar extraction, the inferior alveolar nerve was visualized in 24 (5.7%) extraction sites. Four of the panoramic radiographic signs (darkening of the tooth root, narrowing of the tooth root, interruption of the cortical white lines, and diversion of the canal) were statistically associated with inferior alveolar nerve exposure ($p \leq 0.05$). The sensitivities and specificities of the four radiographic findings ranged from 0.42 to 0.75 and 0.66 to 0.91. The clinicians preoperative estimate of the likelihood of inferior alveolar nerve exposure was statistically associated with increased risk of nerve exposure after impacted mandibular third molar extraction ($p < 0.001$; sensitivity = 0.79; specificity = 0.86).

Panoramic Radiographs and Mandibular Fracture Assessment

Cardinal radiologic signs of alveolar bone fracture are listed in Table 14.2. Nair and Nair (Pittsburg, PA) compared the diagnostic efficacies of panoramic radiographs, plain film mandibular trauma series (comprising an anteroposterior view, a reverse Towne projection, and two lateral obliques), and digitized radiographs for detection of simulated fractures of the mandible [6]. Fractures were induced using blunt trauma to 25 cadaver mandibles. Six observers recorded their interpretations using a five-point confidence rating scale. The data were analyzed using receiver operating characteristic curve analysis. Significant differences based on imaging modalities were found ($p < 0.0015$) in the area under the curves (A_z): panoramic radiograph, 0.8762; mandibular series, 0.7521; panoramic plus anteroposterior radiographs combination, 0.8886; and digitized mandibular radiographic series, 0.7723. Condylar and coronoid fractures were more difficult to detect than those in other areas of the mandible ($p < 0.033$). Intra- and inter-observer agreements were high ($kappa_w$ = 0.81 and 0.76, respectively). It was concluded that panoramic radiographs are adequate for detection of mandibular fractures. Addition of an anteroposterior view augments diagnostic accuracy.

In 2000, Guss et al. (San Diego, CA) stated that the two primary radiographic techniques used in Emergency Medicine for the evaluation of mandibular injury were panoramic radiography (PR) and the standard four-view mandibular radiographic series [7]. A prospective, blind study of 54 patients presenting with acute mandibular injury was used to compare mandibular plain radiographic series with panoramic radiography in detection of mandibular fractures. Two board-certified emergency physicians and a staff radiologist read the series of mandibular series and panoramic radiographs in a randomized fashion without access to clinical information or identifying patient data. The absolute

Table 14.2 Radiologic signs of mandibular fractures

Alveolar bone
• Sharply defined, uncorticated and occasionally jagged radiolucent line in alveolus
• Fracture line(s) mostly horizontal
• Segment of teeth may be displaced
• Widened periodontal ligament spaces
• Possible associated tooth root fractures
Mandibular body
• Radiographic visible line of cleavage if X-ray beam parallels fracture line
• Line of cleavage may be indistinct if X-ray beam is not parallel to fracture line
• Step defect
• Contralateral condylar head frequently fractured
Mandibular condylar
• Condylar head "sheared off" and telescoped inward on itself
• Step defect
• Overlap of trabecular pattern seen as band of increased opacity
• Deviation of mandible to affected side
• Rarely, condylar head maintains integrity

number of fractures present was determined by a neuroradiologist with access to both sets of images simultaneously as well as pertinent clinical information. Thirty patients had 47 mandibular fractures. The sensitivity for fracture detection for each physician was 0.85, 0.77, and 0.89 with mandibular plain radiograph series and 0.79, 0.74, and 0.83 with panoramic radiography ($p \geq 0.51$, $p > 1.00$, and $p > 0.51$, respectively, McNemar's binomial test). The specificity for fracture detection for each physician was 0.88, 0.92, and 0.96 when using the mandibular series and 0.96, 1.00, and 0.92 for panoramic radiographs ($p > 0.625$, $p > 0.50$, and $p = 1.00$, respectively, McNemar's binomial test). Hence, a panoramic radiograph was proven to be equal to a four-radiograph mandibular series in sensitivity and specificity for the detection of mandibular fractures.

Certainly, extensive mandibular fractures through the body of the mandible with segment displacement or comminution are clearly demonstrated on panoramic radiographs (Fig. 14.4.) even though precise patient positioning may be impaired by the patient's injury.

Roles of Computed Tomography and Panoramic Radiology in Mandibular Fracture Detection

A prospective comparison of axial computed tomography (CT), versus a standard mandibular plain radiographic series and panoramic radiographs in the detection of mandibular fractures was made by Markowitz et al. (Los Angeles, CA) [8]. The authors studied 33 mandibular fractures in 21 consecutive patients with standard mandibular series, panoramic radiography, axial CT, and coronal CT. Differences in diagnostic accuracy and sensitivity were calculated for four blinded reviewers. Overall sensitivities of mandibular fracture detection were not statistically significant between the imaging studies. Excluding technically inadequate studies, panoramic radiography was 100% accurate and sensitive. Diagnostic accuracy and sensitivity did not correlate measurably with reviewers' impressions of the quality of a particular exam. Observers using axial CT detected significantly fewer angle fractures than they did with standard radiographs (60% versus 98%, $p = 0.006$) and coronal CT (60% versus 100%, $p = 0.008$).

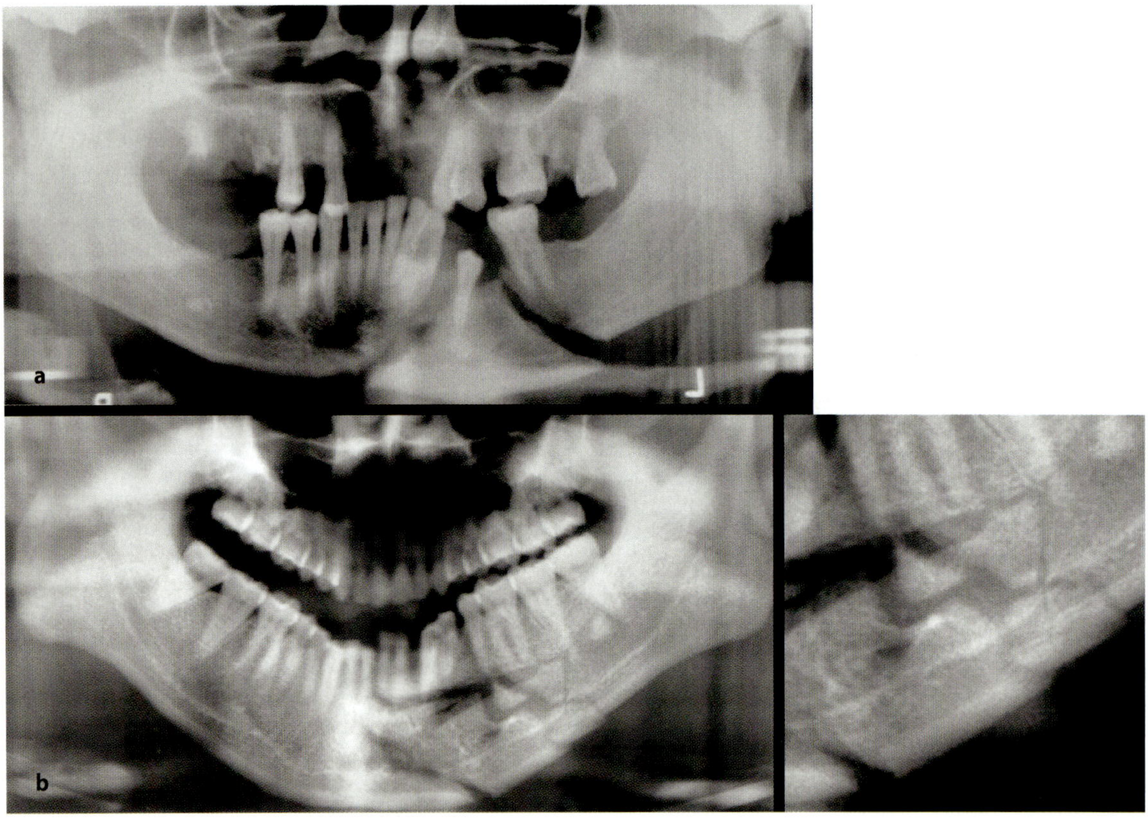

Fig. 14.4 **a** Mandibular fracture (depressed) in left canine/premolar region. Note fracture line and step in cortical outline. **b** Comminuted fracture of left mandibular body (positioning errors are not unusual in trauma victims—the patient's chin was too low and head too far forward in this case)

False-positives were unusual except when observers used plain mandibular radiographs. The clear definition of both coronal and axial CT scans made their analysis simpler than the plain radiographs. Lack of fracture displacement was the single most important factor in missed fractures with all modalities. The authors concluded that in clinically stable and cooperative patients with mandibular trauma, panoramic radiography and coronal CT are recommended to confirm clinical suspicions when the mandibular series is equivocal. To supplement the mandibular series in the uncooperative or multisystem trauma patient, axial CT scans were not found to be beneficial. Moreover, the authors noted that no diagnostic modality obviates the need for a careful physical exam of the patient. An example of the use of cone beam CT demonstrating a mandibular body fracture in axial section and three-dimensional reconstruction is provided by Fig. 14.5.

In 2001, Wilson et al. (Minnesota, USA) reported a prospective study that compared the sensitivity of panoramic tomography to that of multislice helical CT in detection of 73 mandibular fractures in 42 consecutive patients [9]. The study sought to determine the optimal radiologic examination for the diagnosis and operative management of mandibular fractures. The attending surgeons' interpretations of panoramic radiographs and multislice helical CT images in the axial plane were compared with the patients' known surgical findings. A series of questions assessed the relative contribution of the two radiologic examinations in formulating an optimal operative plan for each patient. In the 42 patients studied, the sensitivity of multislice helical CT was 100% for observer detection of mandibular fractures, compared with 86% (36 of 42) for the observers performance in using panoramic radiography ($p = 0.041$). In the six patients where fractures were not noted by the observers using panoramic radiography, operative management was altered because of the additional fractures that were detected on multislice helical CT. Comparing fracture detection by region, seven fractures found on multislice helical CT were not visualized on panoramic radiography—and six of these were in the posterior mandible. Helical CT sufficiently demonstrated details of fractures in 41 of 42 patients; however, in one patient,

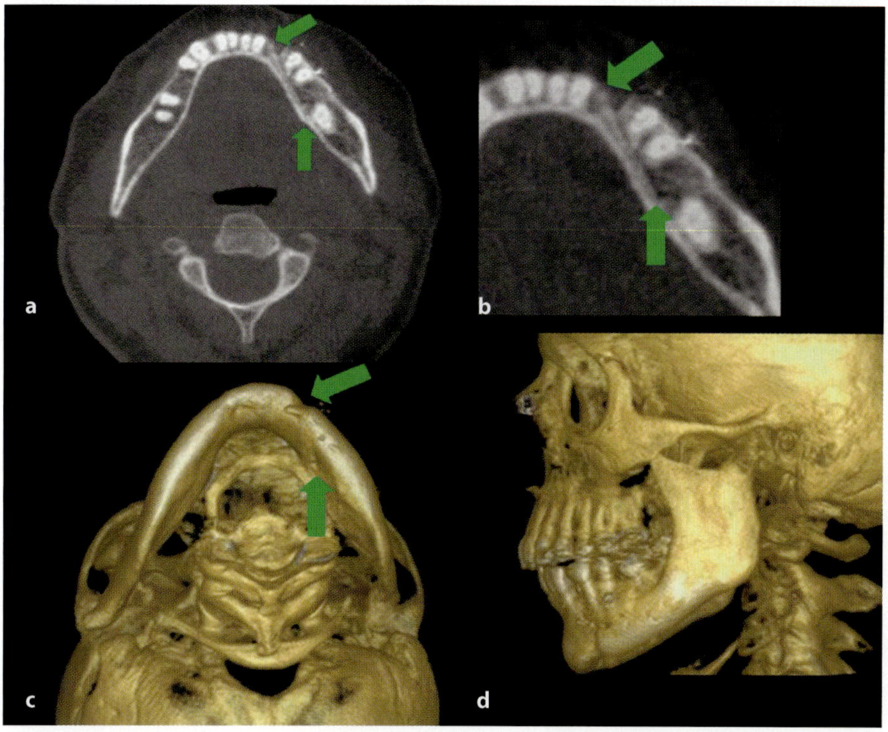

Fig. 14.5 Cone beam computed tomography of mandibular body fracture. **a** Axial section (0.4 mm voxel thickness). **b** Detail from axial slice. **c** Surface rendered 3-D reconstruction: submental view. **d** Surface rendered 3-D reconstruction: lateral view

the nature of a dental root fracture was better delineated by panoramic tomography than with CT. Hence, panoramic radiography can be equal to multislice helical CT for fractures of the body of the mandible and more reliable than multislice helical CT when teeth are in the fracture line, but that multislice helical CT is preferred when there is concern over possible fractures in the mandibular ramus and condyle regions.

Druelinger et al. (Chicago, IL) report that plain radiographs can serve as a springboard, giving direction and orientation to CT when this is indicated [10]. This undoubtedly is also the case for panoramic radiographs.

Roth et al. (2005) compared the identification of mandibular fractures by multislice helical CT and panoramic imaging [11]. They noted that while the introduction of CT in 1972 revolutionized the radiographic evaluation of patients who had experienced facial trauma, panoramic radiography continues to be superior in sensitivity to CT in the identification of mandibular fractures and has been considered the gold standard. On the other hand, for fractures of the maxilla the gold standard is high-resolution multislice helical CT providing multiplanar analysis for detection of fractures of the upper two thirds of the face. In a study by Roth et al. to compare the sensitivity, physician interpretation error, and interphysician agreement of helical CT and panoramic radiography in the identification of mandibular fractures, the number and anatomical location of mandibular fractures identified by helical CT and panoramic radiography was not significantly different. However, the number and location of 96% of fractures identified by multislice helical CT was agreed on by neuroradiologists compared with only 91% of fractures identified by panoramic radiography. Furthermore, the interphysician agreement when no fracture was identified was 96% for multislice helical CT versus only 81% by panoramic radiography. The authors conclude that multislice helical CT now surpasses panoramic radiography for evaluation of mandibular fractures. Nevertheless, an alternative conclusion might be that neuroradiologists need better training in reading panoramic radiographs.

Extensive condylar head displacement subsequent to fracture is obvious on panoramic radiography (Fig. 14.6), however, the beam geometry of panoramic radiography precludes this being the technique of choice where more subtle changes due to trauma to the temporomandibular joint are present. There is often simply too much superimposition of anatomical structures in the temporomandibular joint region when the mouth is closed and standard panoramic radiography is employed.

A comparative study of the sensitivity and specificity of panoramic radiographs with those of coronal CT scans in the diagnosis of mandibular condylar fractures in children was made by Chacon et al. (Seattle, WA) [12]. Medical, dental, and radiographic records of patients who presented between 1995 and 2000 were evaluated for injuries involving the mandibular condyle. The sample included 22 males and 15 females with ages ranging from 2 to 15 years (mean age 8 years). Control subjects matched by age and sex were added. The panoramic radiographs were blocked to allow separate evaluation of each condyle. Representa-

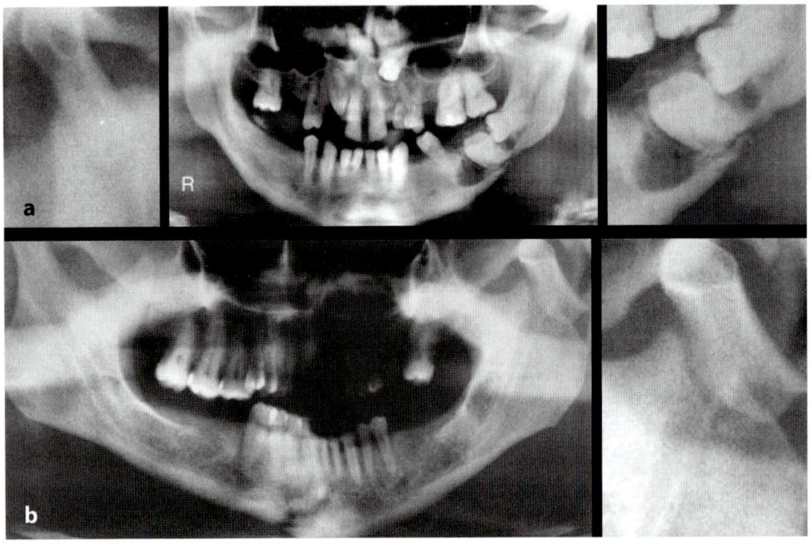

Fig. 14.6. **a** Fracture of right mandibular condyle and at left angle of mandible. **b** Fractures of mandibular symphysis and left condyle

tive images from the CT scans were selected and individually photographed for projection. Both sets of images were evaluated by four groups of examiners: oral and maxillofacial surgeons who regularly deal with pediatric trauma ($n = 2$), community oral and maxillofacial surgeons who had been out of training for at least 5 years ($n = 6$), oral and maxillofacial radiologists ($n = 3$), and oral and maxillofacial surgery residents ($n = 6$). Each image was shown for 20 seconds and the examiners were given three options to choose from: (1) fracture, (2) no fracture, and (3) uncertain. The overall diagnostic accuracy of observers utilizing CT scans was 90% (sensitivity, 92%; specificity, 87%), and that of panoramic radiographs was 73% (sensitivity, 70%; specificity, 77%). Statistical analysis of the results was performed using Chi^2 analysis. The differences for sensitivity measurements using the CT scan were not statistically significant ($p > 0.1$); however, the differences in sensitivity measurements using the panoramic radiographs and the specificity measurements using both the CT and panoramic radiographs were statistically significant ($p < 0.05$). CT scans provided consistently greater accuracy of diagnosis, sensitivity, and specificity than panoramic radiographs in the assessment of children suspected of having condylar fractures. In view of the high rate of false-negative and false-positive results associated with panoramic radiographs, coronal CT scans should be considered the investigation of choice in all patients where fractures involving the temporomandibular joint are suspected.

Pathological Jaw Fracture

Sometimes, very little trauma is needed to cause mandibular fracture. This can be the case where the jaw structure has been eroded or destroyed due to a pathological process such as a large cyst or tumor (Figs. 14.6a, 14.7). In such circumstances, the panoramic radiograph provides radiologic inputs into the eventual diagnosis of the underlying condition, though histopathological analysis of removed tissue is usually essential for deriving the definitive diagnosis.

Foreign Body Detection

On occasion the cause of mandibular fracture is a projectile, such as a bullet. In these circumstances, the projectile might be left behind (Fig. 14.8).Localization of such foreign bodies using panoramic and plain radiographs will require two images be made at a right angle to one another.

Fractures of the Maxilla

The panoramic radiograph is not to be relied upon for detection of fractures in the maxilla; however it can provide adjunctive information, especially when fractures involve teeth and the alveolar bone. The structures of the maxilla outside the dental arch are specifically excluded from a panoramic image area of focus to exclude anatomical noise that would obscure details of the teeth.

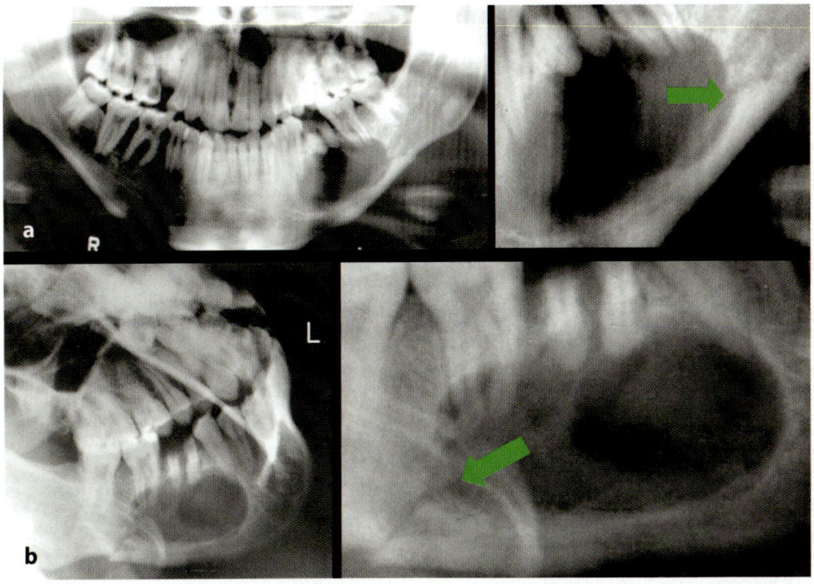

Fig. 14.7 a Pathological fracture associated with large apical periodontal (dental) cyst in left mandibular first molar region. **b** Pathological fracture associated with large apical dental cyst (lateral-oblique view from same patient)

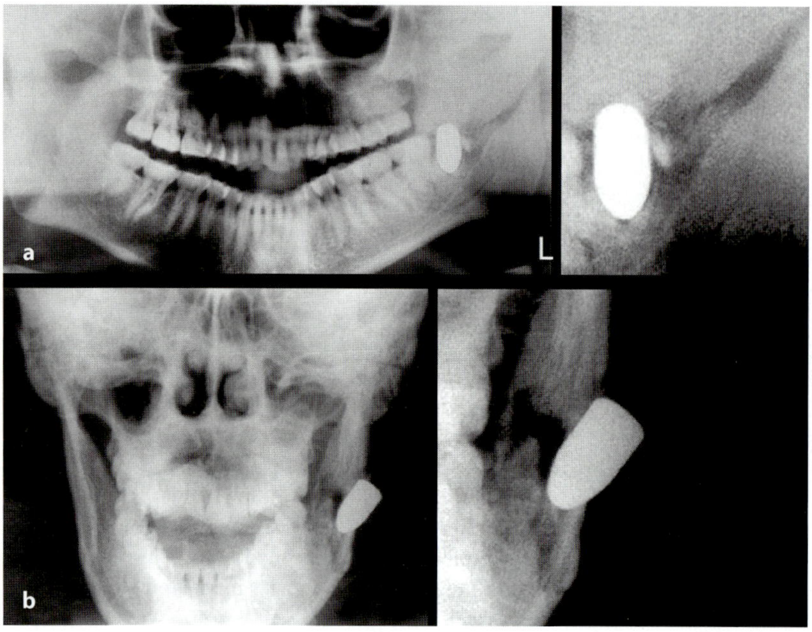

Fig. 14.8 Comminuted fracture of left mandibular ramus caused by gunshot injury. **a** Panoramic radiograph. **b** Posterior-anterior radiograph

Some of these features can, on occasion, be evident using panoramic radiographs (Table 14.3).

Concluding Remarks

Panoramic radiography plays a valuable role in support of maxillofacial surgery for the evaluation of suspected jaw fractures involving teeth, and in assessment of fractures of the mandibular body and angle. Panoramic radiographs should, however, not be relied upon for detecting subtle changes in the temporomandibular joint and condylar head consequent to trauma. To evaluate maxillary trauma, the panoramic radiograph should be considered merely adjunctive to CT. While panoramic radiography is useful in demonstrating changes involving teeth, CT better defines the bony structures of the maxilla. Literature as recent as five years ago found little advantage for CT over plain films; however, technology has improved both for CT and for panoramic radiography.

Table 14.3 Radiologic signs of maxillary fractures

Zygomatic arch fractures
• Together with zygomaticomaxillary fractures, represent 25% of all facial fractures
• Depression of zygomatic arch on submentovertex, Waters' and posterior-anterior views
• Close proximity of coronoid process to zygomatic arch
Zygomaticomaxillary fractures
• Widening of zygomaticofrontal, zygomaticomaxillary, and zygomaticotemporal suture lines
• Step defects at junction of frontal and zygomatic bones, zygoma and maxilla, or zygoma and temporal bone ("tripod" fractures)
• CT used for assessing on nasolacrimal canal, rectus muscles of eye, and possible intracranial hemorrhage
Blow-out fracture of orbital floor
• Force transmitted to thin orbital floor, which generally fractures near infraorbital canal
• Soft tissue swelling over orbital rim
• Opacification of affected maxillary sinus
• Displaced orbital floor ("trap door")
• Polypoid density in roof of maxillary sinus through herniation of orbital contents
• Cheek paresthesia if infraorbital canal involved

Table 14.3 *(continued)* Radiologic signs of maxillary fractures

Le Fort Type I fractures
• Fracture above level of maxillary teeth involving alveolar process, palate, and pterygoid plates
• Clouding of maxillary sinus on one or both sides
• Discontinuity of lateral maxillary sinus walls on plain radiographs
• Sharp horizontal line of cleavage through maxilla, pterygoid plates, and sphenoid
• Canted maxilla relative to cranial base and mandibular teeth
Le Fort Type II fractures
• Pyramidal fracture across nasal bones and frontal processes of maxilla, extending laterally through lachrymal bones, inferior rim of orbit near zygomaticomaxillary suture, lateral walls of maxilla, and pterygoid plates
• Increased width of frontonasal suture
• Radiolucent cleavage lines
• Step defect in orbital rim
• Sinus shadows obscured by hemorrhage
• Disruption in dental occlusion
Le Fort Type III fractures
• Craniofacial disjunction with shearing of facial complex from cranial base. Involves nasofrontal, maxillofrontal, and zygomaticofrontal sutures orbit, ethmoid sinus, and sphenoid sinus floors
• Widened frontonasal, maxillofrontal, zygomaticofrontal, and zygomaticotemporal sutures
• Radiolucent cleavage lines through frontal processes of maxilla, both pterygoid plates and one or both orbital floors
• Sinus shadows obscured by hemorrhage

References

1. Ma'aita J, Alwrikat A. Is the mandibular third molar a risk factor for mandibular angle fracture? Oral Surg Oral Med Oral Pathol Oral Radiol Endod 2000;89:143–146
2. Meisami T, Sojat A, Sandor GK, Lawrence HP, Clokie CM. Impacted third molars and risk of angle fracture. Int J Oral Maxillofac Surg 2002;3:140–144
3. Iida S, Hassfeld S, Reuther T, Nomura K, Muhling J. Relationship between the risk of mandibular angle fractures and the status of incompletely erupted mandibular third molars. J Craniomaxillofac Surg 2005;33:158–163
4. Blaeser BF, August MA, Donoff RB, Kaban LB, Dodson TB. Panoramic radiographic risk factors for inferior alveolar nerve injury after third molar extraction. J Oral Maxillofac Surg 2003;61:417–421
5. Sedaghatfar M, August MA, Dodson TB. Panoramic radiographic findings as predictors of inferior alveolar nerve exposure following third molar extraction. J Oral Maxillofac Surg 2005;63:3–7
6. Nair MK, Nair UP. Imaging of mandibular trauma: ROC analysis. Acad Emerg Med 2001;8:689–695
7. Guss DA, Clark RF, Peitz T, Taub M. Pantomography vs mandibular series for the detection of mandibular fractures. Acad Emerg Med 2000;7:141–145
8. Markowitz BL, Sinow JD, Kawamoto HK Jr, Shewmake K, Khoumehr F. Prospective comparison of axial computed tomography and standard and panoramic radiographs in the diagnosis of mandibular fractures. Ann Plast Surg 1999;42:163–169
9. Wilson IF, Lokeh A, Benjamin CI, Hilger PA, Hamlar DD, Ondrey FG, Tashjian JH, Thomas W, Schubert W. Prospective comparison of panoramic tomography (zonography) and helical computed tomography in the diagnosis and operative management of mandibular fractures. Plast Reconstr Surg 2001;107:1369–1375
10. Druelinger L, Guenther M, Marchand EG. Radiographic evaluation of the facial complex. Emerg Med Clin North Am 2000;18:393–410
11. Roth FS, Kokoska MS, Awwad EE, Martin DS, Olson GT, Hollier LH, Hollenbeak CS. The identification of mandible fractures by helical computed tomography and panorex tomography. J Craniofac Surg 2005;16:394–399
12. Chacon GE, Dawson KH, Myall RW, Beirne OR. A comparative study of 2 imaging techniques for the diagnosis of condylar fractures in children. J Oral Maxillofac Surg 2003;61:668–673

TEST: Panoramic radiology in maxillofacial trauma

1. Impacted third molars predispose to mandibular angle fracture in individuals subjected to maxillofacial trauma.

   True ☐ **False** ☐

2. The panoramic radiograph provides ideal coverage for inspection of the temporomandibular joints for subtle condylar head fractures.

   True ☐ **False** ☐

3. The diagnostic yield of a single panoramic radiograph is approximately equivalent to a full mandibular series of plain radiographs for detection of mandibular fractures.

   True ☐ **False** ☐

4. Computed tomography is preferred over the panoramic radiography for detection of maxillary fractures following facial trauma.

   True ☐ **False** ☐

5. Fractures involving teeth and alveolar bone are often better visualized on panoramic radiographs than on CT scans.

   True ☐ **False** ☐

6. The study of Nair and Nair concerning mandibular fractures involved a retrospective analysis of patient charts and radiographs.

   True ☐ **False** ☐

7. Panoramic radiography can be equal to helical CT for fractures of the body of the mandible and more reliable than helical CT when teeth are involved in the fracture line.

   True ☐ **False** ☐

8. CT scans have been found to provide consistently greater accuracy of diagnosis, sensitivity, and specificity than panoramic radiographs in the assessment of children suspected of having condylar fractures.

   True ☐ **False** ☐

9. Diagnostic accuracy and sensitivity invariably do correlate measurably with reviewers' impressions of the quality of a particular exam.

   True ☐ **False** ☐

10. Extensive fractures through the body of the mandible with segment displacement or comminution are clearly demonstrated on panoramic radiographs even though precise patient positioning may be impaired by the patient's injury.

    True ☐ **False** ☐

Chapter

15

Panoramic Radiographic Detection of Systemic Disease

Arthur H. Friedlander and Keith M. Norman in collaboration with Allan G. Farman, Christoffel J. Nortjé, and Robert E. Wood

Learning Objectives

- Learn through examples how to review panoramic radiographs to screen for early detection of systemic diseases
- Learn how to observe and detect features of systemic diseases when they produce changes in panoramic radiographs
- Understand the limitations of panoramic radiography in detecting systemic diseases

For the purposes of this report, "systemic disease" will be interpreted as conditions that are spread out within the body rather than being localized strictly to the tissues of the oral cavity. Since it would take many volumes to review all such conditions, the intent of this chapter of is to review a few examples where initial panoramic radiographic findings suggest widespread disease of sufficient significance to affect the quality of life or longevity of the patient. The first part of this chapter deals with the possibility of detecting carotid artery calcifications, indicative of cardiovascular disease—the leading cause of death in the US population.

Detection of Carotid Artery Disease and also by Inference, Coronary Artery Disease

Each year more than 700,000 Americans suffer a stroke and 275,000 of these individuals die. Similarly, 1.2 million Americans suffer a myocardial infarct and 220,000 of these are fatal [1]. Common to both disorders is the atherosclerotic process of plaque formation in which fatty substances, cholesterol, platelets, cellular waste products, and calcium are deposited in the inner lining of the carotid and coronary arteries. The presence of an atheromatous plaque in the carotid artery of clinically asymptomatic individuals is often associated with the later development of both cerebrovascular disease [transient ischemic attack (TIA) and stroke] and cardiovascular disease, that is, coronary artery disease (as manifested by angina and myocardial infarction), and death [2–4].

Since 1981, Friedlander and his colleagues have actively promoted panoramic radiography as an aid in detecting patients at risk of stroke [5]. Calcified atherosclerotic lesions at the carotid bifurcation can be seen in the lower corners of the panoramic radiograph adjacent to the cervical spine and hyoid bone (Figs. 15.1–15.3). Such atheromas may appear as a nodular radio-opaque mass or as double radio-opaque vertical lines within the neck. These calcifications are found at the level of the lower margin of the third and the entirety of the fourth cervical vertebra, about 1.5–2.5 cm inferior-posterior to the angle of the mandible [6–8]. The prevalence of these lesions in the general dental population ranges between 3% and 5% [9].

Atherosclerosis is not the only cause of soft tissue calcifications seen anterior to the cervical vertebrae on panoramic radiographs (Fig. 15.4). Care needs to be applied to differentiate carotid calcifications from calcified triticeous or thyroid cartilages, calcified lymph nodes, and non-carotid phleboliths. For this reason, it is important to have an anterior-posterior (AP) radiograph of the neck made using soft tissue exposure settings (Fig. 15.5). Calcifications within the carotid arteries will appear lateral to the spine, whereas calcifications in the thyroid gland, thyroid cartilage, triticeous cartilage or epiglottis will be in the midline, superimposed over the spine. Other calcifications that can be superimposed over the same part of the panoramic film include phleboliths (sclerosing hemangiomata), and calcified acne or lymph nodes. The stylohyoid and stylomandibular ligaments are situated posterior rather than inferior to the mandibular ramus—and therefore should be readily differentiated [10–13].

Different panoramic systems produce non-identical radiographic images. Some machines are likely to be less able to detect carotid calcification than are others. Factors to consider include the positioning of labels with demographic information and date of exposure, lead indicators of the side—and sometimes their ghost images. Unless one can see the anterior outline of the third and fourth cervical vertebrae to the side of the panoramic image, one is probably missing details of the relevant region. Taking a radiograph with the

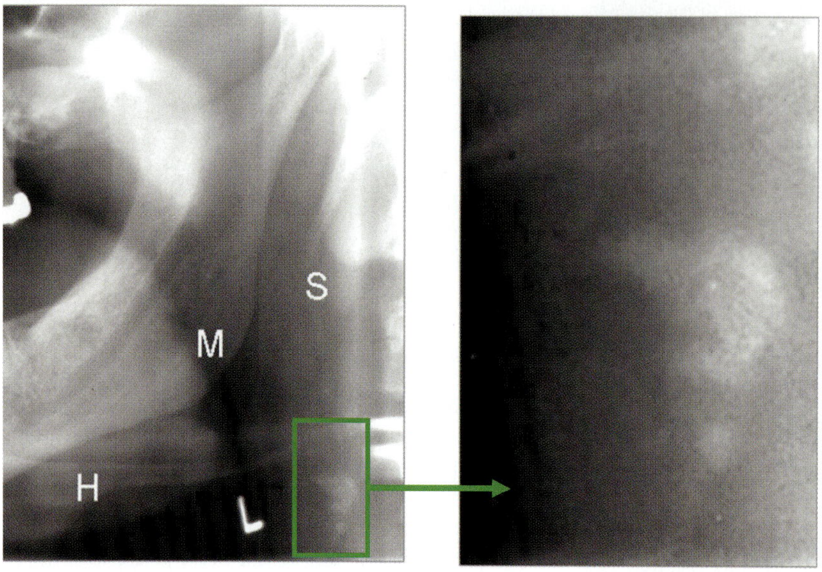

Fig. 15.1 Calcified atheroma (*box* and *detail*) at bifurcation of the left carotid artery. Note relative position of the lesion in relation to angle of the mandible (*M*), styloid process (*S*), and hyoid bone (*H*). The *L* is the laterality marker

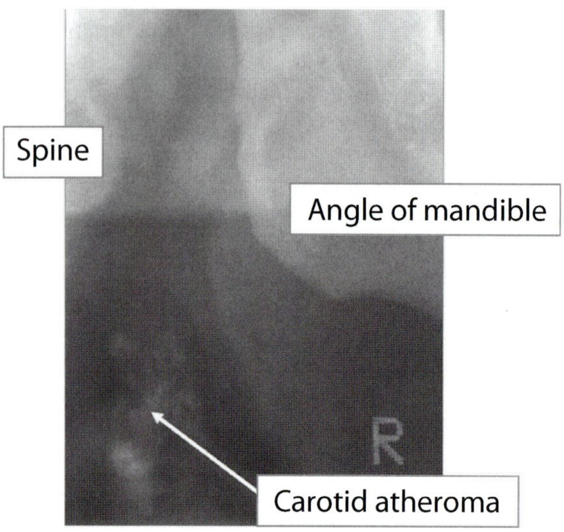

Fig. 15.2 Detail from panoramic radiograph

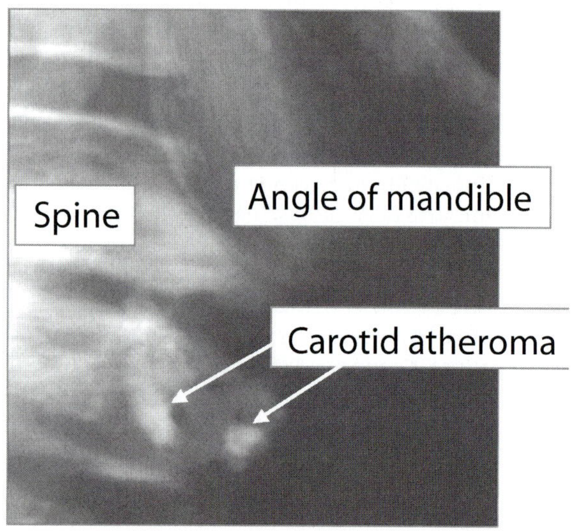

Fig. 15.3 Detail from panoramic radiograph

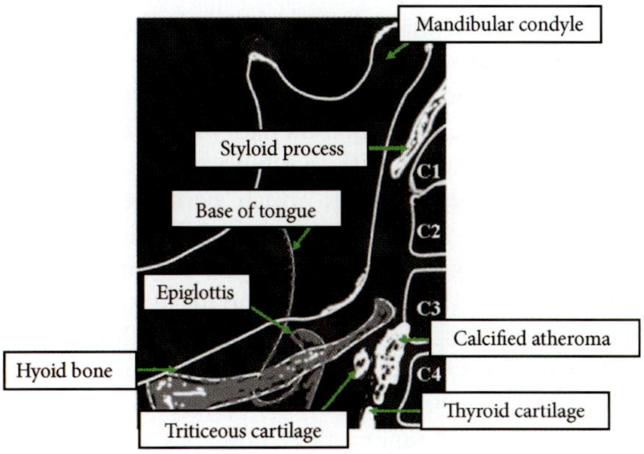

Fig. 15.4 Not every soft tissue calcification in the neck is carotid atheroma. (Diagram modified from Carter LC, Oral Surg Oral Med Oral Pathol Oral Radiol Endod 2000;90:100–110)

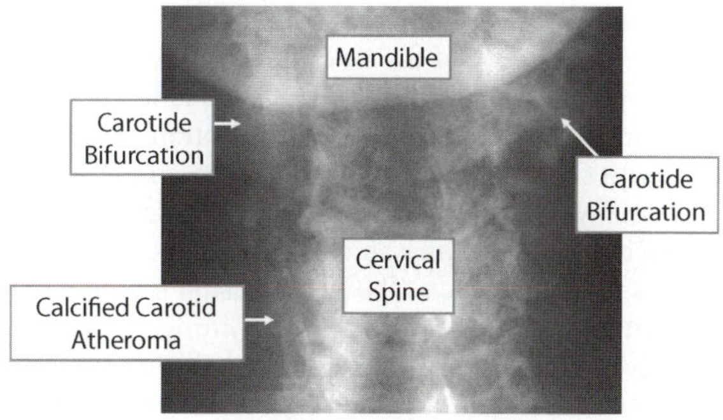

Fig. 15.5 Anterior-posterior (AP) radiograph confirming bilateral deposits of calcified atheroma in the carotid bifurcation region and calcification along the whole length of the right common carotid artery. This radiograph excludes calcification being in a normal midline structure

patient 1 cm anterior and 1 cm superior to the instructions of the manufacturer of the panoramic system would optimize the image for carotid calcification detection—as would underexposure; however, this is not recommended as it is suboptimal for evaluation of the teeth and jaws. The panoramic technique modification described would be best left to follow up to a regularly performed panoramic radiograph.

Viewing conditions are critical to detecting carotid atheromas using panoramic images. The radiograph should be viewed on a view box with a variable rheostat to adjust the intensity of the transmitted light. The ambient lighting should be subdued. A "hot light" is also helpful when looking for carotid calcifications.

Duplex ultrasonography images and spectral analysis (velocity and wave form studies) of the neck and carotid artery distribution were first used by dental researchers Friedlander and Baker [14] in 1994 to confirm the intravascular nature and extent of stenosis caused by radio-opacities initially noted on a panoramic radiograph. Since that time other investigators have incorporated duplex ultrasonography confirmation into their studies [15, 16]. However, it was not until 2005 that dental researchers adopted the Society of Radiologists Ultrasound criteria [17] for diagnosing and grading carotid artery stenosis. Using these criteria, Friedlander et al. [18] demonstrated that 4.2% of 50-year-old neurologically asymptomatic dental patients have an atheroma and that 23% of these atheromas are hemodynamically significant (i.e., the stenosis is 50% or greater) which places the patient at heightened risk of a future stroke.

Factors predisposing carotid atherosclerosis include advancing age, male sex, systolic hypertension, hypercholesterolemia, cigarette smoking, physical inactivity, and obesity [19–21]. In addition, individuals with certain disease states and those who have been exposed to certain therapeutic modalities have an accelerated atherosclerotic process which causes them to have a greater prevalence of calcified carotid atheromas visible on their panoramic radiographs than healthy, age-matched persons.

Friedlander and Maeder (2000) [22] and Friedlander et al. (2002) [23] examined the panoramic radiographs of patients with type 2 diabetes mellitus. They noted that those individuals requiring insulin had an atheroma prevalence rate of 36%, those managed by diet and oral medications had an atheroma prevalence rate of 24%, and non-diabetic age matched controls had an atheroma prevalence rate of 4%. The excessively high prevalence rate of carotid atheromas seen in patients with this disorder arises from diabetes associated hypertension and altered lipid metabolism. Hypertension damages the vessel's endothelial lining permitting large amounts of small, very low-density lipoproteins (VLDL) and low-density lipoproteins (LDL) to enter the arterial wall. These lipoproteins are rapidly oxidized because of the hyperglycemic environment and engulfed by vascular wall macrophages. This process stimulates the macrophage to esterify the lipoproteins, transforming itself into a foam cell. In a mechanism less well-defined, oxidized lipoproteins also are taken up by vascular wall smooth muscle cells, which then also undergo transformation into foam cells. This accumulation of foam cells constitutes the major component of the fatty streak that ultimately becomes the atheromatous plaque. Calcium salts taken up by the lesion during the maturation process correspond to radiopacities seen on the panoramic radiographs.

Friedlander et al. (1999) studied the prevalence of carotid atheromas in patients with obstructive sleep apnea syndrome (OSAS) [24]. Detectable carotid atheromas were found in 22% of the study subjects compared to 4% in age and sex matched controls. This difference was statistically significant. Atheroma formation in individuals with OSAS probably arises from apnea induced hypoxemia which causes central nervous system arousal, a rise in catecholamines and sympathetic activity and results in hypertension. The hypertension disrupts the integrity of the vessel's endothelial lining, rendering it hyperpermeable. Platelets activated during periods of hypoxia pass through the damaged endothelium and elaborate growth factors that cause proliferation of smooth muscle cells in the vessel wall. Low-density lipoproteins oxidized during periods of hypoxia pass through the damaged endothelium and are engulfed by vascular wall macrophages. Foam cells, the major component of an atheroma are then formed from vascular wall macrophages and from vascular wall smooth muscle cells, which have taken up LDL. Calcium salts later absorbed by these lesions correspond to the radiopacities seen on the panoramic radiograph.

Friedlander and Altman (2001) [25] recognizing that more than 60% of the deaths in the USA attributed to stroke occur in postmenopausal women assessed the radiographs of 52 neurologically asymptomatic females with a mean age of 70 years. The radiographs of 16 subjects or 31% exhibited atheromas. This high prevalence rate is in part caused by the low levels of estrogen commonly seen in older postmenopausal women. Reduced levels of circulating estrogen are associated with an increase in lipase activity and a decrease in LDL catabolism, which result in increased levels of LDL cholesterol and reduced levels of high-density lipoprotein (HDL) cholesterol. The LDL is taken up by vascular wall macrophages as previously described and foam cells are formed which constitute the main component of the atheroma.

Kansu et al. (2005) [26] noted that the prevalence rate of calcified carotid artery atheromas on the panoramic radiographs of patients with end-stage renal disease (including those on hemodialysis or post renal transplant) was significantly greater than among age-matched healthy control patients. This high prevalence rate of disease likely results from renal failure (i.e., uremic state) associated hypertension, hyperhomocysteinemia (because of altered metabolism and reduced renal excretion), oxidant stress, elevated levels of lipoprotein (a) and inflammation markers, and disordered calcium phosphorus metabolism [27]. Taken together these factors precipitate the formation of atheromas.

Friedlander and August [28], Friedlander et al. [29], and Friedlander and Freymiller [30] studied the detection by panoramic radiography of radiation-induced accelerated atherosclerosis. The prevalence rate for carotid calcifications in patients who have received, on average, a dose of 60 Gy radiation therapy to the carotid bifurcation was 28%. The prevalence was 5% in a matched sample of non-irradiated patients. This difference was statistically significant. These atheromas likely developed because of radiation injury to the endothelial cells lining the lumen of the carotid artery. This resulted in increased permeability, which permitted circulating LDL to pass into the subendothelial space. In addition, platelets aggregated at the injury site and released growth factors that caused the smooth muscle cells of the vascular wall to hypertrophy. The resultant thickened and elevated lesion is in fact the atheroma, which when calcium salts are absorbed, corresponds to the radiopacity seen on panoramic radiographs.

The clinical significance of identifying neurologically asymptomatic patients with carotid artery atherosclerotic lesions of any extent should not be underestimated. In fact, numerous medical studies have shown that even very early carotid artery lesions are often associated with significant coronary artery disease [31–33]. These findings have been expanded upon by dental researchers (Woodworth et al. [34], Cohen et al. [35,36], Friedlander and Cohen [37]) who have shown that the presence of calcified carotid artery atheromas on panoramic radiographs often heralds future fatal and non-fatal adverse cerebrovascular (stroke, transient ischemic attacks) and cardiovascular events [myocardial infarct, need for revascularization procedures (coronary artery by-pass surgery/coronary artery stent placement), and angina requiring hospitalization]. These associations are not unexpected, given the fact that extracranial carotid artery and coronary artery atherosclerosis are major manifestations of generalized atherosclerosis and have shared risk factors (i.e., age, high levels of LDL cholesterol, elevated triglycerides, diabetes, hypertension, low levels of HDL cholesterol, cigarette smoking, and increased body mass index). It must be noted however that Taneka et al. (2006) conducted a study similar to those administered by Woodworth et al., Cohen et al., and Friedlander and Cohen but could not demonstrate that 80-year-olds with carotid atheromas on their radiographs were at greater risk of future adverse cerebrovascular and cardiovascular events than matched controls without an atheroma [38]. This discrepancy in results may have arisen because Taneka's patients were, on average, 12–25 years older than those assessed by the other groups of investigators.

The public health import of dentists evaluating panoramic radiographs for an incidental finding of a carotid atheroma is likely to be significant given the large numbers of individuals who suffer a stroke and myocardial infarct each year. Thousands of dentists have an opportunity to identify and refer for treatment patients at risk of an adverse vascular event. Specifically, 61% of general dentists and 73% of dental specialists in private practice have panoramic units, and in 1999 (most recent data available) these individuals performed more that

17 million panoramic imaging studies [39]. With many dentists having patient panels of more than 1,000 individuals over age 50, it is likely that approximately 1% or 10 such individuals in their practice may have an undiagnosed hemodynamically significant carotid artery lesion (≥50% stenosis) requiring medical evaluation and possible treatment.

A dentist caring for a patient with a suspected atheroma on his or her radiograph should show the patient the lesion, as well as the lesion's relationship to the course of the internal carotid artery and angle of the mandible. Such a patient should also be informed that these lesions often are markers of generalized atherosclerosis and may be associated with a future stroke and or heart attack. Furthermore, the patient should be given a copy of a written consultation directed to his or her primary care physician that describes the radiographic findings and suggests obtaining a duplex ultrasonography study to confirm the presence and extent of disease. This protocol is consistent with a dentist's professional responsibilities to diagnose oral manifestations of systemic disease and to counsel patients properly about the importance of arranging for and following through with medical consultation [40–43].

The physician will likely attempt to control hypertension, hyperlipidemia, and hyperglycemia, if present, because aggressive control of risk factors has been shown to retard and possibly reverse the atherogenic process and obviate the occurrence of some cerebrovascular accidents and myocardial infarcts. The physician may also suggest carotid artery endarterectomy (or stent placement) because for certain patients surgical removal of the atheroma has proven to be a safe and reliable method of reducing the likelihood of an ischemic stroke.

Osteoporosis

Osteoporosis results in excessive bone porosity and fragility. It is the most common metabolic disease and presents a major public health problem among the elderly, especially amongst postmenopausal Caucasian and Asian women [44]. It is also found in sedentary or immobilized individuals, and in patients on long-term steroid therapy [45]. The asymptomatic progression of osteoporosis, in conjunction with the possibility of catastrophic disability, makes this disorder a major public health priority [46].

Cardinal radiographic features of osteoporosis in the skeleton as a whole include generalized osteopenia that is often most prominent in the spine, thinning and accentuation of the bone cortices, and accentuation of primary and loss of secondary trabeculation. Ancillary radiologic features include spontaneous, atraumatic fracture, especially of the spine, wrist, hip or ribs, basilar invagination in the skull, and granular appearance of bone in the skull [45]. Osteoporosis can lead to pain, especially in the lower back. It can also result in pathological fracture, loss of physical stature, and severe kyphosis.

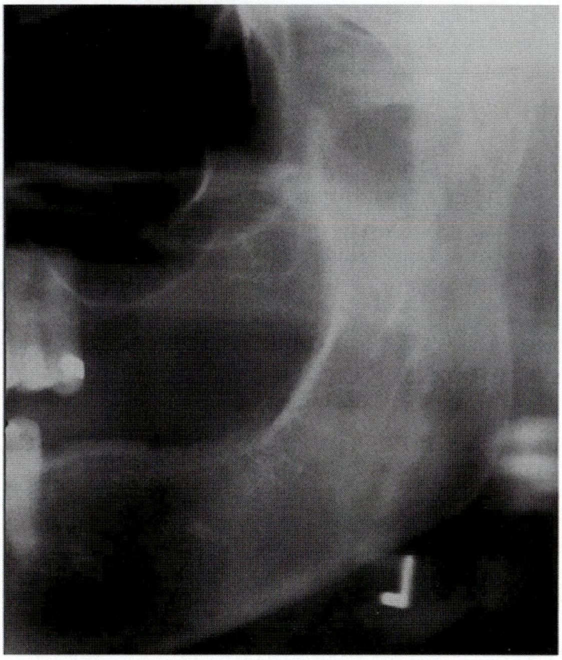

Fig. 15.6 Osteoporosis. Cropped panoramic image shows a relative radiolucency of both jaws with reduced definition of the cortices

Radiologic features of osteoporosis in the jaws (Fig. 15.6) include relative radiolucency of both jaws and reduced definition of the cortices. The accuracy with which panoramic radiographs can be used to assess the likelihood of a person having osteoporosis is still in debate, with evidence being divided, rather than polarized for or against.

Some researchers have concluded that panoramic radiography can be used to assess the likelihood of osteoporosis.

Evidence Supporting Panoramic Radiographs to Screen for Osteoporosis

In 1991, Benson et al. defined a radiomorphometric index of mandibular cortical bone mass, the panoramic mandibular index (PMI) [47]. Differences in the index in a population of 353 adult subjects, equally divided by sex, age (30 years through 79 years), and racial group

(Black, Hispanic, White), were evaluated with respect to side, racial group, sex, age, and combinations of these variables. Blacks were found to have a greater mean PMI than Hispanics or Whites, who were demographically similar. Age-related changes comparing younger and older age groups within each sex and racial group indicated a significant decrease in mean PMI with increasing age in Black and Hispanic women. The mean PMI in white men increased with advancing age.

A retrospective investigation was carried out to determine the strength of association of spinal bone density and the density of selected mandibular sites as determined from panoramic radiographs [44]. Panoramic radiographs of known low bone density and high bone density in women between the ages of 50 and 75 years were evaluated. These radiographs were randomized and then converted to digital images for density analysis. Significant differences were found between the groups at the 95th percentile level. Hence, according to this study, blinded observers should be able to differentiate between persons of high and low bone density using panoramic radiographs.

The relationship between oral signs and osteoporosis was investigated to assess the possibility of using this as an indicator of osteoporosis. Taguchi et al. (1995) [48] studied 64 postmenopausal women aged 50–70 years. Osteoporotic signs consisted of thoracic spine fracture as demonstrated on lateral chest radiographs. Oral signs were the number of teeth present, mandibular cortical width, alveolar bone resorption, and the morphological classification of the inferior cortex on panoramic radiographs. The number of teeth present (N) was highly significantly related to the probability of thoracic spine fracture and was used to derive the probability equation for the presence of thoracic spine fracture: probability value, $p = 1/(1 + e^{-z})$, $Z = 18.68 - 0.29\,\text{Age} - 0.27N$. A probability value, $p > 0.5$ suggested the possibility of thoracic spine fracture. It was concluded that this equation combined with panoramic radiographic findings could serve as a simple and useful tool for dentists to assess the possibility of latent osteoporosis [48].

The usefulness of width and morphology of the inferior cortex of the mandible on panoramic radiographs was evaluated in the diagnosis of postmenopausal osteoporosis [49]. The width and morphology of the mandibular inferior cortex on panoramic radiographs were compared with trabecular bone mineral density of the third lumbar vertebrae measured by dual energy quantitative computed tomography in 29 premenopausal and 95 postmenopausal women. There was a significant negative correlation between the width (Kendall's tau = −0.36, $p < 0.001$) and morphology (Kendall's tau = −0.49, $p < 0.001$) of the mandibular inferior cortex and the third lumbar vertebrae trabecular bone mineral density. Regression analysis showed that significant linear relationships were observed between the third lumbar vertebrae trabecular bone mineral density and age ($p < 0.001$), cortical width ($p < 0.05$), morphology ($p < 0.05$), controlling body mass index, number of teeth present, and menopausal status ($R^2 = 0.42$). The researchers concluded that panoramic radiography can be used to assess the likelihood of osteoporosis.

The value of clinical and radiographic indices in the diagnosis of patients with low skeletal bone mass was investigated among 135 healthy perimenopausal women, aged 45–55 years attending for regular dental treatment [50]. Bone mineral density was measured for the spine and femoral neck, using dual energy X-ray absorptiometry. Each patient's osteoporosis status was calculated according to the World Health Organization criteria for Caucasian women. Each patient received a dental panoramic radiograph, and the width of the inferior mandibular cortex (mental index) was measured. The body mass index and simple calculated osteoporosis risk estimation indices were calculated. The simple calculated osteoporosis risk estimation index was a significant factor in predicting low bone mass, with the weight of the patient being the only significant constituent factor. Mental index, body mass index and simple calculated osteoporosis risk estimation indices were significantly correlated with skeletal bone density. When the logistic regression model included mental index, bone mineral index, and simple calculated osteoporosis risk estimation indices, all three variables were significant predictors of low skeletal bone mass. A thinning of the mandibular cortices (mental index <3 mm) in a normal perimenopausal female was associated with low skeletal bone mass. If, in addition, the patient is underweight (body mass index is below 20 kg/m^2) or has a high simple calculated osteoporosis risk estimation index (= 6) then this assessed increase in risk was found to be reliable in screening for osteoporosis.

Nakamoto et al. (2003) looked into whether untrained general dental practitioners are capable of determining from panoramic radiographs whether women have low bone mineral density [51]. The investigators studied observer agreement and diagnostic efficacy in detecting women with low bone mineral density. This was accomplished when 27 general dental practitioners assessed the appearance (normal or eroded) of the mandibular inferior cortex on dental panoramic radiographs of 100 postmenopausal women who had completed bone mineral density assessments of the lumbar spine and of the femoral neck. Intra- and inter-observer agreements were analyzed with kappa statistics. The diagnostic efficacy (sensitivity, specificity, and predictive values) was analyzed by comparing two groups classified by the mandibular inferior cortex (women with normal and women with eroded mandibular inferior cortex) with those classified by bone mineral density (women with normal bone mineral density and women with osteopenia or osteoporosis). The mean sensitivity and specificity were 77% and 40%, respectively, when bone mineral density of the lumbar spine was used as the standard, and 75% and 39%, respectively, when bone mineral density of the femoral neck comprised the standard. Nineteen of the 21 untrained general dental practitioners presented a moderate to almost perfect intra-observer agreement. It was concluded that dental panoramic radiographs might be used in clinical dental practice to identify postmenopausal women who have undetected low bone mineral density.

Evidence Against Using Panoramic Radiographs to Screen for Osteoporosis

Mohajery and Brooks (1992) conducted a trial to determine whether radiographic changes could be detected in the mandible of patients with mild-to-moderate postmenopausal osteoporosis and whether these changes could be used as a diagnostic tool to differentiate normal from osteoporotic patients [52]. Subjects were classified as either osteoporotic ($n = 21$) or normal ($n = 14$) on the basis of bone density measurements of the lumbar spine and femoral neck, as determined by dual-photon absorptiometry. Mandibular bone density measurements were made on panoramic and periapical radiographs and expressed in terms of millimeters of aluminum equivalent. Thickness of the cortex at the angle of the mandible, sinus floor, and lamina dura of the tooth socket were also measured. There were no significant differences in any of the mandibular measurements between the normal and osteoporotic subjects. Whereas the skeletal bone measurements were correlated with each other, there was no correlation between skeletal and mandibular bone measurements. Women with mild-to-moderate osteoporosis could not be distinguished from women with normal bone density.

The panoramic mandibular index was used in a group of postmenopausal women to determine whether it correlates with bone mineral densities of the femoral neck, lumbar area, and the trabecular and cortical parts of the mandible [53]. Bone mineral density values were measured by dual-energy X-ray absorptiometry of the femoral neck and lumbar area and by quantitative computed tomography of the mandible. Linear correlation of the panoramic mandibular index with all bone mineral density values was weak. However, the low and high index subgroup means were clearly dependent on the bone mineral density variables. The authors concluded that despite significant differences in PMI between osteoporotic subjects and controls, panoramic assessment is not to be advocated as an assessment for osteoporosis.

Watson et al. (1995) investigated whether osteoporotic postmenopausal women show a decrease in mandibular cortical bone height, as measured by the PMI index, when compared with non-osteoporotic postmenopausal women [46]. Seventy-two Caucasian females (33 cases/39 controls), age range 54–71 years, were selected through records and screening via a dual-energy X-ray absorptiometry scan (LUNAR-DEXA). ANOVA analysis indicated no differences in the mean PMI between case and control groups (0.37 ± 0.15 and 0.38 ± 0.13, respectively; $p = 0.69$).

Osteoporosis and Periodontal Disease

A study of 227 healthy postmenopausal women aged 48–56 years was made to determine whether advanced alveolar bone loss, diagnosed by panoramic radiographs plus periodontal probing depths and the number of remaining teeth were correlated with the bone mineral status of the skeleton and cortical bone in the mandible [54]. The results indicated that individuals with high mineral values in the skeleton retained teeth with deep periodontal pockets more readily than did those exhibiting osteoporosis. Individuals with normal or high bone density seem to be best able to retain teeth despite advanced periodontal disease.

Studies have also suggested that osteoporosis and periodontitis are associated diseases. Persson et al. (2002) investigated: (1) the prevalence of self-reported history of osteoporosis in an older, ethnically diverse population; (2) the agreement between panoramic and mandibular cortical index findings and self-reported osteoporosis; and (3) the likelihood of having both a self-reported history of osteoporosis and a diagnosis of periodontitis [55]. Panoramic radiographs and medical histories were obtained from 1,084 female Chinese subjects aged 60–75 years (mean age 68 ± 5 years). Of the panoramic radiographs, 90% were deemed useful for analysis using mandibular cortical index. They were used to grade subjects as not having periodontitis or with one of three grades of periodontitis severity. A positive mandibular cortical index was found in 39% of the subjects, in contrast to 8% self-reported osteoporosis. The intra-class correlation between mandibular cortical index and self-reported osteoporosis was 0.20 ($p < 0.01$). The likelihood of an association between osteoporosis and mandibular cortical index was 3% (95% CI: 1.6, 4.1, $p < 0.001$). Subjects with self-reported osteoporosis and a positive mandibular cortical index had worse periodontal conditions ($p < 0.01$). The Mantel-Haentzel odds ratio for osteoporosis and periodontitis was 1.8 (95% CI: 1.2, 2.5, $p < 0.001$). The prevalence of positive mandibular cortical index was high and consistent with epidemiological studies, but only partly consistent with a self-reported history of osteoporosis with a higher prevalence of positive MCI. Horizontal alveolar bone loss was associated with both positive self-reported osteoporosis and mandibular cortical index findings.

Contrary findings were made by Lundstrom et al. (2001) [56]. The authors examined the periodontal conditions in an age cohort of 70-year-old women comparing an osteoporosis group with a control group with normal bone mineral density. Two hundred and ten women aged 70 years old were randomly sampled from the population register of the community of Linkoping, Sweden. Bone mineral density of the hip was measured by dual energy X-ray absorptiometry. Nineteen women were diagnosed with osteoporosis (bone mineral density <0.640 g/cm^2 in total hip) and 15 of them agreed to participate in the study. As a control group 21 women with normal bone mineral density (bone mineral density >0.881 g/cm^2) were randomly selected from the initial population. The clinical examination included registration of the number of remaining teeth, dental plaque, and periodontal conditions. The examination included a dental panoramic radiograph and vertical bitewings. The subjects completed a questionnaire on general health, age at menopause, concurrent medication, smoking, and oral hygiene habits. No statistically significant differences in gingival bleeding, probing pocket depths, gingival recession, and marginal bone level were found between the women with osteoporosis and those with normal bone mineral density. In conclusion, the study revealed no statistically significant differences in periodontal conditions or marginal bone level between the two groups; however, these results must be interpreted with caution since the compared groups were small.

Diabetes Mellitus

Diabetes mellitus is a common disorder of carbohydrate metabolism through either decreased production of insulin or tissue resistance to the effects of insulin [57]. The former (type 1 diabetes) is insulin-dependent; the latter (type 2 diabetes) is non-insulin-dependent and primarily treated by dietary modification. Taylor et al. (1998) tested the hypothesis that the risk for alveolar bone loss is greater, and bone loss progression more severe, for subjects with poorly controlled type 2 diabetes mellitus compared to individuals without type 2 diabetes or with better controlled disease [58]. The poorly controlled group had glycosylated hemoglobin (HbA1) >9%; the better controlled group had HbA1 <9%. The study was conducted among residents of the Gila River Indian Community. Of 359 subjects aged 15–57 years with less than 25% radiographic bone loss at baseline, 338 did not have diabetes, 14 were better controlled diabetics, and 7 were poorly controlled diabetics. Panoramic radiographs were used to assess interproximal bone level. Bone scores (scale 0–4) corresponding to bone loss of 0%, 1–24%, 25–49%, 50–74%, or >75% were used to identify the worst bone score in the dentition. Change in worst bone score at follow up was specified on a 4-category ordinal scale as no change, or a 1-, 2-, 3-, or 4-category increase over baseline. Poorly controlled diabetes, age, calculus, time to follow up examination, and initial worst bone score were statistically significant explanatory variables in ordinal logistic regression models. Poorly controlled type 2 diabetes mellitus was positively associated with greater risk for a change in bone score (compared to subjects without diabetes). The cumulative odds ratio at each threshold of the ordered response was 11 (95% CI = 2.5, 53.3). When contrasted with subjects with better controlled diabetes, the cumulative odds ratio for those in the poorly controlled group was 5 (95% CI = 0.8, 53.3). The cumulative odds ratio for subjects with better controlled diabetes was 2 (95% CI = 0.7, 6.5), when contrasted to those without diabetes. These results suggest that poorer glycemic control leads to both an increased risk for alveolar bone loss and more severe progression over those without type 2 diabetes mellitus. There may also be a gradient, with the risk for bone loss progression for those with better controlled type 2 diabetes, intermediate between those for poorly controlled diabetes and non-diabetics. Using panoramic radiographs, a case-control study performed on 664 Japanese men aged 46–57 years assessed periodontal disease. This investigation also demonstrated a correlation between the degree of failure of control of type 2 diabetes and the amount of alveolar bone loss [59].

Comparing diabetics to control subjects, a research report from Finland failed to demonstrate an increase in the microflora that could contribute to the increased rate of periodontitis in renal disease, or renal osteodystrophy [60]. The degree of marginal alveolar bone loss has also been assessed in a group of young subjects with type 1 diabetes mellitus [61]. A clear trend toward increased marginal bone loss was seen in the subjects with the poorest controlled diabetes. The subjects with good metabolic control and no complications were no more susceptible to marginal bone loss than non-diabetic controls of the same age.

Hyperparathyroidism

Primary hyperparathyroidism is relatively rare and results from an excess secretion of parathyroid hormones due to a hormone-producing benign or malignant neoplasm [62, 63]. Most persons with primary hyperparathyroidism are over age 60 years. Women are more commonly affected than men [57]. Secondary hyperparathyroidism results in excess secretion of parathyroid hormone due to parathyroid hyperplasia compensating for a metabolic disorder that has resulted in retention of phosphate or depletion of the serum calcium level [46]. Secondary hyperparathyroidism is most commonly found as a complication of end-stage in patients for whom hemodialysis is usually needed.

In Italy, 45 patients afflicted with chronic renal failure (29 men and 16 women; mean age: 48 years) and on hemodialysis for 4–245 months (mean = 67 months) were examined using panoramic images plus radiographs of the skull, hands, shoulders and clavicles, pelvis, and spine [64]. The control group (45 subjects with no renal diseases) was examined only by panoramic radiography. Dental and skeletal radiographs were rated on a 0–6 score and compared to assess possible relationships between skeletal and dental radiographic changes. Twenty-six dialysis patients (58% of all dialysis patients studied) had the following radiographic abnormalities in the jaws: osteoporosis (100%), lamina dura reduction or loss (27%), calcifications of soft tissues or salivary glands (15%), focal osteosclerosis adjacent to tooth roots (12%), and brown tumors (8%). Radiographic abnormalities in the hand, shoulder and pelvis were found in 51% of dialysis patients. In the control group, only 16% had jaw lesions including osteopenia, cortex reduction at the mandibular angles and cyst-like lesions. Caries and periodontal disease experience did not differ between the dialysis group and the controls. It was concluded that panoramic radiography is useful in monitoring renal osteodystrophy, especially to assess the response to therapy such as parathyroidectomy or renal transplantation.

A Bosnian study of panoramic and periapical radiographs of 42 patients receiving hemodialysis and having renal osteodystrophy, demonstrated a progressive increase in periodontal disease, loss of lamina dura, deviation in the trabecular pattern, brown tumor "pseudocyst" formation, and pulp calcifications [65].

The radiologic features of both forms of hyperparathyroidism are similar. These include generalized osteoporosis, unilocular or multilocular cystic radiolucencies in bone (brown tumor), attenuation or loss of lamina dura surrounding the teeth, and calcifications in muscles and subcutaneous tissues (Figs. 15.7, 15.8). It is often considered that histopathological study of a biopsy specimen is the basis for diagnosis of "cystic" lesions of the jaws. Unfortunately, the brown tumor provides no definitive histologic answer. Nuclear medicine or serologic confirmation is usually needed. The brown tumor lesion is composed of fibrous connective tissue containing areas of hemorrhage and foreign body-type multinucleated giant cells. This can be easily confused with other conditions such as the giant cell tumor, foreign body granuloma, aneurismal bone cyst, or osteoclastoma.

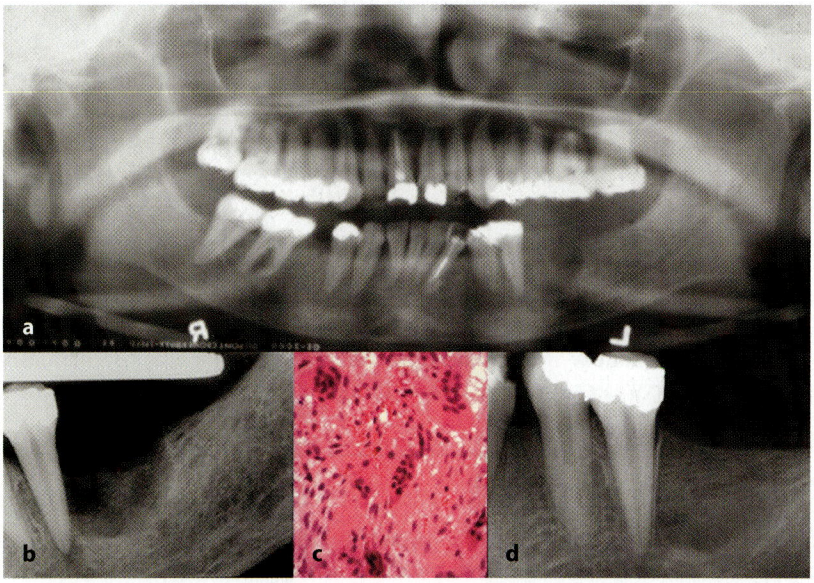

Fig. 15.7 Primary hyperparathyroidism. **a** Panoramic radiograph demonstrating unilocular cystic lesion distal to the left mandibular second premolar. **b** Periapical radiograph showing loss of lamina dura distal to the left mandibular second premolar tooth. **c** Histopathological study of the brown tumor showing numerous multinucleated giant cells. **d** The lesion healed and the lamina dura reconstituted following removal of the parathyroid tumor

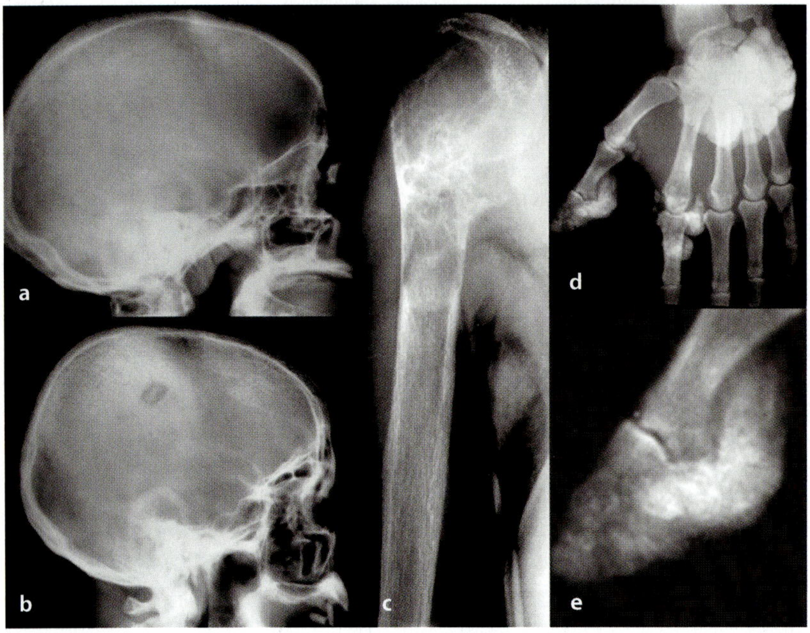

Fig. 15.8 Hyperparathyroidism. **a** Granular appearance of skull in patient having renal osteodystrophy. **b** Solitary "punched-out" radiolucency in calvarium represents a brown tumor in secondary hyperparathyroidism. **c** Right humerus shows coarse internal trabeculation in primary hyperparathyroidism (same case as shown in Fig. 15.7). **d** Metastatic calcifications in hand and wrist of patient with primary hyperparathyroidism. **e** Detail of calcifications adjacent to thumb

It was concluded that panoramic radiography is useful in monitoring renal osteodystrophy, especially to assess the response to therapy such as parathyroidectomy or renal transplantation.

Specific Infections

Not all systemic conditions that can produce jaw lesions are as common as the ones discussed above, but their detection is equally important for the correct treatment to be commenced. In the developed world there had been a decline in advanced lesions from specific infections; however, with a growing population of immune-compromised individuals as a result of the more widespread use of immunosuppressive regimens subsequent to organ transplantation, and through the AIDS-HIV epidemic, a resurgence of previously "vanquished" organisms is possible.

Tuberculosis

Tuberculosis is a specific infection caused by the acid-fast bacillus *Mycobacterium tuberculosis*. Almost all cases arise from pulmonary disease. Involvement of the oral tissues is rare, occurring in less than one in 50 with tuberculosis [45]. Oral tissues are involved through direct inoculation, extension from other infection sites, or hematogenous seeding. Patients with jawbone lesions complain of repeated attacks of "toothache-like" pain and there is usually swelling of the affected area. Sinus tracts develop as the swellings rupture and may drain intraorally or extraorally. Trismus may be present, especially if the temporomandibular joint is involved. Lesions within the jaws (Fig. 15.9) can be rarefactions with ill-defined borders. There may be periosteal new bone formation. Sequestration of necrotic bone can occur. In addition to tuberculous osteomyelitis, calcified lymph upper cervical nodes from tuberculosis may also be detected on panoramic radiographs.

Syphilis

Syphilis is caused by infection with the spirochete *Treponema pallidum*. It can be congenital or acquired after birth. The acquired form can be subclassified into three distinctive stages: primary, secondary, and tertiary. Bone can be affected in congenital syphilis and in both the secondary and tertiary stages of acquired syphilis (Fig. 15.10). The jaws are rarely affected by

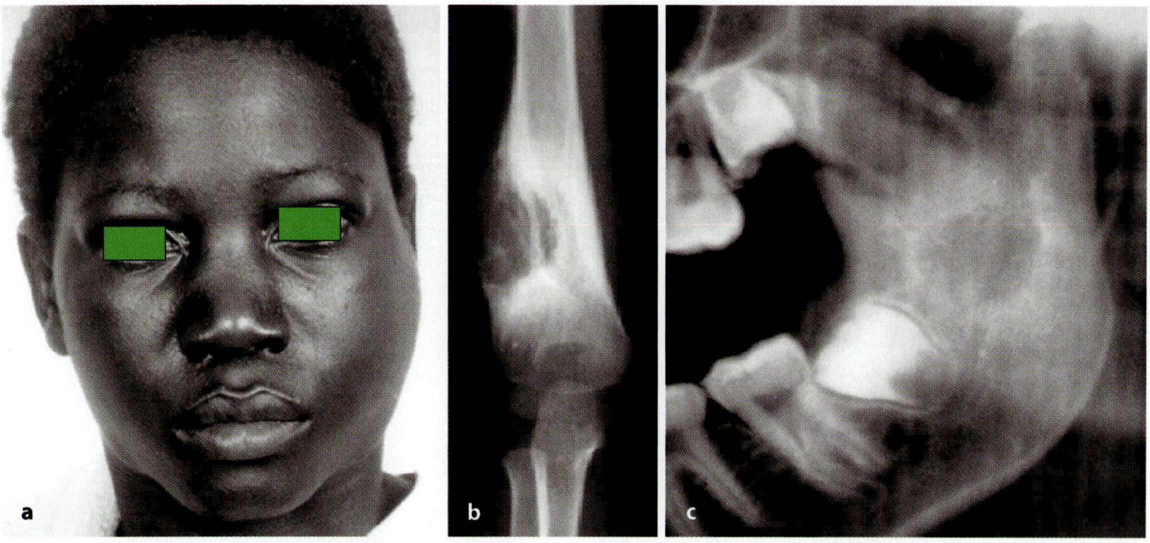

Fig. 15.9 Tuberculous osteomyelitis. **a** Facial swelling is a frequent feature of this uncommon presentation of tuberculosis. **b** Tuberculous osteomyelitis of long bone causing loss of cortical continuity. **c** Detail from panoramic radiograph shows irregular radiolucency below the mandibular notch (tuberculous osteomyelitis)

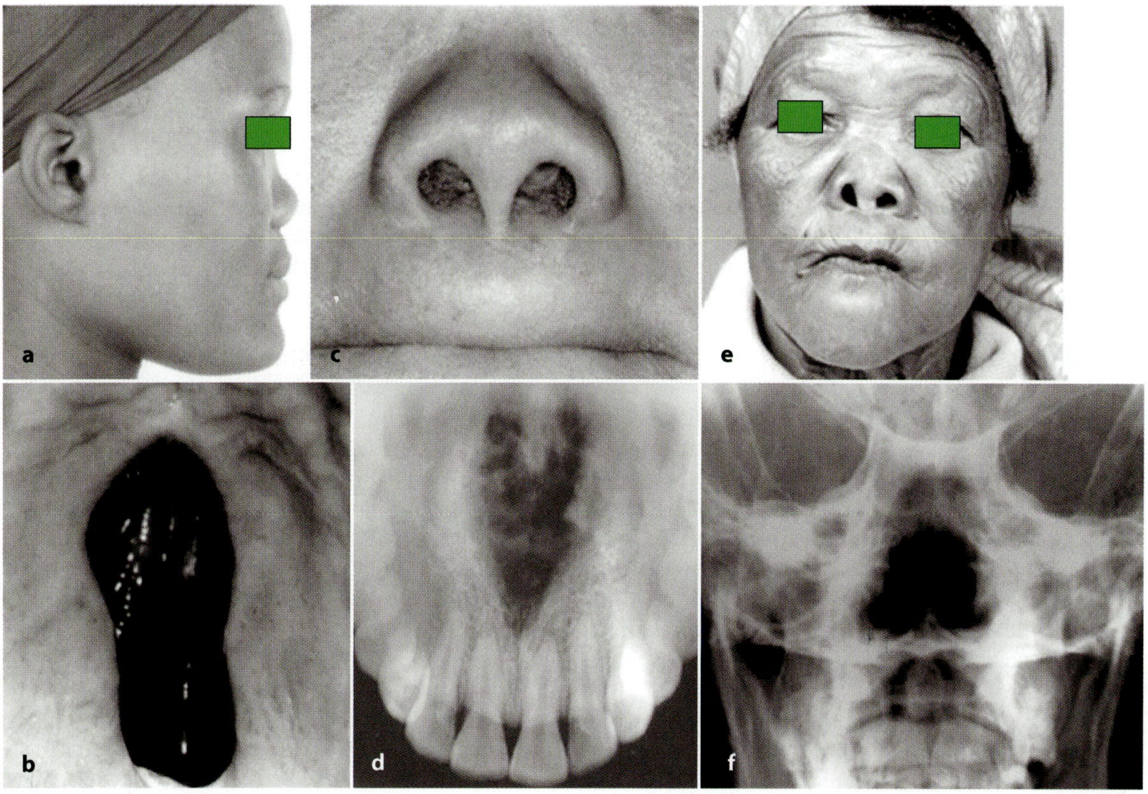

Fig. 15.10 **a–d** Congenital syphilis. (Note deficient bridge of nose.) Lytic lesions in the center of the palate are outside the panoramic focal trough. **e, f** Tertiary syphilis. (Note gummatous destruction in nasal cavity)

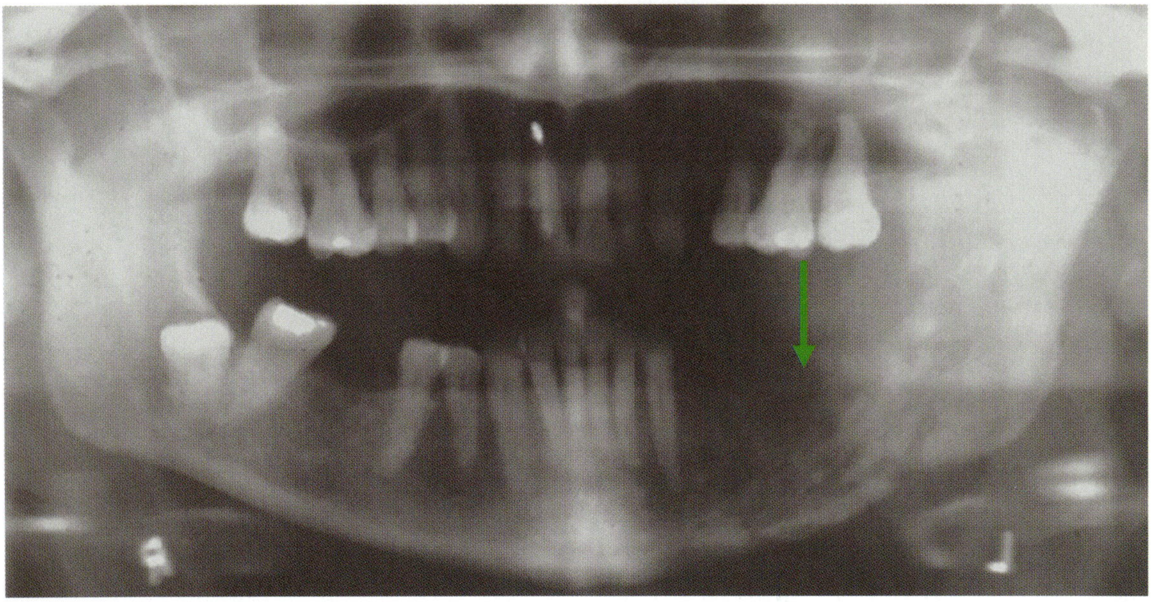

Fig. 15.11 Breast cancer metastasis to left mandibular body. Note "moth-eaten" appearance of the lesion and an associated pathological fracture

syphilis. When they are, the palate is more frequently involved than the mandible. Radiographic features of bone involvement by syphilis include: deposition of subperiosteal new bone along the inferior border of the mandible (syphilitic periostitis); gummatous destruction of bone, especially the palate, resulting in a large radiolucent area; well demarcated destruction along a cortical margin; or multiple radiolucencies with poorly defined margins and sequestration (syphilitic osteomyelitis).

Metastatic Malignancies

The cardinal radiographic signs of metastases to the jaw include a well circumscribed but uncorticated lytic lesion, especially in the posterior mandible, with highly irregular outline, or multiple small areas of bone destruction that gradually coalesce to form large ill-defined areas of bone destruction.

Metastatic tumors to the jaws are rarely reported; however, metastases might well constitute the most common malignant tumors affecting the skeleton [45]. Most metastases to bone are found in the spine, pelvis, skull, ribs, or the humerus. It is reported that approximately one per cent of malignant neoplasms metastasize to the jaws, and metastases comprise about one per cent of all oral malignancies. To qualify as a metastasis, the lesion must be localized to bone as distinguished from direct invasion—and it should be histopathologically verifiable as a metastasis. Most metastases occur in mature individuals over age 50 years.

The process of metastasis occurs by one of three routes: seeding of an adjacent body cavity, lymphatic spread, or hematogenous dissemination. The most common primary sites for tumors metastasizing to the jaws in adults are from organs below the clavicle, namely: breast, kidney, lung, colon, rectum, prostate, stomach, skin, testes, bladder, ovary, and cervix. Above the clavicle, the most frequent primary site for metastases to the jaw is the thyroid gland. In children metastatic disease is extremely rare. When this does occur in childhood, the primary cause is usually a neuroblastoma, retinoblastoma, or Wilms tumor. The clinical presentation of metastatic disease to the jaws is non-specific, including local pain, swelling, numbness, paresthesia of the lip and chin, and loosening or extrusion of the teeth. Pathological fractures may also occur but are considered rare (Fig. 15.11).

The cardinal radiographic signs of metastases to the jaw include a well circumscribed but uncorticated lytic lesion, especially in the posterior mandible, with highly irregular outline, or multiple small areas of bone destruction that gradually coalesce to form large ill-defined areas of bone destruction (Figs. 15.11, 15.12).

Ancillary signs include periapical or periradicular radiolucency or radio-opacity without evidence of pulpal pathology, failure of an extraction socket to heal, generalized loss of the lamina dura, or "floating" teeth.

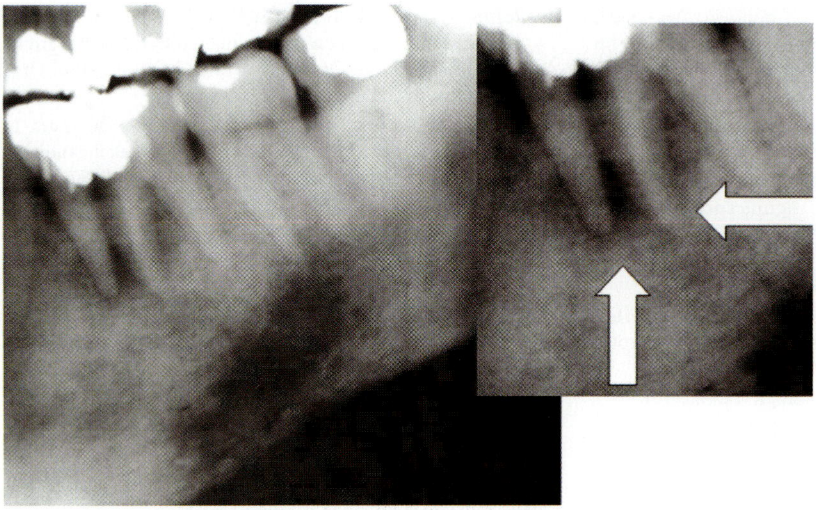

Fig. 15.12 Metastatic carcinoma. Note irregular "moth-eaten" rarefaction adjacent to first molar and second premolar teeth (detail from panoramic radiograph). Using the narrower perspective of a periapical radiograph, this lesion could well be misinterpreted as a simple "endo-perio" case

In a 12-month period, cancer metastatic to the mandible was diagnosed in eight patients at the Oral and Maxillofacial Surgery Clinic of the University of Vienna (1997) [66]. Six of them were presented with pain mimicking toothache, temporomandibular joint disorders, or trigeminal neuralgia, and two showed osteopenic bone lesions on panoramic radiography combined with perimandibular swelling. Anesthesia of the lower lip was the one common clinical feature in all eight cases. Histology revealed breast, lung, renal cancer, and a malignancy of inconclusive origin. Thirty metastases of malignant tumors in jaws were retrospectively studied in the Pathology Department of the Hospital de la Pitié, Paris, France (1991) [67]. They occurred more often in women than in men (17 females:13 males). In 21 cases, the primary cancer was known and had been treated 1–4 years earlier. In the other nine cases, discovery of the bone metastasis led to the discovery of a latent tumor. Clinical signs and symptoms included swelling, pain, loosening of teeth, and labio-mental anesthesia, but rarely pathological fracture. All but two patients had a radiolucent lesion. The metastases almost always involved the mandible (95%), most often in the molar area or angle. Histologically, the majority of lesions were adenocarcinomas from breast (33%) and alimentary canal (stomach, colon). Epidermoid bronchial carcinomas were seen in five cases and malignant melanomas in two cases. Only one sarcoma was involved, and this was from a liposarcoma of the thigh. In all but one patient, the disease was lethal over the short run.

Early detection can lead to appropriate treatment and alleviation of untoward side affects. This is an area where the dentist may well save a life.

Concluding Remarks

While some controversy remains concerning the value of using panoramic radiographs in the screening of systemic diseases, the dentist should be capable of detecting features of such conditions when they produce changes on panoramic radiographs. Such conditions can have a major impact on the quality of life of afflicted patients. Early detection can lead to appropriate treatment and alleviation of untoward side affects. This is an area where the dentist may well save a life.

References

1. American Heart Association. Heart disease and stroke statistics: 2006 update. Dallas: American Heart Association; 2006
2. Executive Committee for Asymptomatic Carotid Atherosclerosis Study. Endarterectomy for asymptomatic carotid artery stenosis. JAMA 1995;273:1421–1428
3. Chimowitz MI, Weiss DG, Cohen SN, Starling MR, Hobson RW 2nd. Cardiac prognosis of patients with carotid stenosis and no history of coronary artery disease. Stroke 1994;25:759–765

4. Cohen SN, Hobson RW, Weiss DG, Chimowitz MI. Death associated with asymptomatic carotid stenosis: long term clinical evaluation. VA Cooperative Study Group 167. J Vasc Surg 1993;18:1002–1009
5. Friedlander AH, Lande A. Panoramic radiographic identification of carotid arterial plaques. Oral Surg Oral Med Oral Pathol 1981;52:102–104
6. Friedlander AH, Golub MS. The significance of carotid artery atheromas on panoramic radiographs in the diagnosis of occult metabolic syndrome. Oral Surg Oral Med Oral Pathol Oral Radiol Endod 2006;101:95–101
7. Farman AG, Farman TT, Khan Z, Chen Z, Carter LC, Friedlander AH. The role of the dentist in detection of carotid atherosclerosis. SADI 2001;56:549–553
8. Ohba T, Takata Y, Ansai T, Morimoto Y, Tanaka T, Kito S, Awano S, Akifusa S, Takehara T. Evaluation of calcified carotid artery atheromas detected by panoramic radiograph among 80-year-olds. Oral Surg Oral Med Oral Pathol Oral Radiol Endod 2003;96:647–650
9. Almog DM, Illig KA, Carter LC, Friedlander AH, Brooks SL, Grimes RM. Diagnosis of non-dental conditions. Carotid artery calcifications on panoramic radiographs identify patients at risk for stroke. N Y State Dent J 2004;70:20–25
10. Carter LC. Discrimination between calcified triticeous cartilage and calcified carotid atheroma on panoramic radiography. Oral Surg Oral Med Oral Pathol Oral Radiol Endod 2000;90:108–110
11. Friedlander AH. Identification of stroke-prone patients by panoramic and cervical spine radiography. Dentomaxillofac Radiol 1995;24:160–164
12. Ahmad M, Madden R, Perez L. Triticeous cartilage: prevalence on panoramic radiographs and diagnostic criteria. Oral Surg Oral Med Oral Pathol Oral Radiol Endod 2005;99:225–230
13. Kamikawa RS, Pereira MF, Fernandes A, Meurer MI. Study of the localization of radiopacities similar to calcified carotid atheroma by means of panoramic radiography. Oral Surg Oral Med Oral Pathol Oral Radiol Endod 2006;101:374–378
14. Friedlander AH, Baker JD. Panoramic radiography: an aid in detecting patients at risk of cerebrovascular accident. J Am Dent Assoc 1994;125:1598–1603
15. Almog DM, Horev T, Illig KA, Green RM, Carter LC. Correlating carotid artery stenosis detected by panoramic radiography with clinically relevant carotid artery stenosis determined by duplex ultrasound. Oral Surg Oral Med Oral Pathol Oral Radiol Endod 2002;94:768–773
16. Bayram B, Uckan S, Acikgoz A, Muderrisoglu H, Aydinalp A. Digital panoramic radiography: a reliable method to diagnose carotid artery artheromas? Dentomaxillofac Radiol 2006;35:266–270
17. Grant EG, Benson CB, Moneta GL, Alexandrov AV, Baker JD, Bluth EI, Carroll BA, Eliasziw M, Gocke J, Hertzberg BS, Katanick S, Needleman L, Pellerito J, Polak JF, Rholl KS, Wooster DL, Zierler RE. Carotid artery stenosis: gray-scale and Doppler US diagnosis. Society of Radiologists in Ultrasound Consensus Conference. Radiology 2003;229:340–346
18. Friedlander AH, Garrett NR, Chin EE, Baker JD. Ultrasonographic confirmation of carotid artery atheromas diagnosed via panoramic radiography. J Am Dent Assoc 2005;136:635–640
19. Pornprasertsuk-Damrongsri S, Thanakun S. Carotid artery calcification detected on panoramic radiographs in a group of Thai population. Oral Surg Oral Med Oral Pathol Oral Radiol Endod 2006;101:110–115
20. Tamura T, Inui M, Nakase M, Nakamura S, Okumura K, Tagawa T. Clinicostatistical study of carotid calcification on panoramic radiographs. Oral Dis 2005;11:314–317
21. Manzi FR, Boscolo FN, de Almeida SM, Haiter Neto F. Panoramic radiography as an auxiliary in detecting patients at risk for cerebrovascular accident (CVA): a case report. J Oral Sci 2003;45:177–180
22. Friedlander AH, Maeder LA. The prevalence of calcified carotid atheromas on the panoramic radiographs of patients with type 2 diabetes mellitus. Oral Surg Oral Med Oral Pathol Oral Radiol Endod 2000;89:420–424
23. Friedlander AH, Garrett NR, Norman DC. The prevalence of calcified carotid artery atheromas on panoramic radiographs of patients with type 2 diabetes mellitus. J Am Dent Assoc 2002;133:1516–1523
24. Friedlander AH, Friedlander IK, Yueh R, Littner MR. The prevalence of carotid atheromas seen on panoramic radiographs of patients with obstructive sleep apnea and their relation to risk factors for atherosclerosis. J Oral Maxillofac Surg 1999;57:516–521
25. Friedlander AH, Altman L. Carotid artery atheromas in postmenopausal women. Their prevalence on panoramic radiographs and their relationship to atherogenic risk factors. J Am Dent Assoc 2001;132:1130–1136
26. Kansu O, Ozbek M, Avcu N, Genctoy G, Kansu H, Turgan C. The prevalence of carotid artery calcification on the panoramic radiographs of patients with renal disease. Dentomaxillofac Radiol 2005;34:16–19
27. O'Hare AM, Rodriguez RA, Bacchetti P. Low ankle-brachial index associated with rise in creatinine level over time: results from the atherosclerosis risk in communities study. Arch Intern Med 2005;165:1481–1485
28. Friedlander AH, August M. The role of panoramic radiography in determining an increased risk of cervical atheromas inpatients treated with therapeutic irradiation. Oral Surg Oral Med Oral Pathol Oral Radiol Endod 1998;85:339–344
29. Friedlander AH, Eichstaedt RM, Friedlander IK, Lambert PM. Detection of radiation induced, accelerated atherosclerosis in patients with osteoradionecrosis by panoramic radiography. J Oral Maxillofac Surg 1998; 56:455–459
30. Friedlander AH, Freymiller EG. Detection of radiation accelerated atherosclerosis of the carotid artery by panoramic radiography. A new opportunity for dentists. J Am Dent Assoc 2003;134:1361–1365
31. Takashi W, Tsutomu F, Kentaro F. Ultrasonic correlates of common carotid atherosclerosis in patients with coronary artery disease. Angiology 2002;53:177–183
32. Oei HH, Vliegenthart R, Hak AE, Iglesias del Sol A, Hofman A, Oudkerk M, Witteman JC. The association between coronary calcification assessed by electron beam computed tomography and measures of extracoronary atherosclerosis: the Rotterdam Coronary Calcification Study. J Am Coll Cardiol 2002;39:1745–1751
33. Chambless LE, Folsom AR, Davis V, Sharrett R, Heiss G, Sorlie P, Howard G, Evans GW. Risk factors for progression of common carotid atherosclerosis: The Atherosclerosis Risk in Communities Study, 1987–1998. Am J Epidemiol 2002;155:38–47

34. Woodworth W, Genco RJ, Carter LC. Calcified carotid artery plaque as a predictor of CVD death (abstract). J Dent Res 2000;79:524
35. Cohen SN, Friedlander AH, Jolly DA, Date L. Carotid calcification on panoramic radiographs: an important marker for vascular risk. Oral Surg Oral Med Oral Pathol Oral Radiol Endod 2002;94:510–514
36. Cohen SN, Friedlander AH, Krauss T, Date L, Jolly DA, Kankar P. Calcifications as a risk factor for vascular disease: a case-controlled study (abstract). Neurology 2002;58(3Suppl):A314
37. Friedlander AH, Cohen SN. Panoramic radiographic atheromas portend adverse vascular events. Oral Surg Oral Med Oral Pathol Oral Radiol Endod 2007 Jan 26; [Epub ahead of print]
38. Tanaka T, Morimoto Y, Ansai T, Okabe S, Yamada K, Taguchi A, Awano S, Kito S, Takata Y, Takehara T, Ohba T. Can the presence of carotid artery calcification on panoramic radiographs predict the risk of vascular diseases among 80-year-olds? Oral Surg Oral Med Oral Pathol Oral Radiol Endod 2006;101:777–783
39. American Dental Association's Survey Center. The 2000 Survey of Dental Practice: Characteristics of Dentists and Their Patients. Chicago, IL: American Dental Association; 2002
40. Grimes RM, Richards E, Flaitz CM. Avoiding malpractice for non-dental conditions. The example of the human immunodeficiency virus. J Am Dent Assoc 2001;132:499–507
41. Almog DM. Time for dentistry to step up to the plate. N Y State Dent J 2005;71:11
42. Roldan-Chicano R, Onate-sanchez RE, Lopez-Castano F, Cabrerizo-Merino MC, Martinez-Lopez F. Panoramic radiograph as a method for detecting calcified atheroma plaques. Review of literature. Med Oral Patol Oral Cir Buca 2006;11:E261–E266
43. Barkhuysen R, Berge SJ, van Damme PA. Non ordinary radiopacity on a panoramic radiograph. Ned Tijdschr Tandheelkd 2006;113:148–149
44. Mohammad AR, Alder M, McNally MA. A pilot study of panoramic film density at selected sites in the mandible to predict osteoporosis. Int J Prosthodont 1996;9:290–294
45. Farman AG, Nortjé CJ, Wood RE. Oral and maxillofacial diagnostic imaging. St Louis: Mosby-Year Book; 1993
46. Watson EL, Katz RV, Adelezzi R, Gift HC, Dunn SM. The measurement of mandibular cortical bone height in osteoporotic vs. non-osteoporotic postmenopausal women. Spec Care Dentist 1995;15:124–128
47. Benson BW, Prihoda TJ, Glass BJ. Variations in adult cortical bone mass as measured by a panoramic mandibular index. Oral Surg Oral Med Oral Pathol 1991;71:349–356
48. Taguchi A, Tanimoto K, Suei Y, Otani K, Wada T. Oral signs as indicators of possible osteoporosis in elderly women. Oral Surg Oral Med Oral Pathol Oral Radiol Endod 1995;80:612–616
49. Taguchi A, Suei Y, Ohtsuka M, Otani K, Tanimoto K, Ohtaki M. Usefulness of panoramic radiography in the diagnosis of postmenopausal osteoporosis in women. Width and morphology of inferior cortex of the mandible. Dentomaxillofac Radiol 1996;25:263–267
50. Horner K, Devlin H, Harvey L. Detecting patients with low skeletal bone mass. J Dent 2002;30:171–175
51. Nakamoto T, Taguchi A, Ohtsuka M, Suei Y, Fujita M, Tanimoto K, Tsuda M, Sanada M, Ohama K, Takahashi J, Rohlin M. Dental panoramic radiograph as a tool to detect postmenopausal women with low bone mineral density: untrained general dental practitioners' diagnostic performance. Osteoporos Int 2003;14:659–664
52. Mohajery M, Brooks SL. Oral radiographs in the detection of early signs of osteoporosis. Oral Surg Oral Med Oral Pathol 1992;73:112–117
53. Klemetti E, Kolmakov S, Heiskanen P, Vainio P, Lassila V. Panoramic mandibular index and bone mineral densities in postmenopausal women. Oral Surg Oral Med Oral Pathol 1993;75:774–779
54. Klemetti E, Collin HL, Forss H, Markkanen H, Lassila V. Mineral status of skeleton and advanced periodontal disease. J Clin Periodont 1994;21:184–188
55. Persson RE, Hollender LG, Powell LV, MacEntee MI, Wyatt CC, Kiyak HA, Persson GR. Assessment of periodontal conditions and systemic disease in older subjects. I. Focus on osteoporosis. J Clin Periodontol 2002;29:796–802
56. Lundstrom A, Jendle J, Stenstrom B, Toss G, Ravald N. Periodontal conditions in 70-year-old women with osteoporosis. Swed Dent J 2001;25:89–96
57. Neville BW, Damm DD, Allen CM, Bouquot JE. Oral and maxillofacial pathology. Philadelphia: Saunders; 1995
58. Taylor GW, Burt BA, Becker MP, Genco RJ, Shlossman M. Glycemic control and alveolar bone loss progression in type 2 diabetes. Ann Periodontol 1998;3:30–39
59. Marugame T, Hayasaki H, Lee K, Eguchi H, Matsumoto S. Alveolar bone loss associated with glucose tolerance in Japanese men. Diabet Med 2003;20:746–751
60. Collin HL, Uusitupa M, Niskanen L, Kontturi-Narhi V, Markkanen H, Koivisto AM, Meurman JH. Periodontal findings in elderly patients with non-insulin dependent diabetes mellitus. J Periodontol 1998;69:962–966
61. Tervonen T, Karjalainen K, Knuuttila M, Huumonen S. Alveolar bone loss in type 1 diabetic subjects. J Clin Periodontol 2000;27:567–571
62. Morano S, Cipriani R, Gabriele A, Medici F, Pantellini F. Recurrent Brown tumors as initial manifestation of primary hyperparathyroidism. An unusual presentation. Minerva Med 2000;91:117–122
63. Migita H, Ohno A. Oral bony lesion in a patient with medical history of hyperparathyroidism. Int J Oral Surg 1979;8:67–70
64. Scutellari PN, Orzincolo C, Bedani PL, Romano C. Radiographic manifestations in teeth and jaws in chronic kidney insufficiency. Radiol Med (Torino) 1996;92:415–420
65. Ganibegovic M. Dental radiographic changes in chronic renal diseases. Med Arh 2000;54:115–118
66. Glaser C, Lang S, Pruckmayer M, Millesi W, Rasse M, Marosi C, Leitha T. Clinical manifestations and diagnostic approach to metastatic cancer of the mandible. Int J Oral Maxillofac Surg 1997;26:365–368
67. Auriol M, Chomette G, Wann A, Guilbert F. Metastases of malignant tumor in the jaw. Analysis of 30 case reports. Rev Stomatol Chir Maxillofac 1991;92:155–159

TEST: Panoramic radiographic detection of systemic disease

1. Type 1 diabetes is non-insulin-dependent and primarily treated by dietary modification.

   True ☐ **False** ☐

2. When malignant metastases to the jaws occur in childhood, the most frequent. primary sites are the stomach, bladder, and liver.

   True ☐ **False** ☐

3. Involvement of the oral tissues by tuberculosis is rare, occurring in less than 1 in 50 with tuberculosis.

   True ☐ **False** ☐

4. Osteoporosis can lead to pathological fracture, loss of physical stature, and severe kyphosis.

   True ☐ **False** ☐

5. Secondary hyperparathyroidism results in excess secretion of parathyroid hormone due to compensating for a metabolic disorder that has resulted in retention of phosphate or depletion of serum calcium.

   True ☐ **False** ☐

6. Studies have reported lip paresthesia to be an unusual feature of metastases to the mandible.

   True ☐ **False** ☐

7. The value of using panoramic radiographs in screening for osteoporosis remains debatable.

   True ☐ **False** ☐

8. Syphilis is caused by infection with the spirochete *Treponema pallidum* and may be associated with bone changes both in congenital and acquired forms.

   True ☐ **False** ☐

9. Brown tumors of hyperparathyroidism are definitively diagnosed by basic histologic analysis.

   True ☐ **False** ☐

10. Dual-energy X-ray absorptiometry is used to assess bone mineral density.

    True ☐ **False** ☐

Panoramic Radiology: Oncologic Dentistry Considerations

16

Allan G. Farman
in association with Zafrulla Khan

Learning Objectives

After studying this article, the reader should be able to:

- Define oncologic dentistry
- Understand role played by panoramic radiology in helping to obviate serious side effects of cancer treatment by facilitating early detection and treatment of complications to therapy
- Describe the radiographic signs of osteoradionecrosis

Panoramic radiology can serve as an important input supporting the practice of oncologic dentistry. Not only are panoramic radiographs of value in the determination of the distribution of detected malignancies, they are also important (1) for planning dental treatment in preparation of the oral cavity prior to chemotherapy and radiation to reduce subsequent complications of cancer therapies; (2) for early detection of maxillofacial complications of cancer therapy when they do occur; and (3) to assist in detection of recurrent tumors within the maxillofacial complex. The dentist knowledgeable in oncologic dentistry can greatly assist in improving quality of life outcomes for many cancer patients receiving systemic chemotherapy, and also for patients receiving head and neck radiation therapy and/or surgery to treat head and neck tumors.

A comprehensive oral and dental screening should be part of the pretreatment workup of patients with cancer, especially those who have head and neck tumors (Fig. 16.1) [1–3]. This screening needs to be performed by a dentist who is familiar with the pathological process of disease and the type of treatment being rendered; and who comprehends the seriousness associated with eradicating malignancy. It has been estimated that as many as 400,000 out of 1 million patients newly diagnosed with malignancies in the US each year develop oral complications of cancer treatment, especially from systemic chemotherapy, but also from head and neck radiation therapy [4]. The trend toward people maintaining their teeth longer coupled with the rising age of the population suggest that dentists will be frequently treating patients with cancer, and should be informed about aspects of oncologic care that will affect oral health [4]. Unfortunately, however, when the cancer curricula of US dental schools was investigated in 1999, it was found that deficits in oncologic dentistry education included failure to provide practical clinical oncology experience in diagnosis, the decision-making process, referral procedures, management of oral complications of cancer therapy, and maxillofacial rehabilitation; and psychosocial training in oncology [5].

This chapter is intended as a primer for practitioners, most of whom undoubtedly will need to deal with cancer patients. The panoramic radiograph should be viewed as central to diagnosis, treatment planning, and follow up in such patients.

What is Oncologic Dentistry?

Oncologic dentistry consists of the oral and dental care of patients receiving treatment for cancer, especially when that treatment involves systemic chemotherapy or radiation to the head and neck region. The oncologic dentist is responsible for: (1) assuring that the oral cavity is prepared to reduce potential side effects of treatment; (2) educating the cancer patient as to the possible short-term and long-term complications, no matter what anti-cancer therapies are used; (3) training the cancer patient in oral hygiene methods and therapeutics needed to preserve oral health; (4) where necessary fabricating intraoral shields and positioners for radiation therapy; (5) provision of services to correct surgical defects consequent to cancer treatment (often requiring special training in maxillofacial prosthodontics); and (6) long-term follow up, evaluation, and treatment of the cancer patient for complications of therapy—always with an eye to the possibility of cancer recurrence [1–3, 6–10]. The oncologic dentist should provide the timeline for the surgeon, medical oncologist, and radiation oncologist in which all necessary dental treatment will be completed [1]. The oncologic dentist plays an important role in the prevention, stabilization, and treatment of oral and dental problems that can compromise the

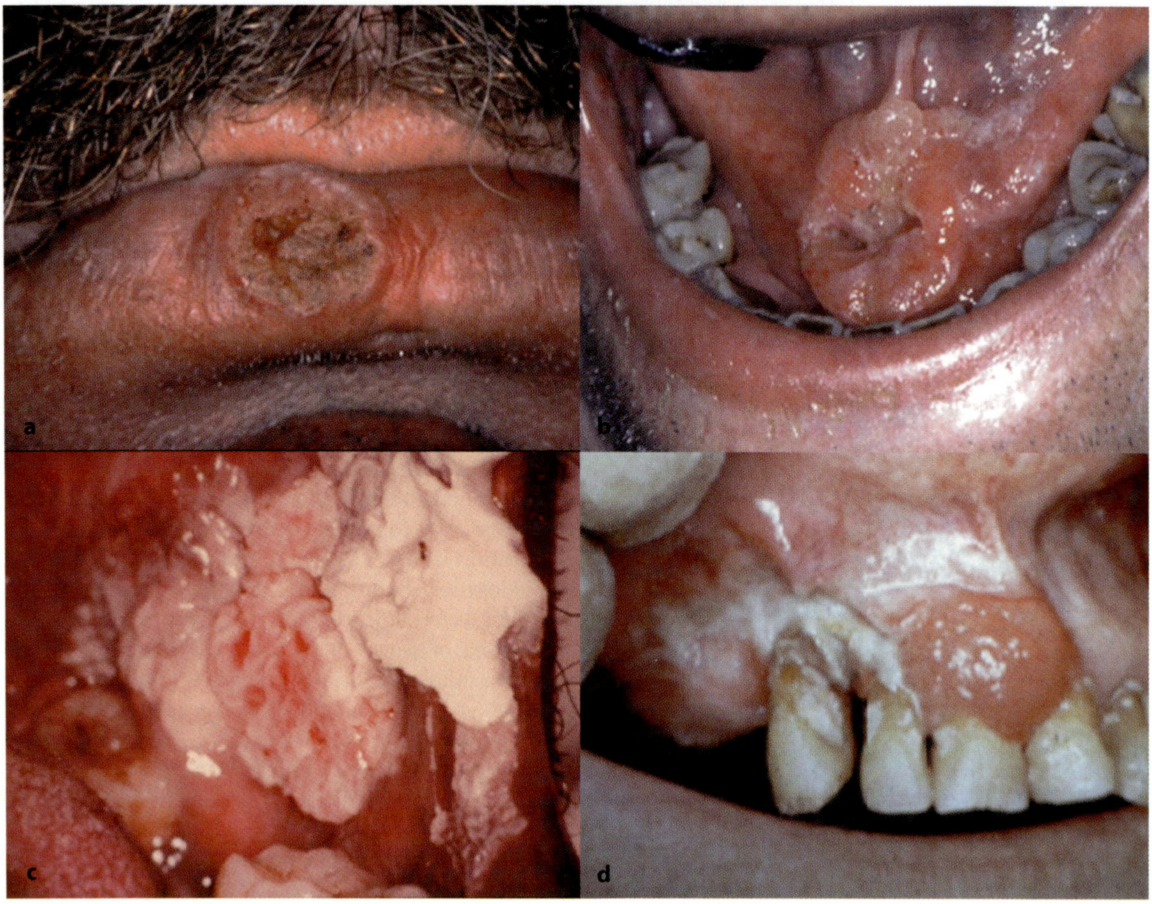

Fig. 16.1 Clinical features of moderately advanced oral squamous cell carcinoma. **a** Lower lip: keratotic ulcer with the inner portion white due to moistening from saliva. **b** Floor of mouth. **c** Buccal mucosa of a patient from the Indian subcontinent: mixed leukoplakia and erythroplakia (white and red patches). **d** Gingival carcinoma in a pipe smoker

cancer patient's health and quality of life during and after the cancer treatment.

Moizan et al. (2003) sent a questionnaire to 164 practitioners caring for head and neck cancer patients to question dental treatment provision [11]. The absence of a dental consultation was considered a serious problem that could impair preventive care and prosthetic rehabilitation, potentially reducing life quality.

The frequency of oral cancer as a percentage of all cancers varies tremendously from geographic region to geographic region. In the USA and Europe, oral cancer represents approximately 3–5% of all cancers, whereas in the Indian subcontinent the proportion can be one third or more. Oral cancers found in the US and European populations are most frequent on the lower lip due to solar radiation and floor of the mouth and upper aerodigestive tract through smoking habits. Lesions of the cheek mucosa are more common in persons from India, perhaps due in part to the habit of chewing betel nut combined with tobacco and slaked lime. Figure 16.1 illustrates typical clinical features of fairly advanced oral squamous cell carcinomas. Approximately 85% of all upper aerodigestive tract malignancies are squamous cell carcinomas.

The panoramic radiograph is a vital tool in the hands of the oncologic dentist (Figs. 16.2, 16.3). In addition to sometimes providing the first evidence of maxillofacial cancer, the panoramic radiograph provides a valuable overview of the baseline conditions of the teeth and jaws. This baseline can help in pre-therapy dental treatment planning, and also acts as a baseline source of comparison for subsequent panoramic radiographs made during post-therapy evaluations. As the oral cavity can be extremely sore and friable during and initially following radiation or chemotherapy, the extraoral nature of the panoramic radiographic approach is more readily facilitated than the use of intraoral series of radiographs. Further, the wider anatomic scope of

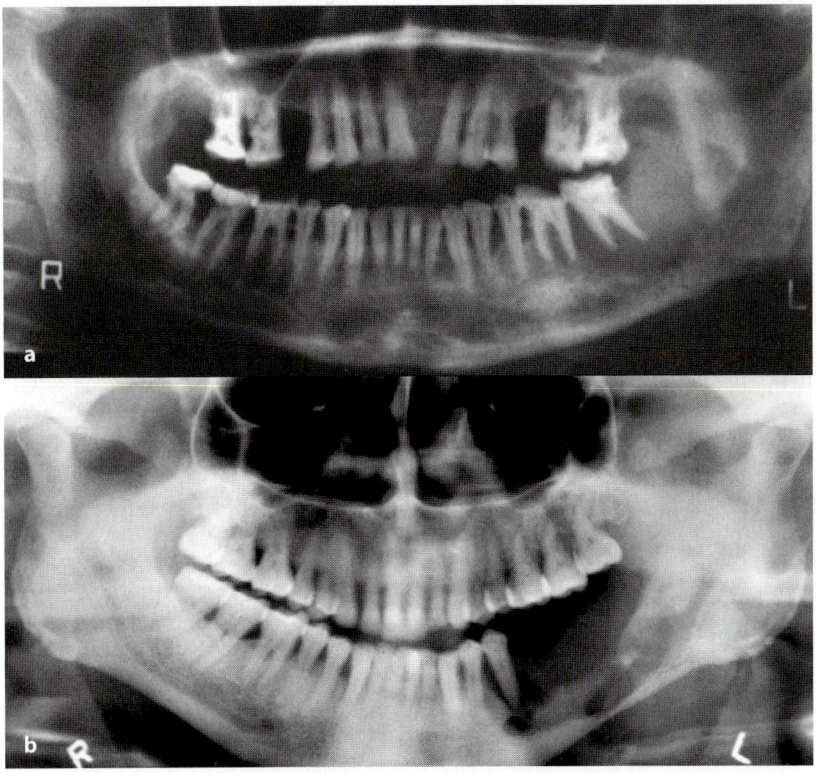

Fig. 16.2 **a**, **b** Panoramic radiographs from patients having advanced oral cancer with secondary invasion of the mandible. Note the "saucerization" of the upper surface of the left side of the mandible in both of these cases. Both cases also show "floating teeth" where supporting bone has been destroyed. Case (**b**) shows invasion of the mandibular canal

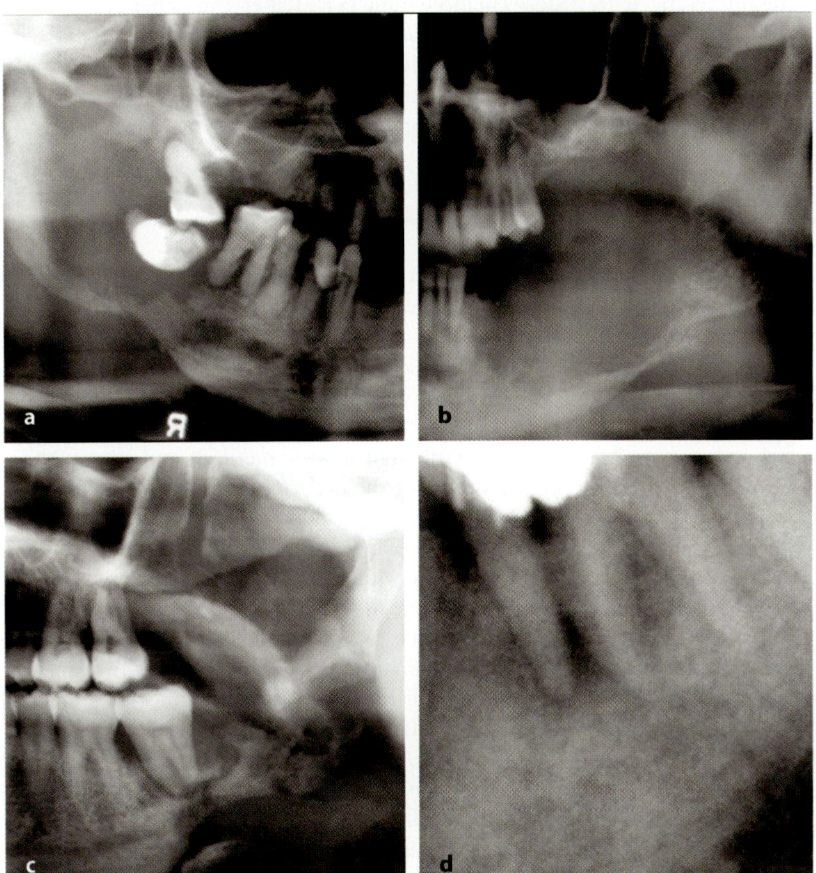

Fig. 16.3 Panoramic radiograph details. **a, b** Invasion of the mandible from intraoral cancer. Saucerization has extended almost to the lower border of the mandible in these cases, and both mandibles have undergone pathological fracture. **c**, **d** Malignancies central within the mandible. Case **c** also shows a pathological fracture and involvement of the mandibular canal. Case (**d**) is metastatic breast cancer and demonstrates irregular erosion arising centrally within the mandible

the panoramic radiograph can be of value in detecting changes that would be excluded in periapical radiography. Of particular concern are dental infections that can be exacerbated during therapy, and occasionally may precursor osteoradionecrosis. The oncologic dentist also needs to look for tumor recurrences, metastatic lesions (Fig. 16.3d), and second primary tumors that might occur following cancer treatment [12].

Cancer Therapy Effects on Oral Tissues

Radiation therapy and chemotherapy are particularly effective in destroying rapidly dividing cells, hence their value in cancer treatment [13]. The tissues of the oral mucosa, the salivary glands, and blood vessels can be damaged as the result of such therapies. Head and neck cancer patients often experience unwanted oral effects that have both short-term and long-term implications.

Oral Mucositis

Oral mucositis is a common side effect of radiation and certain chemotherapy agents (Figs. 16.4, 16.5). Luglie et al. (2002) made a longitudinal evaluation of 30 patients undergoing antineoplastic chemotherapy with 5-fluoruracil at the Department of Oncology of the University of Sassari, Italy [14]. The study lasted one year. The research subjects underwent professional oral hygiene, were educated in home oral hygiene, and prescribed antibacterial rinses. The control group of 33 patients was not provided supplemental dental services. Visible plaque and gingival bleeding were recorded for each patient. The mucosa was evaluated according to the WHO index. The values of the bleeding and plaque indices were considerably diminished between the first and the last visit, in nearly all the patients; the incidence of oral mucositis in the treated group was 20%, while in the control group it was 66%. It was concluded that professional and home oral hygiene and the use of antibacterial rinses (chlorhexidine), can reduce the incidence of oral mucositis as a side effect of chemotherapy [14].

Xerostomia

Xerostomia, commonly called "dry mouth," is not infrequent among patients who have been treated with head and neck radiation therapy [15]. It can also be a side effect of certain medications, and of connective tissue or immunological disorders (e.g., Sjögren syndrome). Xerostomia from radiation therapy often is associated with a reduction in salivary flow. Complications of xerostomia include increased dental caries—"radiation caries" (Fig. 16.6), infections, and difficulty with the use of removable dentures [15]. Remedies for xerostomia usually are palliative, but could be minimized by using radiation shields and positioners to shield normal tissues.

Periodontal Disease

Marques and Dib (2004) studied periodontal changes in patients undergoing head and neck radiation therapy in Sao Paulo, Brazil [16]. Clinical periodontal parameters (probing depth, clinical attachment level, gingival recession, plaque index, and bleeding on probing) were assessed on 27 patients before and 6–8 months following radiation therapy. The greatest changes occurred in clinical attachment level: overall, 70% of the patients showed a loss, with 92% of these evidencing loss in the mandible. Attachment loss was directly related to the field of radiation and was greater when the jaws were actually included in the irradiated area. It was concluded that periodontal status should be evaluated prior to and following radiation therapy in the head and neck region to help ensure that periodontal health is maintained in oncology patients. The infected periodontium can act as a focus for systemic infection in cancer patients suffering neutropenia as a result of high-dose chemotherapy [17]. Raber-Durlacher et al. (2002) conclude that assessment of a patient's periodontal condition before the onset of profound neutropenia is critical to the diagnosis and the management of potentially life-threatening infections [17].

Osteonecrosis

Late complications such as osteoradionecrosis are attributed to radiation therapy (see Figs. 16.5–16.8) [18–20]. The long-term problems largely arise from blood vessel damage, essentially endarteritis obliterans, reducing tissue vascularity (Figs. 16.8, 16.9). The interpretation of data derived from particular series can be difficult due to the different scoring methods and classification systems used for the evaluation of post-radiation bone damage [19]. The incidence of osteoradionecrosis in head and neck cancer patients treated with radiation therapy, varies widely in the literature from 0.4% to 56% [19]. Although osteoradionecrosis occurs typically in the first three years after radiation therapy, patients probably remain at indefinite risk. Factors that may be associated with the risk of osteoradionecrosis include treatment-related variables such as radiation therapy dose, field size, and volume of the mandible irradiated with a high dose; patient-related variables such as periodontitis, pre-irradiation bone surgery, oral hygiene, alcohol and tobacco abuse, and dental extraction following radiation therapy; and tumor-related factors such as lesion size and lesion proximity to bone.

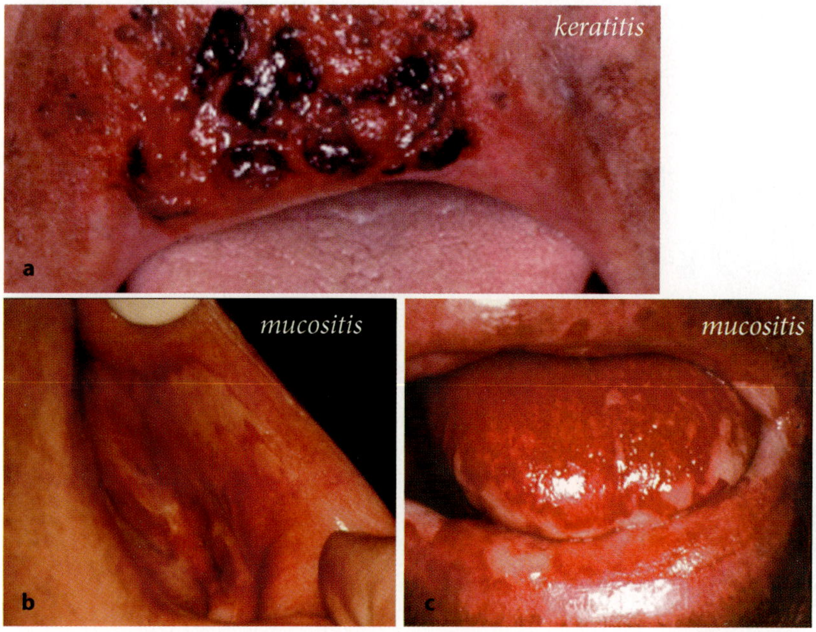

Fig. 16.4 Post-irradiation keratitis (**a**) and mucositis (**b, c**)

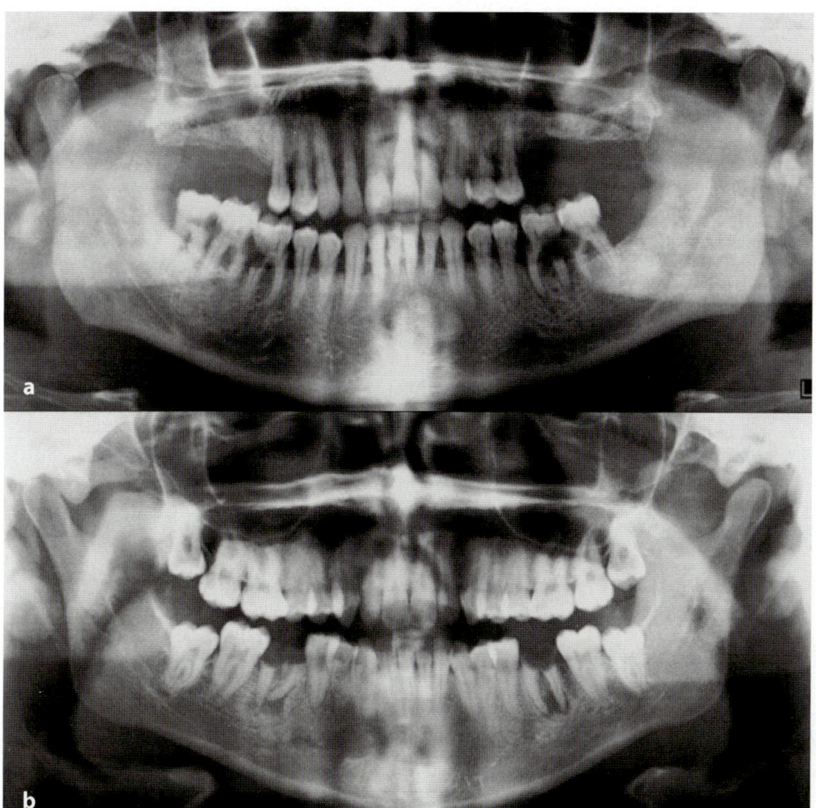

Fig. 16.5 **a**, **b** Patients having oral cancer not infrequently have extensive dental disease due to neglect. Periodontal disease and dental caries can lead to complications if not attended to in advance of cancer therapy

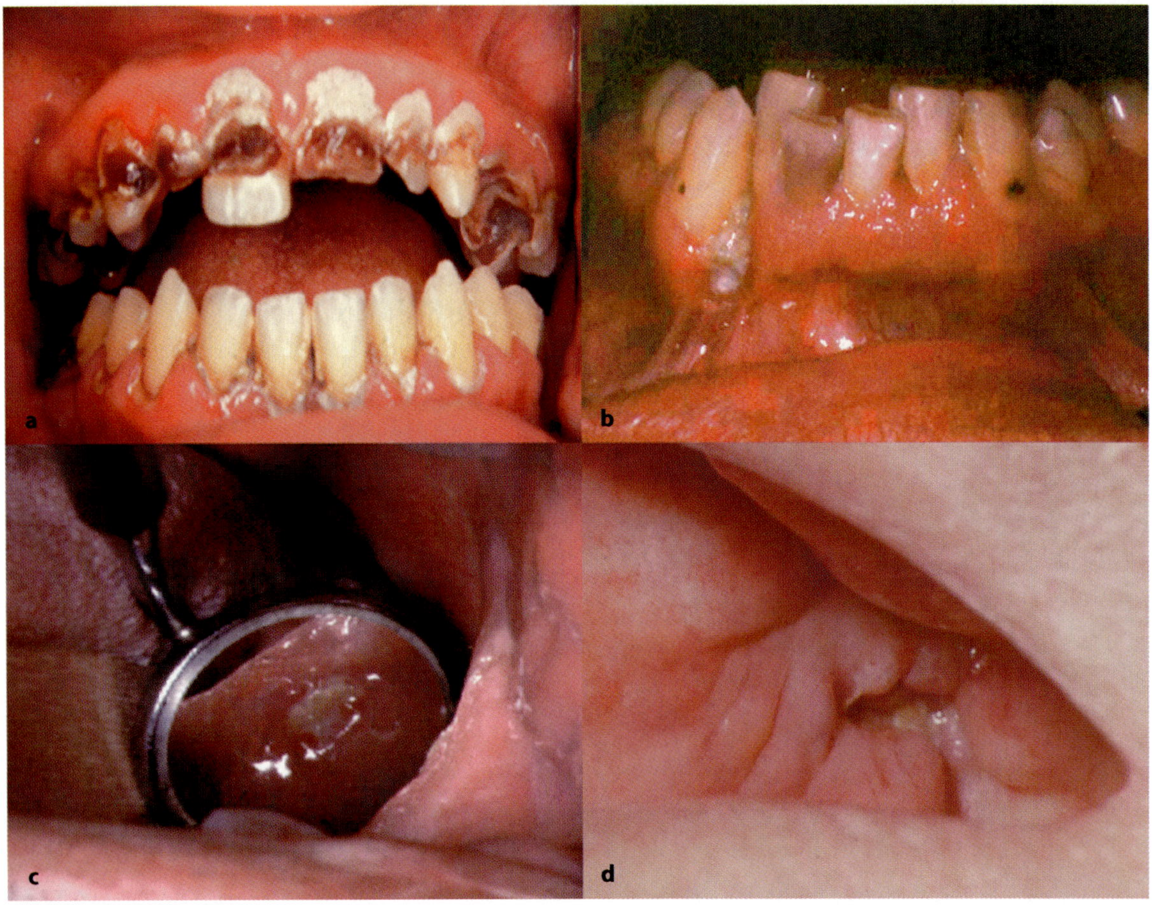

Fig. 16.6 "Radiation caries" can result from reduced salivary flow (**a**). Necrotic bone sequestration is an ominous sign of osteoradionecrosis post-radiation of the jaws (**b–d**)

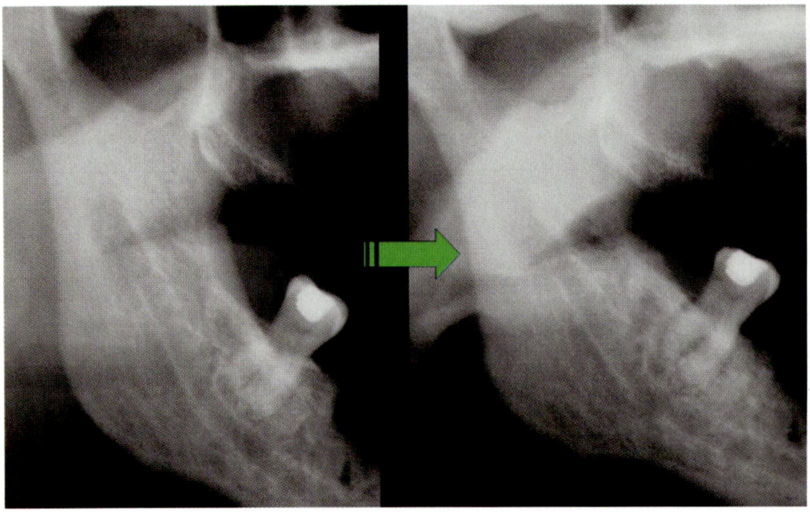

Fig. 16.7 Details from panoramic radiographs. Progress of osteoradionecrosis 6 months (*left*) and 2 years (*right*) following radiation therapy. Note increased dimensions of patches of sclerotic bone and widening of the periodontal ligament space around the mandibular molar over the follow up period

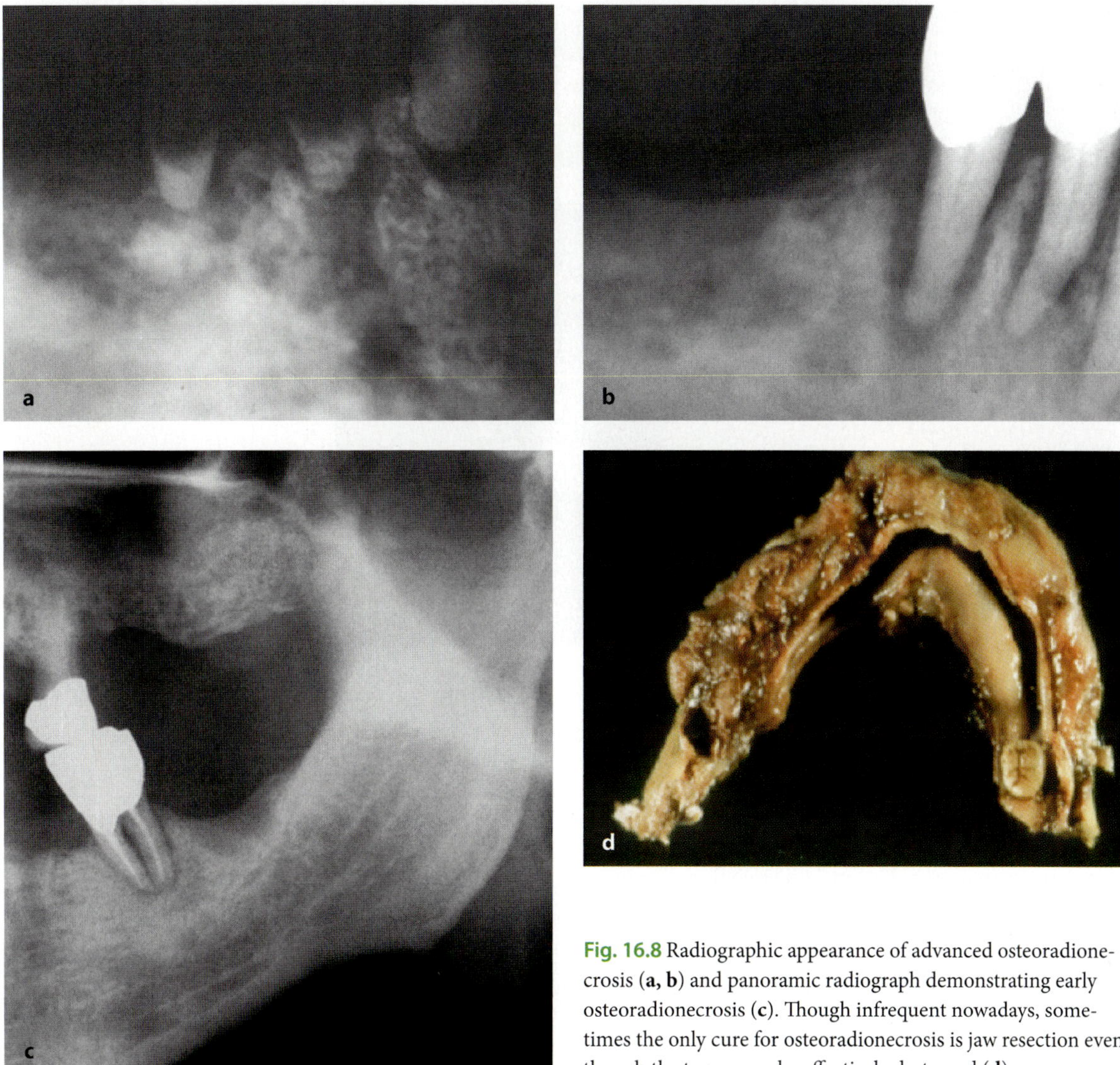

Fig. 16.8 Radiographic appearance of advanced osteoradionecrosis (**a, b**) and panoramic radiograph demonstrating early osteoradionecrosis (**c**). Though infrequent nowadays, sometimes the only cure for osteoradionecrosis is jaw resection even though the tumor can be effectively destroyed (**d**)

In a recent study, the incidence of osteoradionecrosis of the jaws after irradiation using modern three-dimensional planning as well as hyperfractionation or moderately accelerated irradiation was evaluated and compared with the incidence in earlier times [21]. Studer et al. (2004) reviewed the records of 268 head and neck cancer patients irradiated between 1 January 1980 and 31 December 1998 with a dose to the mandible of at least 60 Gy. All patients had computerized dose calculation with isodose charts. The long-term cumulative incidence of osteoradionecrosis needing mandibular resection after conventional fractionation was 6.2% (60–66.6 Gy target dose) or 20.1% (66.6–72.0 Gy target dose); 6.6% after hyperfractionated irradiation with a target dose 72.0–78.8 Gy; no case after concomitant boost irradiation according to the MD Anderson Cancer Center (Houston, TX) regime with a dose of 63.9–70.5 Gy; and ~17% (small patient number) after 6 × 2 Gy/day or 7 × 1.8 Gy/day and a total target dose of 66–72 Gy. Comparison of the incidence of osteoradionecrosis during the period 1980–90 with the period 1990–98 showed a decrease in risk to approximately 5% using modern three-dimensional techniques as well as hyperfractionation or moderately accelerated fractionation [21].

Oh et al. (2004) carried out a chart review in an attempt to establish whether unerupted third molars should be removed or left in place in patients requiring radiation therapy for cancer [22]. Patients were divided into two groups on the basis of pre-irradiation extraction. Group 1 comprised patients who had impacted third molars extracted before radiation therapy ($n = 55$). Group 2, comprised patients in whom impacted third molars were left in place ($n = 38$). Before radiation therapy, 99 impacted third molars were extracted from the 55 patients in Group 1, while 55 impacted third molars were left in place in the 38 patients in Group 2. Only

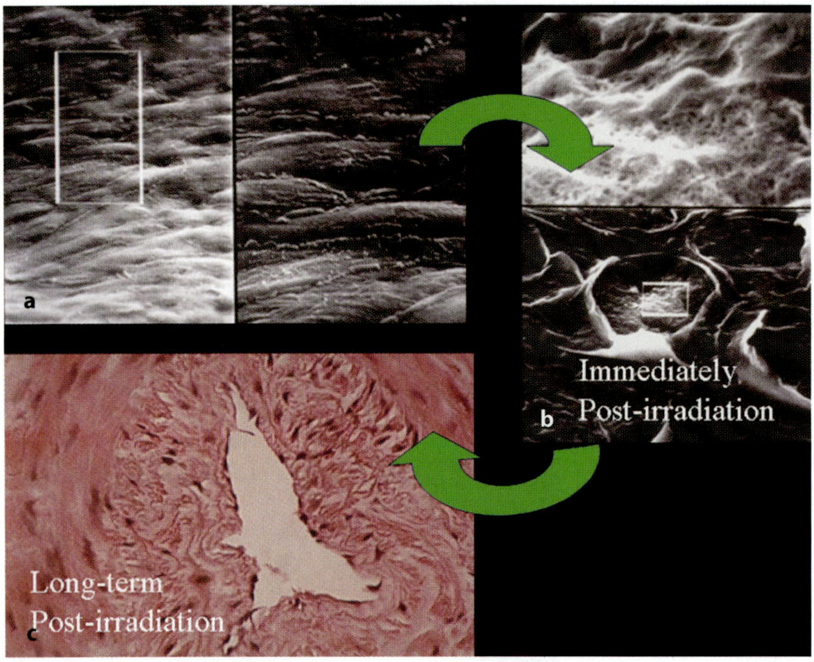

Fig. 16.9 Vascular changes are key to post-irradiation complications. The normal and immediately post-irradiated endothelial cell linings of a rabbit artery are illustrated in the scanning electron micrographs, (**a**) and (**b**), respectively. Long-term changes are luminal narrowing due to endarteritis obliterans (**c**); hematoxylin and eosin-stained histologic slide

four patients (two from Group 1 and two from Group 2) subsequently developed osteoradionecrosis; hence, no notable difference in the incidence of osteoradionecrosis could be attributed to prophylactic removal of unerupted third molars prior to radiation therapy.

Sulaiman et al. (2003) investigated irradiated head and neck patients to evaluate those patients who developed osteoradionecrosis through dental extraction [23]. Of 1,194 patients with a history of radiation to the head and neck treated at Memorial Sloan-Kettering Cancer Center, 187 had subsequent dental extractions and only 4 of these developed osteoradionecrosis. It could be concluded that healthy teeth should be retained in patients undergoing radiation therapy.

Osteonecrosis is not only a complication of radiation therapy; it can also occur with certain chemotherapeutic regimens [24]. Ruggiero et al. (2004) reported from the Long Island Jewish Medical Center, New York that long-term use of bisphosphonates, widely used in the management of metastatic disease to the bone and in the treatment of osteoporosis, can also result in osteonecrosis. The necrosis detected is otherwise typical of osteoradionecrosis. Between February 2001 and November 2003, 63 patients were identified with refractory osteomyelitis and a history of chronic bisphosphonate therapy (56 had received intravenous bisphosphonates for at least 1 year and 7 patients were on chronic oral bisphosphonate therapy) [24]. Typical presentation was either a non-healing extraction socket or an exposed jawbone refractory to conservative debridement and antibiotic therapy. Biopsy showed no evidence of metastatic disease. The majority of the patients required surgical removal of the necrotic bone. In view of the widespread use of chronic bisphosphonate therapy, the observation of an associated risk of osteonecrosis of the jaw should alert practitioners to monitor for this potential complication. Early diagnosis might reduce morbidity resulting from advanced destructive lesions of the jawbone. Periodic panoramic radiography is warranted in such patients.

Local application of high concentrations of fluoride gel as well as good oral hygiene are the most appropriate measures to implement for prevention of dental caries and other complications in patients treated by radiation or chemotherapy [6, 25]. Pasquier et al. (2004) carried out a systematic review on the peer reviewed literature from 1960 to 2004 concerning the use of hyperbaric oxygen therapy in the treatment of radiation-induced lesions [18]. They concluded that, while more controlled randomized trials are needed, the level of evidence supports use of hyperbaric oxygen therapy for treatment of osteoradionecrosis, and in prevention of osteoradionecrosis after dental extractions. A parallel systematic review concluded that there is a lack of reliable clinical evidence for or against the use therapeutic use of hyperbaric oxygen for irradiated dental implant patients [26].

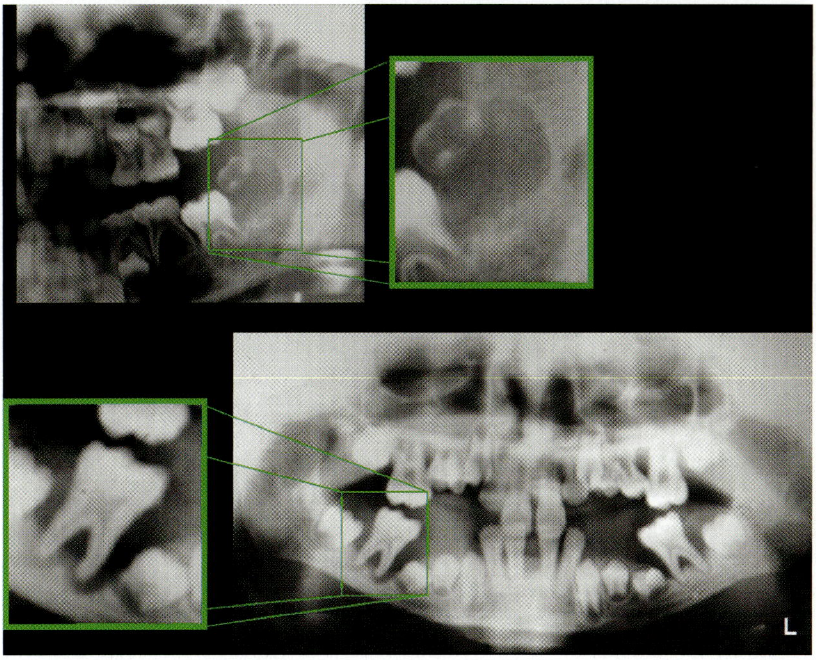

Fig. 16.10 Panoramic radiographic features of two cases of acute leukemia in children: displacement of developing tooth (*upper*); causing dramatic loss of periodontal support of affected teeth (*lower*)

Childhood Therapy

While childhood malignancies are comparatively uncommon, they do occur and can sometimes be detected on panoramic radiographs. By way of example, Fig. 16.10 illustrates two different panoramic radiographic presentations of acute leukemia. Many childhood malignancies respond well to chemotherapy. Treatment for malignancies, in childhood—particularly if radiation therapy is employed—can affect growth and development. Radiation to the jaws during the period of tooth formation, though comparatively rare these days, can lead to hypodontia and teeth with stunted roots (Fig. 16.11).

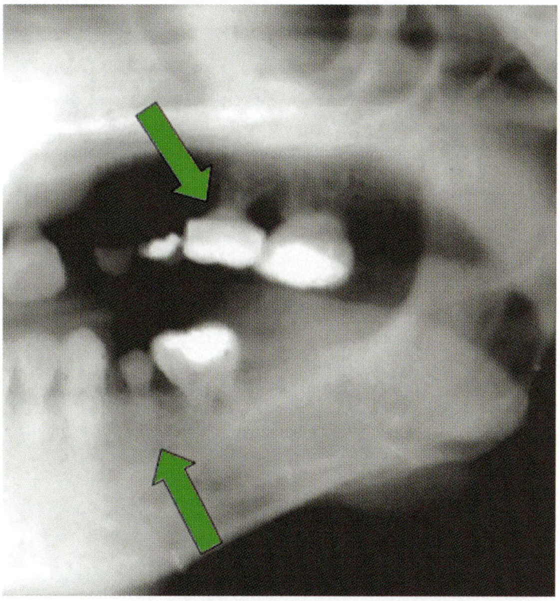

Fig. 16.11 Stunted roots and missing teeth are possible complications of irradiation during childhood (detail from panoramic radiograph)

Oguz et al. (2004) investigated the late effects of chemotherapy treatment for childhood non-Hodgkin's lymphomas on oral health and dental development [27]. Thirty-six long-term survivors were included in this study and 36 volunteers with similar age and sex distribution served as controls. Both groups underwent a complete oral and dental examination for decayed, missing, and filled teeth and tooth surfaces, gingival and periodontal health according to standard periodontal and plaque indices, enamel defects and discolorations, root malformations, eruption status, agenesis, premature apexifications, and microdontia. Non-Hodgkin's lymphoma patients had significantly higher plaque index, more enamel discolorations, and root malformations than did the controls, oral and dental disturbances that may be attributed to the chemotherapy regimens. It should be noted that patients with non-Hodgkin's lymphoma sometimes receive limited (mantle field) neck radiation.

Dental Restorations Affecting Radiation Therapy Planning and Application

Fuller et al. (2004) studied dose effects of metallic dental alloys in the field of head and neck irradiation. They used intensity modulated radiation therapy for base of tongue squamous cell carcinoma [28]. Significant artifact on computed tomography was induced by metallic alloy, non-removable dental restorations in both the mandible and maxilla. Simultaneously with intensity modulated radiation therapy, thermoluminescent dosimeters were placed in the oral cavity. After a series of three treatments, the data from the thermoluminescent dosimeters and software calculations were analyzed. Analysis of mean *in vivo* thermoluminescent dosimetry revealed differentials from software predicted dose calculation that fell within acceptable dose variation limits. Intensity modulated radiation therapy dose calculation software proved to be a relatively accurate predictor of dose attenuation and augmentation due to dental alloys within the treatment volume, as measured by intraoral thermoluminescent dosimetry.

Dental Outcomes

Allison et al. (1999) studied the relationship between dental status and health-related quality of life in upper aerodigestive tract cancer patients [29]. The investigation aimed to investigate the hypothesis that dental status is a predictor of quality of life. A cross-sectional study design was used with a sample of 188 subjects. Data were collected on socio-demographic, disease, treatment, and dental status. Linear multiple regression analysis was used to determine those variables with a significant independent association with quality of life. Two multivariate models were developed each containing age, sex, employment status, cancer site, and disease stage, plus either the dental status category "partially dentate with no prosthesis" (F-value = 7.31; $p < 0.0001$; $r^2 = 0.20$) predicting a significantly worse health-related life quality, or the dental status category "edentulous with prostheses" (F-value = 7.56; $p < 0.0001$; $r^2 = 0.20$) predicting a significantly better quality of life. Furthermore, the "partially dentate with no prosthesis" group reported significantly more "problems with their teeth" (ANOVA, $p = 0.0004$), significantly more "trouble eating" (ANOVA, $p = 0.024$), and significantly more "trouble enjoying their meals" (ANOVA, $p = 0.01$). The results of this study indicate that dental status has an important effect on health-related quality of life in post-therapeutic upper aerodigestive tract cancer patients (Fig. 16.12).

Most head and neck cancer patients are treated with high-dose radiation therapy to the oral cavity and surrounding structures. Significant side effects occur in

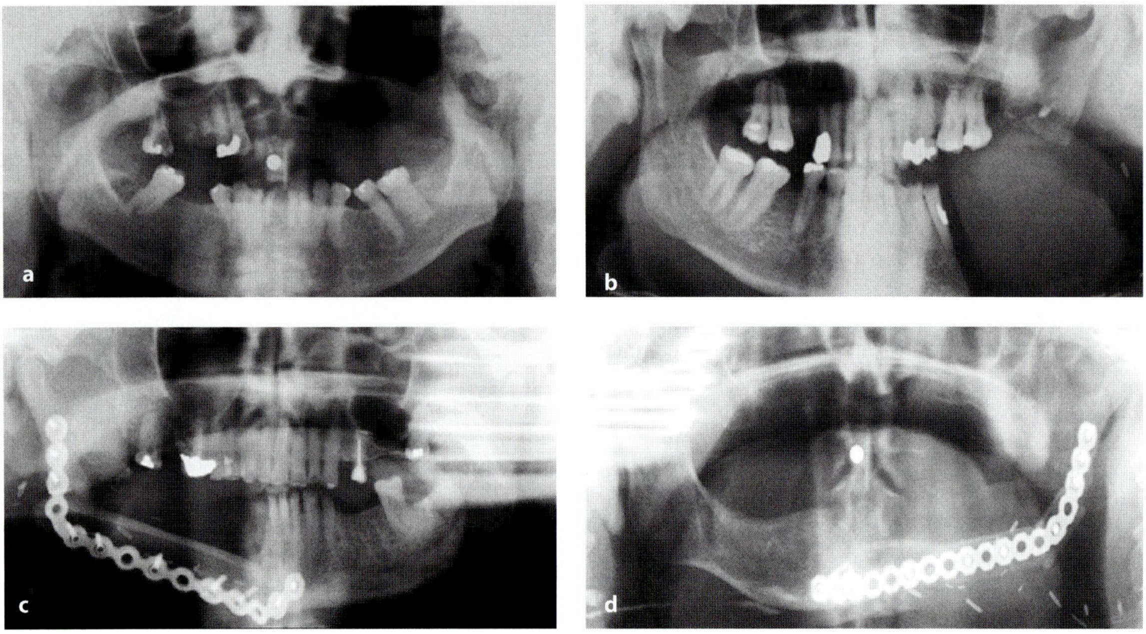

Fig. 16.12 Defects left by surgical resection need to be repaired both surgically and by maxillofacial prostheses: hemimaxillectomy (**a**); hemimandibulectomy prior to surgical reconstruction (**b**); hemimandibulectomy following surgical reconstruction (**c, d**)

both the acute phase and in the long term. A dedicated multidisciplinary team of oncologist, head and neck surgeon, oncologic dentist/dentist, nurse, dietician, physical therapist, social worker, and in some instances a plastic surgeon, a maxillofacial prosthodontist, and a psychologist are needed to provide the optimal supportive care for such patients [30].

Osseointegrated implants used in the rehabilitation of patients who have undergone head and neck surgery have provided a reliable means of retaining intraoral and extraoral prostheses [1]. With close communication between the head and neck surgeon and oncologic dentist, and careful patient selection, optimized outcomes are more likely. The panoramic radiograph is central to planning pre-cancer treatment dental approaches, and in the long-term follow-up of head and neck cancer patients.

References

1. Maureen S. The expanding role of dental oncology in head and neck surgery. Surg Oncol Clin N Am 2004;13:37–46
2. Harrison JS, Dale RA, Haveman CW, Redding SW. Oral complications in radiation therapy. Gen Dent 2003;51:552–561
3. Huber MA, Terezhalmy GT. The head and neck radiation oncology patient. Quintessence Int 2003;34:693–717
4. Meraw SJ, Reeve CM. Dental considerations and treatment of the oncology patient receiving radiation therapy. J Am Dent Assoc 1998;129:201–205
5. Rankin KV, Burzynski NJ, Silverman S Jr, Scheetz JP. Cancer curricula in U.S. dental schools. J Cancer Educ 1999;14:8–12
6. Barillot I, Horiot JC. Prevention of caries and osteoradionecrosis in patients irradiated in oncology. Critical review. Rev Belge Med Dent 1999;54:205–207
7. Cengiz M, Ozyar E, Ersu B, Akyol FH, Atahan IL. High-dose-rate mold brachytherapy of early gingival carcinoma: a clinical report. J Prosthet Dent 1999;82:512–514
8. Oelgiesser D, Levin L, Barak S, Schwartz-Arad D. Rehabilitation of an irradiated mandible after mandibular resection using implant/tooth-supported fixed prosthesis: a clinical report. J Prosthet Dent 2004;91:310–314
9. Taniguchi H. Radiation therapy prostheses. J Med Dent Sci 2000;47:12–26
10. Schiodt M, Hermund NU. Management of oral disease prior to radiation therapy. Support Care Cancer 2002;10:40–43
11. Moizan H, Meningaud JP, Giumelli B, Herve C; Head and Neck Cancer Committee. Committee on cancer of the upper aerodigestive tract and survey on buccodental aspects. Report of 164 teams. Rev Stomatol Chir Maxillofac 2003;104:5–9
12. Marsiglia H, Haie-Meder C, Sasso G, Mamelle G, Gerbaulet A. Brachytherapy for T1-T2 floor-of-the mouth cancers: the Gustave-Roussy Institute experience. Int J Radiat Oncol Biol Phys 2002;52:1257–1263
13. Shaw MJ, Kumar ND, Duggal M, Fiske J, Lewis DA, Kinsella T, Nisbet T. Oral management of patients following oncology treatment: literature review. Br J Oral Maxillofac Surg 2000;38:519–524
14. Luglie PF, Mura G, Mura A, Angius A, Soru G, Farris A. Prevention of periodontopathy and oral mucositis during antineoplastic chemotherapy. Minerva Stomatol 2002;51:231–239
15. Guggenheimer J, Moore PA. Xerostomia: etiology, recognition and treatment. J Am Dent Assoc 2003;134:61–69
16. Marques MA, Dib LL. Periodontal changes in patients undergoing radiation therapy. J Periodontol 2004;75:1178–1187
17. Raber-Durlacher JE, Epstein JB, Raber J, van Dissel JT, van Winkelhoff AJ, Guiot HF, van der Velden U. Periodontal infection in cancer patients treated with high-dose chemotherapy. Support Care Cancer 2002;10:466–473
18. Pasquier D, Hoelscher T, Schmutz J, Dische S, Mathieu D, Baumann M, Lartigau E. Hyperbaric oxygen therapy in the treatment of radio-induced lesions in normal tissues: a literature review. Radiother Oncol 2004;72:1–13
19. Jereczek-Fossa BA, Orecchia R. Radiation therapy-induced mandibular bone complications. Cancer Treat Rev 2002;28:65–74
20. Reuther T, Schuster T, Mende U, Kubler A. Osteoradionecrosis of the jaws as a side effect of radiation therapy of head and neck tumour patients: a report of a thirty year retrospective review. Int J Oral Maxillofac Surg 2003;32:289–295
21. Studer G, Gratz KW, Glanzmann C. Osteoradionecrosis of the mandible in patients treated with different fractionations. Strahlenther Onkol 2004;180:233–240
22. Oh HK, Chambers MS, Garden AS, Wong PF, Martin JW. Risk of osteoradionecrosis after extraction of impacted third molars in irradiated head and neck cancer patients. J Oral Maxillofac Surg 2004;62:139–144
23. Sulaiman F, Huryn JM, Zlotolow IM. Dental extractions in the irradiated head and neck patient: a retrospective analysis of Memorial Sloan-Kettering Cancer Center protocols, criteria, and end results. Oral Maxillofac Surg 2003;61:1123–1131
24. Ruggiero SL, Mehrotra B, Rosenberg TJ, Engroff SL. Osteonecrosis of the jaws associated with the use of bisphosphonates: a review of 63 cases. J Oral Maxillofac Surg 2004;62:527–534
25 Piret P, Deneufbourg JM. Mandibular osteoradionecrosis: sword of Damocles of radiation therapy for head and neck cancers? Rev Med Liege 2002;57:393–399
26. Coulthard P, Esposito M, Worthington HV, Jokstad A. Therapeutic use of hyperbaric oxygen for irradiated dental implant patients: a systematic review. J Dent Educ 2003;67:64–68
27. Oguz A, Cetiner S, Karadeniz C, Alpaslan G, Alpaslan C, Pinarli G. Long-term effects of chemotherapy on orodental structures in children with non-Hodgkin's lymphoma. Eur J Oral Sci 2004;112:8–11
28. Fuller CD, Diaz I, Cavanaugh SX, Eng TY. In vivo dose perturbation effects of metallic dental alloys during head and neck irradiation with intensity modulated radiation therapy. Oral Oncol 2004;40:645–648
29. Allison PJ, Locker D, Feine JS. The relationship between dental status and health-related quality of life in upper aerodigestive tract cancer patients. Oral Oncol 1999;35:138–143
30. Specht L. Oral complications in the head and neck radiation patient. Introduction and scope of the problem. Support Care Cancer 2002;10:36–39

TEST: Panoramic radiology: oncologic dentistry considerations

1. It is always necessary to extract all teeth prior to radiation therapy in head and neck cancer patients.

   True ☐ **False** ☐

2. Osteonecrosis can be found in patients following certain chemotherapeutic regimens.

   True ☐ **False** ☐

3. In the USA as many as 400,000 patients treated for cancer each year can show oral complications.

   True ☐ **False** ☐

4. Antibacterial rinses (e.g., chlorhexidine) can reduce the incidence of oral mucositis as a side effect of antineoplastic chemotherapy.

   True ☐ **False** ☐

5. Periodic panoramic radiographs can help in the early detection of tumor recurrence or jaw complications from radiation therapy.

   True ☐ **False** ☐

6. Most head and neck cancer patients are treated with high-dose radiation therapy to the oral cavity and surrounding structures.

   True ☐ **False** ☐

7. Dental Schools in the USA generally provide a high-quality practical experience in oncologic dentistry in the dental curriculum.

   True ☐ **False** ☐

8. Osseointegrated implants used in the rehabilitation of patients who have undergone head and neck surgery have provided a reliable means of retaining intraoral and extraoral prostheses.

   True ☐ **False** ☐

9. Dental status has not been found to have any important effect on health-related quality of life in post-therapeutic upper aerodigestive tract cancer patients.

   True ☐ **False** ☐

10. Systematic review has indicated a lack of reliable clinical evidence for or against the therapeutic use of hyperbaric oxygen for irradiated dental implant patients.

    True ☐ **False** ☐

Cephalometric Attachments Are Not Only of Value for Orthodontic Assessment

Allan G. Farman

17

Learning Objectives

After reviewing this chapter, the reader will:

- Be made familiar with the variety of extraoral projections possible with a cephalometric attachment to the panoramic system

Panoramic radiographic systems can be combined with a cephalometric ("ceph") attachment for performance of skull projections. A cephalostat is commonly used to standardize patient positioning for lateral cephalograms used in orthodontic assessment. What is not always remembered is that the cephalometric radiograph is simply a standardized skull radiograph. Panoramic machines with "ceph" attachments can actually be used for producing a variety of plain images to evaluate the skull and jaws. In every case it is possible to use a 10 inch x 8 inch detector with indirect exposure X-ray film with screens within a cassette or photostimulable phosphor plates. There are also systems that use a scanning or "single shot" solid-state detector. For the purpose of this chapter the term "detector" will be used to encompass all of these modalities.

The aim of this chapter is to briefly overview representative standard head image projection techniques and outlines the key uses of each. It should be cautioned that while the cephalostat is valuable for the purpose of positioning the patient for orthodontic assessment, the head holder should preferably be removed or extended away from the head when making standard head images for other purposes as the shadow cast from this device may occasionally obscure diagnostic information.

Lateral Skull Projection

In the absence of signs and symptoms of disease, plain image extraoral radiographs are rarely selected except for cephalometric analysis for orthodontic purposes. The lateral cephalometric radiograph is made with a long source to midsagittal plane of 60 inches (152.4 cm) to minimize magnification distortion that would otherwise mean the tissues of the side of the head nearest the beam source would be magnified much more than those closest the detector. In the USA, it is a tradition to have the left side of the face closest to the detector—elsewhere the right side is sometime chosen to be closest to the detector (Fig. 17.1). The detector is generally placed at a standard distance from the head, frequently 10–15 cm. The midsagittal plane is parallel to the cassette. The cassette is perpendicular to the beam with the central ray of the beam directed 2 cm above and 2 cm anterior to the external auditory meatus. The head is stabilized in a cephalostat with ear rods and perhaps a pointer to the bridge of the nose. The natural head position is used with the mouth closed. To achieve this position a mirror in front of the patient can help. The patient is instructed to look straight into their eyes in the mirror.

The cephalometric radiograph is a special case of lateral skull radiograph (Fig. 17.2). Lateral skull radiographs, other than cephalograms, do not need specific source to detector distances, as precise measurements are usually unnecessary. Actually, leaving the cephalostat away from the patient's head might be desirable to prevent its shadow confusing the radiographic features (Fig. 17.3). Lateral skull radiographs can be used to evaluate possible fractures to the skull, jaws, or cervical spine, to evaluate structural changes in the calvarium in systemic disease, or to evaluate suspected local pathological processes to the skull, jaws, and pituitary fossa/sella turcica.

Posterior-Anterior (PA) Projection

The acronym "PA" is frequently misused in dentistry to signify a periapical intraoral radiograph. Strictly speaking, radiologically "PA" is restricted to posterior-anterior projections as opposed to "AP" or anterior-posterior projection. Conventionally, the point of entry of the X-ray beam is listed first and the exit point (that closest to the detector) is listed second. PAs are preferred to APs for dental purposes as the structures closest to the detector are clearer due to less beam scatter and lower magnification distortion.

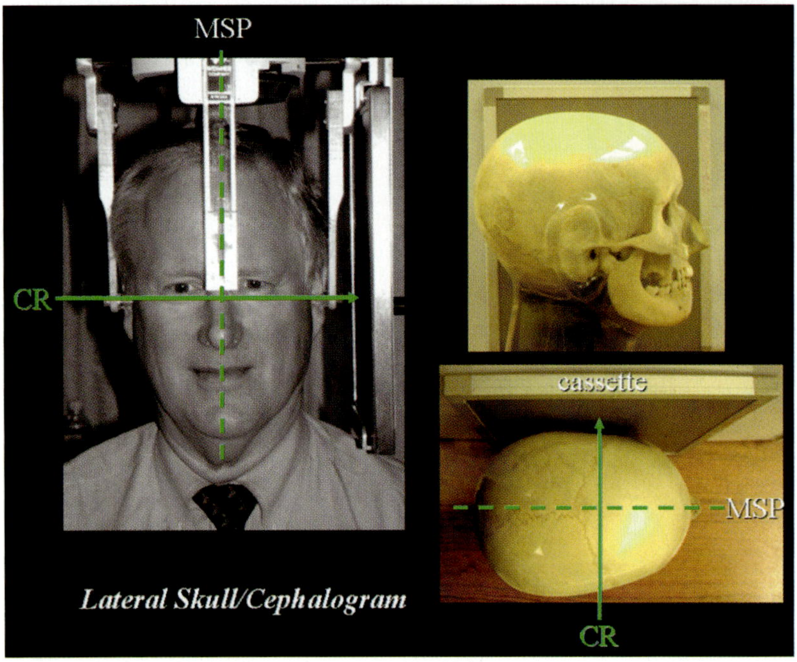

Fig. 17.1 Lateral skull projection. The use of a cephalostat makes the radiographic image a cephalogram suitable for orthodontic analysis. *CR* Central ray, *MSP* midsagittal plane. The left side of the face is toward the cassette

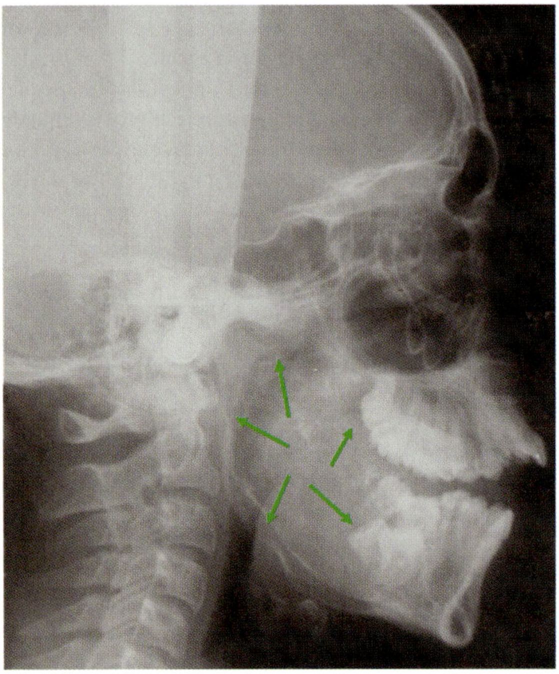

Fig. 17.2 Lateral cephalogram of a patient with cherubism. Note that the multilocular radiolucency of mandibular ramus (*arrows*) spares the mandibular condyle. Unerupted molar teeth are displaced forward

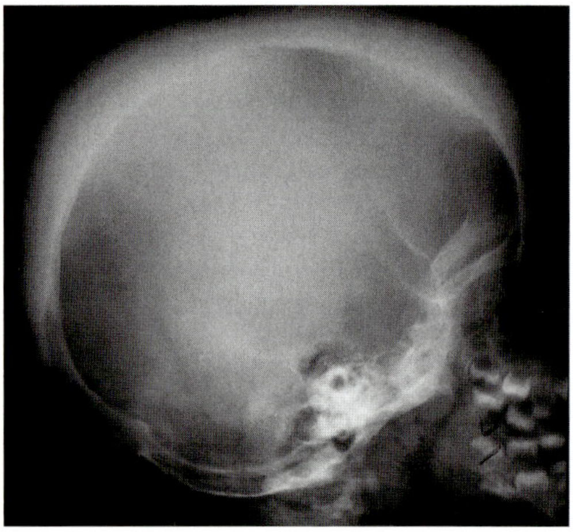

Fig. 17.3 Lateral skull radiograph of patient having Cooley anemia. There is a granular thickening of calvarium. This is not a cephalogram as no cephalostat is evident

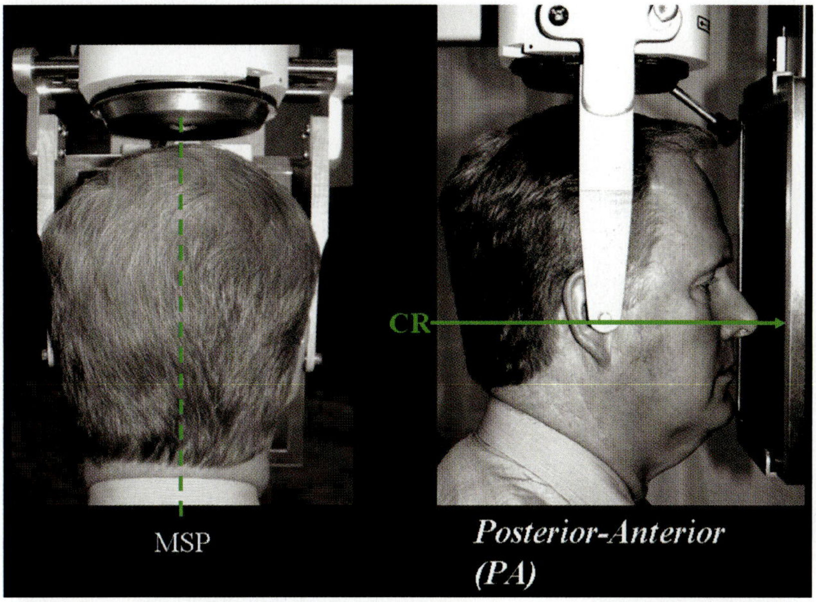

Fig. 17.4 Posterior-anterior (PA) projection. The use of a cephalostat makes the radiographic image a cephalogram suitable for orthodontic analysis. *CR* Central ray, *MSP* midsagittal plane

For the PA, the patient is positioned facing the detector with the tragus-canthal line parallel to the floor and the forehead and nose touching the cassette (Fig. 17.4). The X-ray beam is perpendicular to the detector and parallel to the midsagittal plane. The beam enters at the center of the external occipital protuberance and exits at the bridge of the nose.

Indications for the PA skull projection include orthodontic evaluation of jaw asymmetry, detection of fractures or foreign bodies following trauma, to evaluate structural changes in the calvarium in systemic disease, or to evaluate suspected local pathological processes to the skull and jaws (Figs. 17.5, 17.6). It can be used in combination with the lateral skull radiograph to assist in localization of structures or foreign bodies.

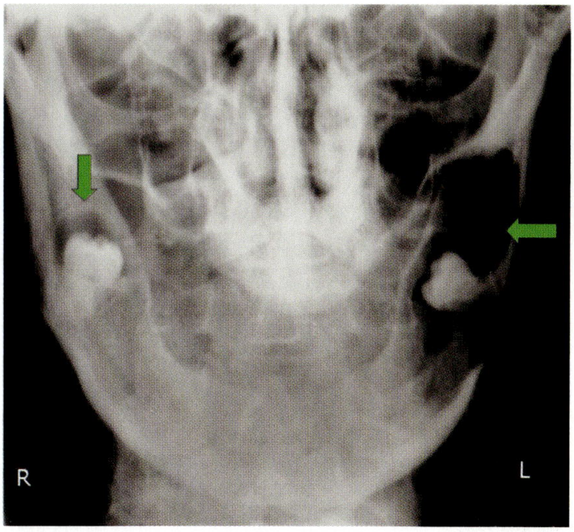

Fig. 17.5 PA view. Image detail demonstrates bilateral mandibular dentigerous cysts (*arrows*) in this otherwise edentulous patient

Occipitomental Projection (Waters' Technique)

The Waters technique is a posterior-anterior projection with the skull and beam inclined to prevent superimposition of the highly radio-opaque petrous temporal bones over the maxillary sinuses. The resulting film can be used to inspect the outline of the orbital ridges and floor, the frontal sinus, the maxillary sinuses, the zygomatic arches, the odontoid process of the second cervical vertebra, and the mandible.

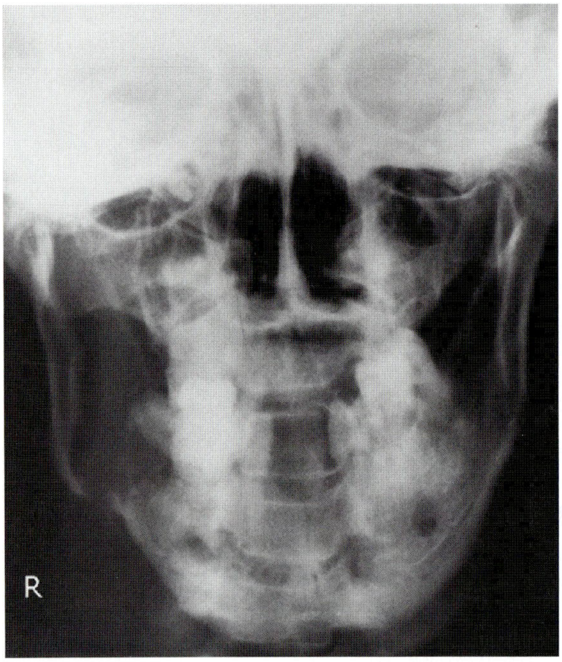

Fig. 17.6 PA view of squamous cell carcinoma involving the right mandible showing pathological fracture. Note the saucerized erosion typical of an extrabony origin to the lesion

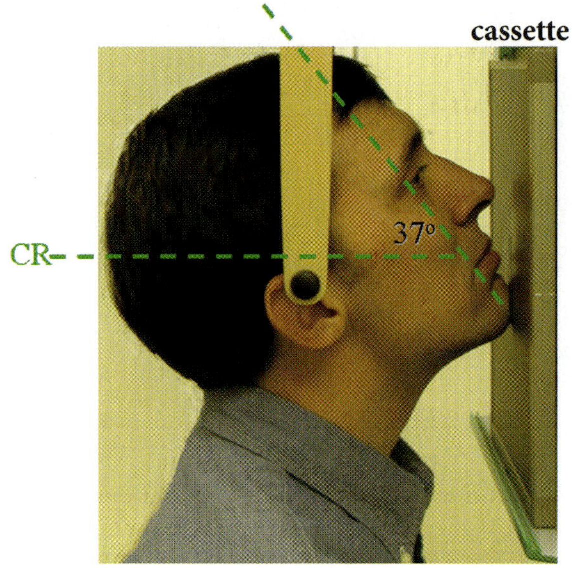

Fig. 17.7 Waters (occipitomental) projection. *CR* Central ray

The patient is positioned with the midsagittal plane perpendicular to the plane of the digital detector or film cassette (Fig. 17.7). The patient's chin rests on the cassette and the nose is about 1 inch (3 cm) from the cassette. The tragus-canthal line approximates 37° to the central ray, with the central ray perpendicular to the cassette and centered at the level of the maxillary sinuses.

The resulting image is valuable for evaluation of the lateral and medial walls of the maxillary sinus and to determine a possible fluid level indicative of sinusitis (Fig. 17.8) or soft tissue proliferations within the sinus. It is also of value as the preliminary view to inspect for possible fractures affecting the zygomatico-maxillary complex. Referral of the patient for further evaluation using computed tomography is advised when fractures are detected.

Reverse Towne Projection

The patient faces the detector cassette with the forehead resting on the cassette, the nose one inch (2.54 cm) away from the cassette, and the mouth open (to bring the condyles to the crest of the articular eminences). The beam is perpendicular to the detector and parallel to the patient's midsagittal plane. The central ray passes through a point midway between the external auditory meati (Fig. 17.9).

This projection is used to demonstrate the coronal aspect of the mandibular condyles to evaluate for possible condylar fractures (and medio-lateral displacement; Fig. 17.10) following trauma. It is also useful for evaluating the posterior wall of the maxillary sinus, the nasal septum, the mandibular rami, and the styloid processes.

Submentovertex Projection

The submentovertex projection provides a plan or cross-sectional view of the head, providing information on the medio-lateral aspects of the zygomatic arch, mandibular condyles, the sphenoid, ethmoid, and maxillary sinuses, and the mastoid air cells and an assessment of mandibular symmetry. It provides a clear view of the foramina in the base of the skull such as foramen ovale, foramen spinosum, and foramen magnum.

The patient faces the X-ray source with the head and neck hyper-extended backward, and the vertex of the skull placed on the detector cassette (Figs. 17.11, 17.12).

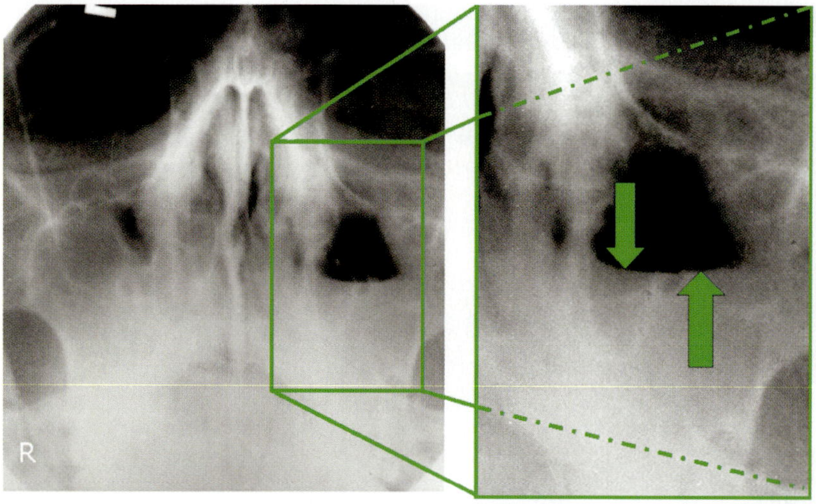

Fig. 17.8 Acute sinusitis: Waters view shows opaque right maxillary sinus with classic air-fluid level in the left (*arrows*)

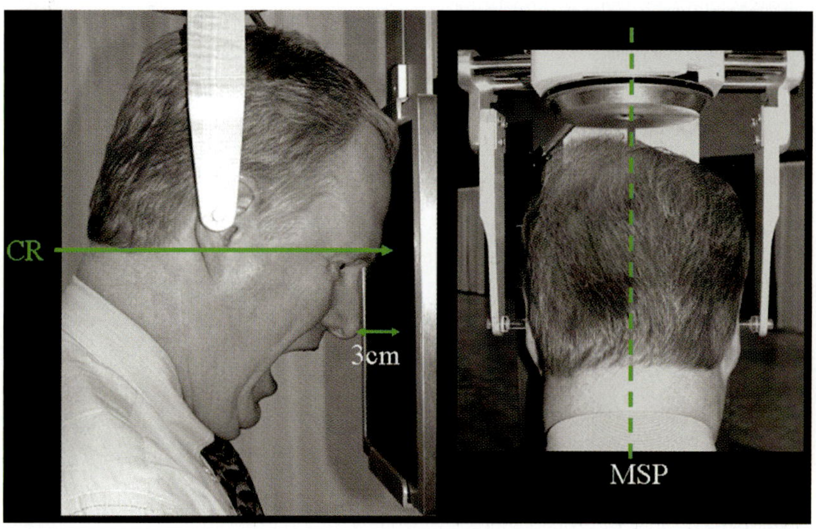

Fig. 17.9 Reverse Towne projection. The patient faces the cassette with the forehead touching the cassette, the nose 3 cm from the cassette and the mouth open. The cephalostat is best kept out of the image for this projection. *CR* Central ray, *MSP* midsagittal plane

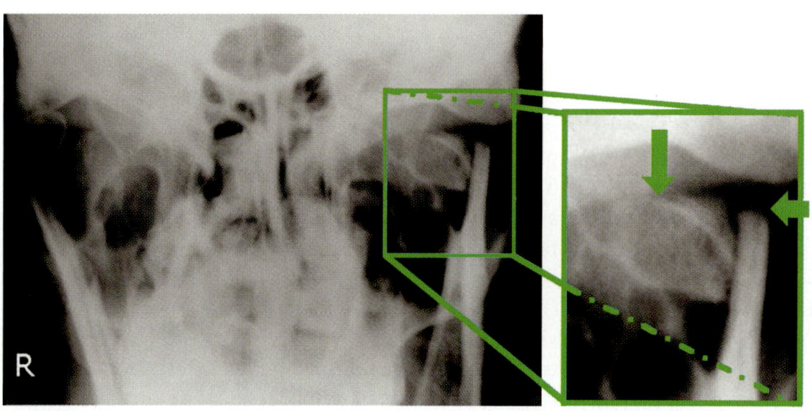

Fig. 17.10 Reverse Towne projection demonstrating fracture of left mandibular condyle with medial displacement of mandibular condylar head (*arrows* in *detail*)

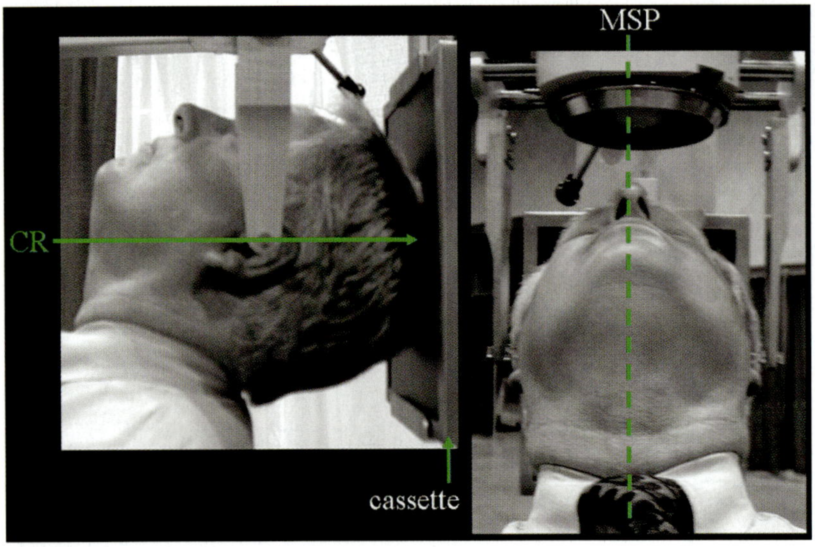

Fig. 17.11 Submentovertex projection. *CR* Central ray, *MSP* midsagittal plane

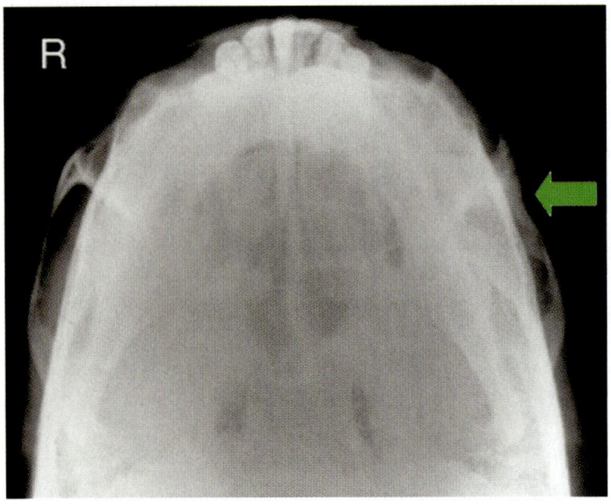

Fig. 17.12 Submentovertex projection demonstrating depressed fracture of left zygomatic arch. This projection is sometimes known as a "jug-handle" projection in view of the appearance of the normal zygomatic arch as demonstrated on the right side of the image

The tragus-canthal line is perpendicular to the floor and parallel to the cassette. The X-ray beam enters the midline between the condyles below the chin (the "submento-", component of the projection's name) and exits the vertex of the skull.

Lateral-Oblique Projection of the Jaws

The lateral-oblique provides a plain image projection of the posterior dental arches on one side of the patient at a time. To a great extent this projection has been replaced by the panoramic dental image. For a view of the posterior jaw segments, the patient is positioned with head rotated toward the cassette, and tilted to achieve a negative beam angulation of −15° to −20° resulting in a the beam entering approximately 1 inch (2.54 cm) below the angle of the mandible on the X-ray tube side (Figs. 17.13–17.15). The projection can be used to provide a full-thickness view of the posterior dental arch to evaluate impacted third molar teeth, fractures of the mandibular body, or pathoses affecting the jaws.

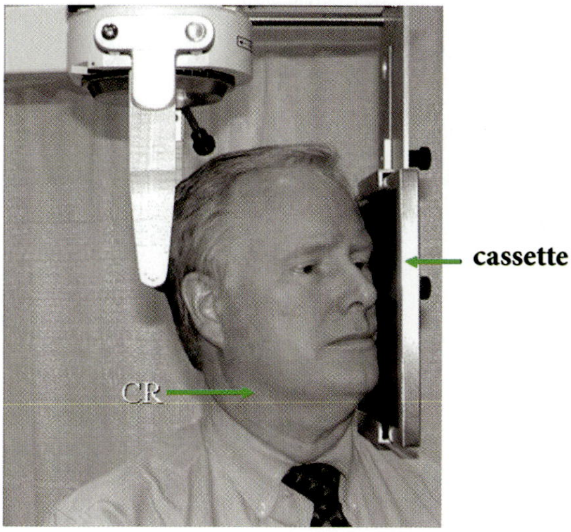

Fig. 17.13 Lateral-oblique projection of the jaw. The lateral-oblique projection often necessitates the cassette being held by the patient to achieve the desired X-ray beam angulation. *CR* Central ray

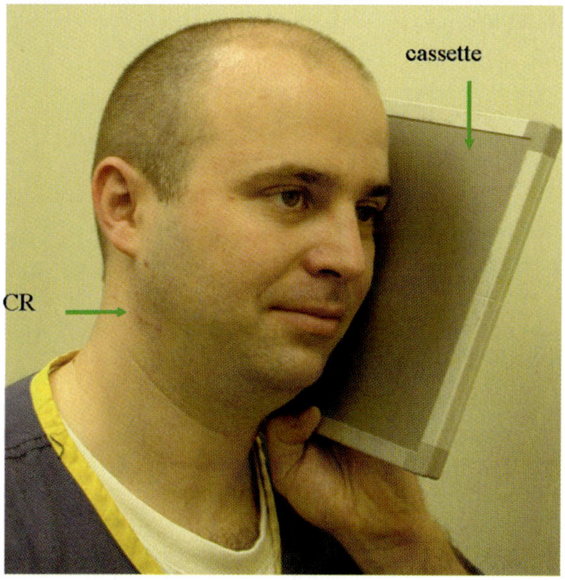

Fig. 17.14 Alternate positioning of cassette for lateral-oblique projection (hand held rather than held by cassette holder

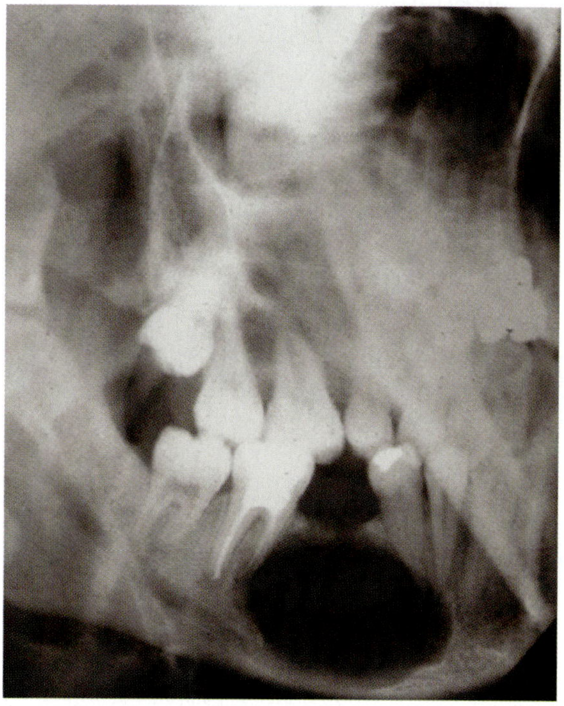

Fig. 17.15 Lateral-oblique radiograph of a patient with a large residual cyst in the mandible

TEST: Extraoral projections using the cephalometric projection

1. The radiographic projection most suited to examination of the maxillary sinuses is:
   (a) Reverse Towne
   (b) Occipitomental
   (c) Lateral skull
   (d) Lateral-oblique

2. The most frequent size used for skull radiographs made using a pan-ceph unit is:
   (a) 5 × 7 inches (12.7 × 17.8 cm)
   (b) 12 × 6 inches (30.5 × 15.2 cm)
   (c) 10 × 8 inches (25.4 × 20.3 cm)
   (d) None of the above

3. Approximately how far should the patient's nose be from the detector when making a Reverse Towne radiograph?
   (a) 0 cm (touching cassette)
   (b) 1.5 cm
   (c) 2.5 cm
   (d) 10 cm

4. A projection used to inspect for a possible zygomatic arch fracture is:
   (a) Waters view
   (b) Submentovertex
   (c) PA
   (d) More than one of the above

5. In radiological terms "PA" is the acronym for:
   (a) Posterior-anterior
   (b) Periapical intraoral projection
   (c) Both (a) and (b)

6. Of the following, the most appropriate projection for examining impacted third molar teeth is the:
   (a) Submentovertex
   (b) Lateral skull
   (c) Waters'
   (d) Lateral-oblique

7. The submentovertex projection can be used to evaluate the foramen ovale, foramen spinosum and foramen magnum.

   True ☐ **False** ☐

8. The X-ray source distance for lateral cephalometry is generally:
   (a) 16 inches (40.6 cm)
   (b) 30 inches (76.2 cm)
   (c) 50 inches (127.0 cm)
   (d) 60 inches (152.4 cm)

9. For lateral cephalometry in the USA the right side of the patient's face is next to the detector/cassette.

   True ☐ **False** ☐

10. The point of entrance of the beam for the posterior-anterior projection is the:
    (a) External occipital protuberance
    (b) Articular eminence
    (c) Skull vertex
    (d) Nasal bridge

Chapter

18 Selected Abstracts

Allan G. Farman

Learning Objectives

This chapter provides a selected overview of recent contributions to the literature concerning panoramic radiography that in themselves are insufficient to include in separate chapters. It is added for the purpose of adding completeness and currency of knowledge.

Dental Caries Assessment

Dental caries: **For detection of occlusal dental caries, no statistical significance was demonstrated between panoramic and bitewing radiography.**

Thomas MF, Ricketts DN, Wilson RF. Occlusal caries diagnosis in molar teeth from bitewing and panoramic radiographs. Prim Dent Care 2001;8:63–69. [From the Division of Conservative Dentistry, Kings College, London, UK]

Previous studies implying that panoramic radiographs are inferior to bitewing radiographs for caries diagnosis lacked validation. This study used an electronic caries meter (ECM II, LODE, Groningen, The Netherlands) to validate occlusal caries diagnoses made from bitewing and panoramic radiographs. Forty-nine Army recruits were examined with the electronic caries meter, and had bitewing and panoramic radiographs made. In total, 299 molar occlusal surfaces were available for examination. Seven examiners viewed the bitewing and panoramic radiographs on two separate occasions and rated each occlusal surface for dentin caries using a five interval scale (1: almost definitely no caries, 2: probably no caries, 3: unsure, 4: caries probably present, and 5: caries almost definitely present). To determine intrarater reliability, repeat measures were made on 20% of the radiographs at two further separate sittings. Electronic caries meter conductance readings greater than 9 were taken to indicate dentin caries. Examiner decisions that caries was probably and definitely considered to be present were taken as positive diagnoses. Bitewing and panoramic radiographs provided sensitivity values of 25% and 19% and specificity values of 93% and 97%, respectively. Receiver operating characteristic analysis was also performed. No statistically significant difference in diagnostic quality was proven between the panoramic and bitewing radiographs. Intra-examiner reproducibility was found to be poor to moderate (Kappa values for bitewing radiographs = 0.31–0.44, and for panoramic radiographs = 0.07–0.54). In conclusion, no difference in overall diagnostic performance was proven between bitewing and panoramic radiographs for the diagnosis of occlusal surface dentin caries.

Commentary: *Neither intraoral nor panoramic radiographs are ideal for the detection of dental occlusal caries, a condition that benefits from careful visual inspection of the mouth by the clinician.*

Periodontal Disease Assessment

Periodontal disease: **Panoramic radiography is the most frequently used X-ray method for assessment of periodontal disease at dental schools in the UK and Ireland.**

Tugnait A, Clerehugh DV, Hirschmann PN. Survey of radiographic practices for periodontal disease in UK and Irish dental teaching hospitals. Dentomaxillofac Radiol 2000;29:376–381. [From the Department of Periodontology, Leeds Dental Institute, Leeds, UK]

The objective of this paper was to assess current radiographic practices for the management of patients having periodontal disease. All dental teaching programs in the United Kingdom and Ireland were sent a questionnaire on radiographic equipment and radiograph selection currently used for assessment of patients with destructive periodontal diseases. Opinions were recorded for advantages and disadvantages of the most frequently used radiographic views. A 100% response rate was achieved. All programs used panoramic and specific periapical radiographs as one of their radiographic regimes for patients with periodontal disease. Of the respondents, 53% most frequently made panoramic and selected periapical radiographs, 24% made full mouth periapical radiographic series most often, and 18% took a panoramic radiograph alone. In conclusion, more than 70% of dental teaching programs in the UK and Ireland make panoramic radiographs, with or without selected periapicals, to assess periodontal status.

Commentary: *While a paralleling intraoral radiographic technique and vertical bitewings are usually considered standard for periodontal assessment, the panoramic radiograph also has utility in terms of providing an overview of periodontal status.*

Endodontics

Endodontic assessment: **Panoramic radiographs can be used to evaluate the treatment outcomes for endodontic restorations.**

Lupi-Pegurier L, Bertrand MF, Muller-Bolla M, Rocca JP, Bolla M. Periapical status, prevalence and quality of endodontic treatment in an adult French population. Int Endod J 2002;35:690–697. [From the Department of Public Health, University of Nice, France]

This study used panoramic radiographs to determine the periapical status and the quality of root-canal treatment amongst an adult population attending a dental school. Patients who attended the dental school in Nice, France for the first time during 1998 were included. The survey involved 344 patients: 180 females and 164 males. Panoramic radiographs, made by a trained radiology assistant, were used in this study. The periapical areas of all teeth with the exception of third molars were examined and the technical quality of root fillings was evaluated for both apical extension and density. Statistical analyses were conducted using ANOVA, Chi-square, Fisher's PLSD and Cohen's Kappa tests. Males had significantly fewer natural remaining teeth than females ($p < 0.03$). Similarly, the average number of root-filled teeth was lower for males ($p < 0.01$). Non root-filled teeth ($n = 6{,}126$) had significantly fewer signs of periapical pathology than root filled teeth ($n = 1{,}429$) (1.7% vs. 31.5%, $p < 0.0001$). Many root-canal treatments were technically unsatisfactory in terms of quality and treatment outcome. There was a significant correlation between the presence of periapical pathology and inadequate root-canal fillings ($p < 0.001$).

Commentary: *The panoramic radiograph can be a useful adjunct to intraoral radiographs as the patient who requires endodontic treatment in one tooth is also likely to have other endodontically related lesions.*

Selection Criteria

Panoramic diagnostic yield: **Optimization of the diagnostic yield from panoramic radiographs requires a systematic approach with special attention to high yield areas.**

Monsour PA. Getting the most from rotational panoramic radiographs. Aust Dent J 2000;45:136–142. [From the Queensland Diagnostic Imaging, Holy Spirit Hospital, Brisbane, Australia]

Rotational panoramic radiography is an invaluable tool in modern dentistry. To use the full potential of this resource the entire radiograph must be examined in a systematic way to extract the great wealth of information available. A framework should be applied for the development of a systematic method to examine panoramic radiographs. The essential elements are that all areas of the radiograph should be examined and that there are a number of high yield areas with regard to pathology that require special attention.

Commentary: *All radiographs that are selected for examination of a patient must be carefully observed in their entirety rather than simply viewed in the context of the patient's chief complaint.*

Film selection: **Both Kodak Ektavision and Agfa OrthoLux did well in standard sensitometric tests and in the perceived clarity of image features.**

Wakoh M, Nishikawa K, Kobayashi N, Farman AG, Kuroyanagi K. Sensitometric properties of Agfa Dentus OrthoLux, Agfa Dentus ST8G, and Kodak Ektavision panoramic radiographic film. Oral Surg Oral Med Oral Pathol Oral Radiol Endod 2001;91:244–251. [From the Department of Oral and Maxillofacial Radiology Tokyo Dental College, Chiba, Japan]

This study compares the panoramic imaging qualities of Kodak Ektavision, Agfa OrthoLux, and Agfa ST8G panoramic radiographic films in combination with Kodak versus Agfa intensifying screens. The density response and resolution of panoramic radiographic film/intensifying screen combinations was evaluated by means of Hurter and Driffield curves, modulation transfer function, and noise equivalent quanta. Image clarity of selected anatomical structures was also rated. The ISO speed for the Agfa OrthoLux film/screen combinations was the fastest, and the Kodak Ektavision system was the slowest. The average gradient for the Agfa ST8G system was relatively steep in comparison with those for the other film/screen combinations indicating a narrower recording latitude. The modulation transfer function for the Kodak Ektavision film (a measure of spatial resolution) was higher than those for the Agfa films, irrespective of the screen combination used. The noise equivalent quanta for the Agfa ST8G film/screen combinations was lower than that for the other film/screen combinations tested. The noise equivalent quanta of the Kodak Ektavision film/screen combinations was well within the high-frequency range; whereas Agfa OrthoLux combined with either the Kodak Ektavision imaging screen or the Kodak Lanex Regular imaging screen produced a noise equivalent quanta similar to that of the Kodak Ektavision film/screen combinations in the low-frequency range. Agfa OrthoLux was perceived to provide clearer images of the selected anatomical details than Agfa ST8G, and the Agfa OrthoLux/Agfa Ortho Regular 400 combination was not significantly different from the Kodak Ektavision/Kodak Lanex Regular combination in terms of perceived image quality. Agfa OrthoLux is an improvement over Agfa ST8G in film speed, spatial resolution, granularity, and perceived diagnostic image quality. The Agfa OrthoLux/Agfa Ortho Regular 400 combination; however, did not exceed the Kodak Ektavision film/Kodak Ektavision imaging screen combination in terms of resolution, granularity, and perceived image quality.

Commentary: *When using traditional analog film radiography it is important to use film and screens that are matched. From a radiation safety viewpoint, the fastest receptor consistent with diagnostic radiographs of high diagnostic quality should be utilized.*

Safety and Risk

Risk assessment: **The risk from radiation used in making a panoramic radiograph is less than one in a million. It is of a similar magnitude to the risks associated with public road traffic encountered on the way to the examination.**

Jung H. The radiation risks from X-ray studies for age assessment in criminal proceedings. Rofo Fortschr Geb Rontgenstr Neuen Bildgeb Verfahr 2000;172:553–556. [From the Institute of Biophysics, Hamburg University, Germany]

Age estimation for forensic purposes is usually based on a panoramic radiograph of the teeth or a radiograph of the left hand. Procedure mortality risks were calculated using both the risk coefficients of International Committee for Radiation Protection and the mass ratio of radiation-exposed portion to total organ. For a panoramic radiograph the following doses were used: bone surface and red bone marrow 0.25 mGy, skin on the neck 0.56 mGy, thyroid gland 0.053 mGy. For a radiation dose of 0.15 mGy was adopted. Mortality risks obtained were 1.8×10^{-7} for a panoramic radiograph and 5.1×10^{-8} for a radiograph of the hand. By comparison, it was estimated that the calculated risks is approximately equivalent to the mortality risks associated with public road traffic during less 2.5 hours or one hour, respectively. The calculated radiation risks are of similar magnitude to the risks the person is exposed to from transportation accidents on the way to the examination.

Commentary: *Risk from radiation imparted during panoramic radiography can be considered very low when there is a diagnostic need to conduct the procedure.*

Radiation-associated meningioma: **Full-mouth series performed 15–40 years ago, when radiation exposure from full-mouth series was greater than it is now, were associated with an increased risk of meningioma. No increased risk to meningioma was observed with panoramic radiographs, cephalograms, or bitewings.**

Longstreth WT Jr, Phillips LE, Drangsholt M, Koepsell TD, Custer BS, Gehrels JA, van Belle G. Dental X-rays and the risk of intracranial meningioma: a population-based case-control study. Cancer 2004 1;100:1026–1034. [From the Department of Neurology, University of Washington, Seattle, USA]

Ionizing radiation is a likely cause of intracranial meningioma. The authors investigated whether the risk of intracranial meningioma was associated with past dental radiographic procedures; specifically, posterior bitewings, full-mouth series, and lateral cephalometric and panoramic radiographs. A population-based case-control study was made among residents of various counties in western Washington State. Case patients ($n = 200$) each had an incident of intracranial meningioma that was confirmed histologically. Random digit dialing and Medicare eligibility lists were used to identify two control subjects to be age- and sex-matched to each case patient. Exposures were determined during an in-person interview. The authors compared self report and dental records in a subset of study participants. Of the 4 dental radiographic procedures evaluated, only the full-mouth series (specifically, = 6 over a lifetime) was associated with a significantly increased risk of meningioma (odds ratio, 2.06; 95% confidence limits, 1.03–4.17). However, evidence for a dose-response relation was lacking (p for trend = 0.33). The risk was elevated with the aggregate number of full-mouth series in 10-year periods from approximately 15–40 years before diagnosis, with significant elevations in the 10-year periods beginning 22–30 years before diagnosis. The risks in these analyses were even greater when only women were considered.

Commentary: *Risk from radiation imparted during dental radiography has been assessed by retrospective analy-*

sis of populations. Care should be taken when reviewing such studies to remember that doses of radiation have been substantially reduced in comparison with the past. Nevertheless, radiographs should only be made if needed for diagnostic purposes and the dose should be kept to that minimally required to produce images of excellent diagnostic quality.

Dosage: **It is possible to reduce radiation dose by substituting solid-state imaging devices for analog film during panoramic radiography; however, dose savings from solid-state panoramic imagers are not as large as found when changing to digital imaging for intraoral radiography.**

Visser H, Hermann KP, Bredemeier S, Kohler B. Dose measurements comparing conventional and digital panoramic radiography. Mund Kiefer Gesichtschir 2000;4:213–216. [From the Abteilung Parodontologie, Georg-August-Universitat Gottingen, Germany]

This study measured and compared patient exposure by digital and conventional panoramic radiography. Dose measurements were carried out on an anthropomorphic phantom, which was specially developed for dental radiography. Panoramic radiographs were made with three different conventional devices and two solid state digital devices. Exposure conditions followed clinical routine. The energy dose was measured at 28 places inside and on the surface of the phantom by using a set of 108 thermoluminescence detectors. Additionally, exposure time, tube voltage, central-beam dose, and dose-area products were measured. The effective doses were calculated on the basis of the absorbed doses. In each case, the highest energy doses were recorded at the parotid gland, the mandibular angle, the submandibular gland, and the skin in the neck. Panoramic radiographs made with the conventional units yielded effective doses in the range of 16–21 μSv, the digital units yielded 5–14 μSv. Hence, in comparison with conventional techniques, patient exposure was reduced by solid state digital panoramic radiography. The extent of dose reduction depended on the device employed and was generally smaller than the dose reduction that can be achieved by digital imaging devices in intraoral radiography.

Commentary: *The radiation dose imparted during panoramic radiography is to some extent dependent on the quantum efficiency of the detector.*

Digital Imaging

Third molar assessment: **Digital panoramic radiography proved equal to film imaging for assessing unerupted third molar teeth.**

Benediktsdottir IS, Hintze H, Petersen JK, Wenzel A. Accuracy of digital and film panoramic radiographs for assessment of position and morphology of mandibular third molars and prevalence of dental anomalies and pathologies. Dentomaxillofac Radiol 2003;32:109–115. [From Department of Oral Radiology, Royal Dental College, University of Aarhus, Denmark]

This study compared the accuracy of digital and film panoramic radiographs for determining (1) the position and shape of mandibular third molars before surgical removal and (2) the prevalence of dental anomalies and pathologies. Three hundred and eighty-eight third mandibular molars were available for examination. Position and morphology of third molars observed on film radiographs and on digital panoramic images from five different systems were recorded by two observers and were compared with surgeons' findings at the time of the operation. One observer further recorded the prevalence of dental anomalies and pathologies using both imaging modalities. Few differences were found between the digital and film based panoramic systems in the assessment of accuracy of position and morphology of mandibular third molars. The prevalence of dental anomalies and pathoses determined with the two modalities was similar. The five digital panoramic systems evaluated in this study were evaluated to be equally as useful for third molar treatment planning and diagnosis of dental anomalies and pathologies as conventional film-based panoramic radiographs.

Commentary: *It can be concluded that digital panoramic systems have a similar diagnostic yield to those using analog film as the detector.*

Soft versus hard copy: **Digital panoramic images were judged to have better quality when viewed on the computer monitor than when printed; however, diagnostic utility was found to be comparable when it came to viewing anatomic features.**

Guerrant GH, Moore WS, Murchison DF. Diagnostic utility of thermal printed panographs compared with corresponding computer monitor images. Gen Dent 2001;49:190–196. [From the Wilford Hall USAF Medical Center, Lackland AFB, Texas, USA]

Digital panoramic radiographs can be either viewed on computer monitors or archived as thermal or laser prints. To compare the available diagnostic information from thermal print images to that of corresponding computer monitor images, four calibrated evaluators performed a qualitative analysis of 13 specified anatomic features in 60 pairs of digital panoramic images presented in random order on a computer monitor and as thermal printed images. Each anatomic site as rated both for subjective diagnostic quality and diagnostic utility using a nominal scale. Computer monitor images more often were subjectively judged to have better quality. Within the parameters of this study, both formats had acceptable diagnostic utility for the majority of the anatomic features evaluated.

Commentary: *When using digital radiography, image quality is best when using a well-calibrated computer monitor display rather than prints.*

Dental Implants

Dental implants: **The panoramic radiograph is considered by some to be a standard for treatment planning dental implants.**

Dula K, Mini R, van der Stelt PF, Buser D. The radiographic assessment of implant patients: decision-making criteria. Int J Oral Maxillofac Implants 2001;16:80–89. [From the Department of Oral Surgery, University of Berne, Switzerland]

Indications for the most frequently used imaging modalities in implant dentistry are proposed based on clinical need and biologic risk to the patient. To calculate the biologic risk, the authors carried out dose measurements. A panoramic radiograph plus a series of four conventional tomographs of a single-tooth space in the molar region were calculated to carry respectively 5% and 13% of the risk from computed tomography. The authors indicate that panoramic radiography is considered the standard radiographic examination for treatment planning of implant patients, because it imparts a low dose while giving the best radiographic survey. They state that periapical radiographs are used to elucidate details or to complete the findings obtained from the panoramic radiograph. Other radiographic methods, such as conventional film tomography or computed tomography, are applied only in special circumstances, film tomography being preferred for smaller regions of interest and computed tomography being justified for the complete maxilla or mandible when methods for dose reduction are followed. During follow-up, intra-oral radiography is considered the standard radiographic examination, particularly for implants in the anterior maxilla. In patients requiring more than five periapical images, a panoramic radiograph is preferred.

Commentary: *Panoramic and intraoral radiographs provide only a two-dimensional view. Three-dimensional radiologic assessment of potential dental implant sites is preferable in most instances. Cone beam volumetric computed tomography is perhaps the modality of choice for dental implant planning.*

Implantology: **Panoramic radiography was proven to be equal to intraoral radiography for the assessment of peri-implant bone loss in the anterior mandible.**

Zechner W, Watzak G, Gahleitner A, Busenlechner D, Tepper G, Watzek G. Rotational panoramic versus intra-oral rectangular radiographs for evaluation of peri-implant bone loss in the anterior atrophic mandible. Int J Oral Maxillofac Implants 2003;18:873–878. [From the Department of Oral Surgery, University of Vienna, Austria]

In patients with atrophic mandibles, elevation of the floor of the mouth often prevents intra-oral rectangular radiography for longitudinal follow-up studies, while extraoral techniques such as panoramic radiographs have been perceived to produce distorted views of the interforaminal region. In this study, intra-oral and panoramic radiographs were compared for their accuracy in evaluating peri-implant bone loss. In a recall program, 22 patients with 88 screw-type implants (44 MKII and 44 Frios) were followed. Interforaminal marginal bone loss was evaluated by panoramic radiography and by using intra-oral radiographs. In addition, pocket depth, periodontology test readings, and bleeding on probing were recorded. For statistical analysis, the Spearman coefficient of correlation was used. The effects on bone loss and clinical variables were computed with a mixed model and the Bland and Altman method. Computed as least square means, the mean difference between panoramic radiographs (2.4 ± 0.2 mm for MKII implants and 1.6 ± 0.2 mm for Frios implants) and intra-oral radiographs (2.6 ± 0.2 mm and 1.4 ± 0.2 mm, respectively) was 0.2 mm (range, 0.1 to 0.8 mm). In this study, the two imaging techniques were comparable clinically in terms of the precision with which they could be used to measure marginal bone loss. Hence, for highly atrophic mandibles with unfavorable imaging conditions, rotational panoramic radiographs can be a useful alternative to intra-oral radiographs for evaluating peri-implant bone loss.

Commentary: *It should be noted that panoramic and intraoral radiographs provide only a two-dimensional view. Three-dimensional radiologic assessment of potential dental implant sites is preferable in most instances.*

A method was devised for using panoramic radiographs to assess the space availability for miniscrew implants used in orthodontics. It appears that adequate space for placement is rarely available in the attached gingiva.

Schnelle MA, Beck FM, Jaynes RM, Huja SS. A radiographic evaluation of the availability of bone for placement of miniscrews. Angle Orthod 2004;74:832–837. [From Ohio State University, Columbus, Ohio, USA]

Monocortical screws are used to improve anchorage for application of orthodontic forces. It is clinically advantageous for such miniscrews to be placed in attached mucosa. A study was conducted to determine radiographically the most coronal interradicular sites for placement of miniscrews in orthodontic patients and to determine if orthodontic alignment increases the number of sites with adequate interradicular bone for placement of these screws. Following Institutional Review Board approval, 60 panoramic radiographs (30 pre-treatment and 30 post-treatment) of orthodontic patients were obtained from an archival database. Selection criteria included minimal radiographic distortion and complete eruption of permanent second molars. Interradicular sites were examined with a digital caliper for presence of 3–4 mm of bone to the designated horizontal bone location for implant placement. If 3–4 mm of bone existed, then a vertical measurement from the cemento-enamel junction to the initial measurement point was made. The magnification inherent in panoramic radiographs was estimated. Ninety-five per cent confidence intervals were calculated for the vertical distances from the cemento-enamel junction to the horizontal bone location. Bone stock for placement of screws was found to exist primarily mesial to maxillary first molars and both mesial and distal to mandibular first molars. Adequate bone space was typically located more than halfway down the root length, which is likely to be covered by movable mucosa. Inability to place miniscrews in attached gingiva could necessitate design modifications to decrease soft tissue irritation.

Commentary: *Panoramic and intraoral radiographs provide only a two-dimensional view. Three-dimensional radiologic assessment of potential dental implant sites is preferable in most instances. Further, no radiographic method can make up for inherent complications in implant design related to the desired positioning.*

Prosthodontics

Edentulous ridge assessment: Laboratory data suggests that serial panoramic radiographs are suitable for assessing the progression of maxillary ridge resorption.

Kreisler M, Schulze R, Schalldach F, d'Hoedt B, Behneke A, Behneke N. A new method for the radiological investigation of residual ridge resorption in the maxilla. Dentomaxillofac Radiol 2000;29:368–375. [From the Department of Oral Surgery, Johannes Gutenberg-University, Mainz, Germany]

The authors present a method for assessing residual ridge resorption in the edentulous maxilla. Defined experimental and reference areas in the maxilla were drawn on transparent film laid over a panoramic radiograph and digitized. Bone areas were measured with an integrated planimetry program and expressed as a ratio. The effect of positioning errors on reliability of the method was investigated using dry skulls. The correlation between the change in ratio and actual bone loss was examined by progressively reducing the height of an artificial residual ridge on one skull. The coefficient of variation for the absolute ratio in different head positions was <0.05 and its correlation coefficient of the change in the ratio and the degree of resorption was $r^2 \geq 98.3\%$ ($p = 0.0001$). Comparison of the experimental area with the reference area on serial panoramic radiographs appears suitable for the assessment of residual ridge resorption in the maxilla.

Commentary: *It is much easier to effect precise repositioning of a skull in vitro than of a patient in vivo. Care should be made to keep to the same panoramic system as magnification and distortion differ between systems as well as being influenced by patient positioning.*

Orthodontics

Apical root resorption: Panoramic radiographs made before and following orthodontic treatment has been used to assess apical root resorption.

McNab S, Battistutta D, Taverne A, Symons AL. External apical root resorption following orthodontic treatment. Angle Orthod 2000;70:227–232. [From Queensland University of Technology, Brisbane, Australia]

The association of appliance type and tooth extraction with the incidence of external apical root resorption of posterior teeth following orthodontic treatment was investigated using pre- and post-treatment panoramic radiographs. The study comprised 97 patients. A 4-level ordinal scale was used to rate apical external root resorption. The analysis was mutually adjusted for the effects of age at the start of treatment, pre-treatment overbite and overjet, use of headgear, tooth extraction, and type of appliance. The incidence of such resorption was positively associated with tooth position ($p < .001$), appliance type ($p = .038$), and extractions ($p = .001$). The incidence of resorption was 2.3 times higher for Begg appliance treatment compared with edgewise, and it was 3.7 times higher where extractions had been performed than when they were not.

Commentary: *Caution should be taken when attempting to use the panoramic radiograph for assessment of tooth root resorption, especially in the anterior segments of the jaws. Poor positioning of the patient within the cephalostat—or simply marked jaw size discrepancies—can take the tooth apices outside the image layer or focal trough.*

This can lead to the impression of root resorption that is not actually present. (See Chapter 10 for use of panoramic radiographs in orthodontics.)

Orthodontics: Premolar extraction reduces the probability of third molar impaction.

Kim TW, Artun J, Behbehani F, Artese F. Prevalence of third molar impaction in orthodontic patients treated nonextraction and with extraction of 4 premolars. Am J Orthod Dentofacial Orthop 2003;123:138–145. [From the Department of Orthodontics, Seoul National University, Korea]

This study tested the hypothesis that premolar extraction treatment is associated with mesial movement of the molars concomitant with an increase in the eruption space for the third molars, thereby reducing the frequency of third molar impaction. Panoramic or periapical radiographs, lateral cephalograms, and study models made before (Time 1) and after (Time 2) treatment and a minimum of 10 years postretention (Time 3) of 157 patients were selected from the Department of Orthodontics of the University of Washington, Seattle. Treatment for 105 patients included extraction of four premolars; the other 53 (controls) had been treated without extraction. Student *t*-tests were applied to the data for statistical comparison. For the controls, third molar impaction was found to be more common than in patients who had undergone premolar extraction ($p < .01$), there was less mesial movement of the molars from Time 1 to Time 2 ($p < .01$), and a smaller retromolar space was found on average at Time 2 ($p < .001$) in both arches. Moreover, molar movement was more mesial from Time 1 to Time 2 both in the maxilla ($p < .01$) and in the mandible ($p < .05$), and the retromolar space was larger in both arches ($p < .001$) of the patients with eruption than in those with impaction of third molars. The results support the hypothesis that premolar extraction reduces the frequency of third molar impaction due to increased eruption space afforded by mesial movement of the molars during space closure.

Commentary: *Panoramic radiographs can be used sequentially to assess the impact of dental extractions on subsequent eruption of adjacent teeth. (See Chapter 10 for use of panoramic radiographs in orthodontics.)*

Panoramic radiography was used to assess the successful outcome of third molars replacing extracted second molar teeth.

De-la-Rosa-Gay C, Valmaseda-Castellon E, Gay-Escoda C. Spontaneous third-molar eruption after second-molar extraction in orthodontic patients. Am J Orthod Dentofacial Orthop 2006;129:337–344. [From the School of Dentistry, University of Barcelona, Spain]

A retrospective study was made to assess the eruption of third molars by using panoramic radiographs and to identify the variables associated with unsuccessful eruption. The subjects were 48 patients who had 128 permanent second molars extracted during or before orthodontic treatment. Their ages at extraction were 11 to 23 years. The position of the third molars was assessed from panoramic radiographs made prior to second-molar extraction and after third-molar eruption. The median time of eruption was three to four years (interquartile range, 2 years). A successful final position for the third molar was defined as eruption with proximal contact with the adjacent first molar and an angle between these two teeth of no more than 35°. 96% of the maxillary and 66% of the mandibular third molars erupted in positions considered to be "good" in terms of successful replacement of the extracted second molars. Most cases designated unsuccessful were due to excessive mesial tilting or lack of proximal tooth contact.

Commentary: *This study demonstrates that panoramic radiographs can be used sequentially to assess the impact of dental extractions on subsequent eruption of adjacent teeth. (See Chapter 8 for use of panoramic radiographs in orthodontics.)*

Premolar extraction: Panoramic radiology was used to assess the effects of first premolar extraction on the angulation of third molar teeth.

Saysel MY, Meral GD, Kocadereli I, Tasar F. The effects of first premolar extractions on third molar angulations. Angle Orthod 2005;75:719–722 [From the Department of Oral Surgery, Hacettepe University, Ankara, Turkey]

This study determined the relationship between the inclinations of second and third molar teeth during a two to two and a half year period in patients treated orthodontically both with and without premolar extractions. Records of 37 first premolar extraction cases and 33 non-extraction cases were examined. Pre-treatment and post-treatment panoramic radiographs were analyzed. Angles were measured between the long axis of the third molar and the occlusal plane and between the long axis of the third molar and the long axis of the second molar. Changes in third molar angulations from pre-treatment to post-treatment for two groups were compared using the Mann-Whitney U-test. Statistical analysis revealed that mandibular third molars showed an improvement in angulation relative to the occlusal plane in the first premolar extraction group.

Commentary: *Panoramic radiographs can be used sequentially to assess the impact of dental extractions on subsequent eruption of adjacent teeth. This study confirms the findings of the previous abstracted study. (See above.)*

Third molar eruption assessment: Sequential panoramic radiographs can be used to evaluate eruption of third molars following extraction of second molar teeth.

Orton-Gibbs S, Crow V, Orton HS. Eruption of third permanent molars after the extraction of second permanent molars. Part 1: Assessment of third molar position and size. Am J Orthod Dentofacial Orthop 2001;119:226–238. [From St. Helier Hospital, Surrey, UK]

The eruptive path of third molars after extraction of second molars was examined in 63 patients. Panoramic radiographs from the start and the end of active treatment and three or more years after treatment were assessed. Study models were used to compare the size of the second and third molar teeth and to assess the final position of the third molars following eruption. All third molars erupted; none became impacted. During eruption, maxillary third molar crowns uprighted and maintained their angulation as they came into occlusion. Mandibular third molar crowns continued to upright significantly mesiodistally after active treatment, with space closure being the result of horizontal translation rather than mesial tipping. Further uprighting occurred once occlusion was established although few became as upright as the second molars they replaced. Mandibular third molar roots were frequently curved distally, thus the third molar crown position was invariably better than the overall tooth angulation would suggest by 16.5° on average. Model analysis (Richardsons' scoring system) showed 96% of mandibular and 99% of maxillary third molars erupted into an acceptable position. The mesiodistal size of third molars was suitable to replace second molars. On average, mandibular third molars were 0.55 mm larger and maxillary third molars were 0.70 mm smaller than second molars.

Commentary: *Panoramic radiographs can be used sequentially to assess the impact of dental extractions on subsequent eruption of adjacent teeth. (See Chapter 8 for use of panoramic radiographs in orthodontics.)*

No statistical difference was found between ABO standardized methods for assessing orthodontic treatment success and a visual index applied subsequent to the ABO analysis.

Scott SA, Freer TJ. Visual application of the American Board of Orthodontics Grading System. Aust Orthod J 2005;21:55–60. [From the School of Dentistry, University of Queensland, Australia]

Assessment of orthodontic treatment outcomes has traditionally been accomplished using the subjective opinion of experienced clinicians. Reduced subjectivity in the assessment of orthodontic treatment can be achieved with the use of an occlusal index. To implement an index for quality assurance purposes is time-consuming and subject to the inherent error of the index. Quality assessment of orthodontic treatment on a routine basis has been difficult to implement in private practice. This study was to investigate whether a clinician can accurately apply the American Board of Orthodontics Objective Grading System by direct visual inspection instead of measuring individual traits. A random sample of 30 cases was selected, including pre-treatment and post-treatment maxillary and mandibular study casts and panoramic radiographs. The cases were examined and scored with the standardized measuring gauge according to the protocol provided by the American Board of Orthodontics. The records were re-examined six weeks later and the individual traits scored by visual inspection. There were no significant differences between the pre- and post-treatment American Board of Orthodontics gauge and visual inspection scores. The authors suggest that occlusal traits defined by the American Board of Orthodontics Objective Grading System might be accurately assessed by visual inspection. The visual index score provides a simple and convenient method for critical evaluation of treatment outcome by a clinician.

Commentary: *This study might have produced stronger evidence if the sequence of evaluation had been reversed for half of the cases included in the study. (See Chapter 8 for use of panoramic radiographs in orthodontics.)*

Growth and Maturity

Age determination: Standard criteria have been developed using panoramic radiographs for the assessment of biologic age in Swedish children and adolescents.

Nystrom M, Aine L, Peck L, Haavikko K, Kataja M. Dental maturity in Finns and the problem of missing teeth. Acta Odontol Scand 2000;58:49–56. [From the Department of Pedodontics and Orthodontics, University of Helsinki, Finland]

Development of teeth was studied from 2,483 dental panoramic radiographs of 1,651 healthy subjects ranging in age from 2 to 25 years. Dental maturity was assessed using a method based on developmental stages of seven left mandibular teeth. Sex-specific tables were developed of maturity as a function of chronological age and of ages as a function of maturity scores. Percentile graphs for visual evaluations of dental maturity in children and adolescents were also developed. Since maturity scales do not tolerate any missing data, the authors developed linear regression models for predicting the formation stages of each of the seven mandibular teeth. It was easiest to predict the formation stage of the mandibular first molars (correct in 87% within the study material) and most difficult to predict the formation stage of second molars and second premolars (correct in 69% and 70%, respectively).

Commentary: *The panoramic radiograph is perhaps the most efficient method for judging tooth development stages. (See Chapter 9.)*

Dental age assessment: Panoramic radiography provides an excellent means of assessing the dental age of patients; however, there is a need to develop separate assessment standards for different population groups.

Davidson LE, Rodd HD. Interrelationship between dental age and chronological age in Somali children. Community Dent Health 2001;18:27–30. [From the Department of Child Dental Health, University of Sheffield, UK]

This cross-sectional study compared dental age with chronological age in Somali children under 16 years of age and age- and sex-matched white Caucasian children, all resident in Sheffield, England. The sample group comprised 162 subjects: 84 Somali and Caucasian boys (mean age 10.6 years) and 78 Somali and white Caucasian girls (mean age 11.2 years). The dental age was assessed for each subject using existing panoramic radiographs. Comparisons of the difference between dental age and chronological age were made for each sex and both ethnic groups. Independent sample *t*-tests were employed for statistical analysis. The level of significance was set at $p < 0.05$. The mean difference between dental age and chronological age was found to be: 1.0 years for Somali boys, 0.2 years for Caucasian boys, 1.2 years for Somali girls, and 0.5 years for Caucasian girls. The difference between dental and chronological age was significantly greater in Somali subjects than in Caucasian children. The authors conclude that Somali children are more dentally advanced than their Caucasian peers. This finding underlines the need for population-specific dental development standards for accurate dental age assessment.

Commentary: *While the panoramic radiograph is an efficient method for judging tooth development stages, ethnicity should be factored when relating this information to age assessments. (See Chapter 9.)*

Lateral cephalograms: Cervical vertebral morphology can be used to accurately assess skeletal maturity.

San Roman P, Palma JC, Oteo MD, Nevado E. Skeletal maturation determined by cervical vertebrae development. Eur J Orthod 2002;24:303–311. [From the Department of Orthodontics, Complutense University, Madrid, Spain]

This study investigated the validity of using cervical vertebral radiographic assessment to predict skeletal maturation. Left hand-wrist and lateral cephalometric radiographs of 958 Spanish children from 5 to 18 years of age were studied. The classification of Grave and Brown was used to assess skeletal maturation from the hand-wrist radiograph. Cervical vertebrae maturation was evaluated with lateral cephalometric radiographs using the stages described by Hassel and Farman and by Lamparski. A new method to evaluate the cervical maturation by studying the changes in the concavity of the lower border, height, and shape of the vertebral body was created. Correlation coefficients were calculated to establish the relationship between skeletal maturation values obtained by the three classifications of vertebral and skeletal maturation measured at the wrist. All correlation values obtained were statistically significant ($p < 0.001$). In the population investigated, the new method was as accurate as the Hassel and Farman classification and superior to the Lamparski classification.

Commentary: *Continued development and education of the profession regarding cervical vertebral indices for skeletal aging seems warranted. (See Chapter 9.)*

Stylohyoid ossification: Ossification within the stylohyoid chain is demonstrable on panoramic radiography. Such ossification advances with increased patient age.

Krennmair G, Lenglinger F, Lugmayr H. Variants of ossification of the stylohyoid chain. Rofo Fortschr Geb Rontgenstr Neuen Bildgeb Verfahr 2001;173:200–204. [From the Oral and Maxillofacial Surgery Clinic, University of Vienna, Austria]

Panoramic radiographs of 380 patients (including 718 radiographs clearly depicting the regions of the stylohyoid chains), were subdivided into four age groups (= 20 years, 21–40 years, 41–60 years, > 60 years), and were reviewed and examined for the incidence, length and location(s) of ossifications in the stylohyoid chains. Elongation of the styloid process or ossification of the stylohyoid ligament was found in 221 (30.8%) of the reviewed stylohyoid chains. With increasing age, there was an increase in the prevalence and length of stylohyoid ossifications ($p < 0.01$). A significant linear correlation between the length of the stylohyoid ossifications and age was only found in the young age group (= 20 years; $p < 0.01$). In this age group, there was also a predominance of isolated locations of ossification in the superior stylohyoid segment. With increasing patient age, the presence of ossifications in the middle and inferior stylohyoid segments and combinations of ossified variations were prominent. The authors conclude that stylohyoid ossification shows age-related differences in incidence, length and topography.

Commentary: *Care should be taken when using the panoramic radiograph to assess calcification of the stylohyoid ligament. The image layer/focal trough is designed to demonstrate the dentition, and to a lesser extent the temporomandibular joint. The stylohyoid ligament might not be clearly demonstrated.*

Oncologic Dentistry

Oral cancer: Panoramic radiography is a useful adjunct in evaluation of bone invasion by gingival squamous cell carcinoma.

Gomez D, Faucher A, Picot V, Siberchicot F, Renaud-Salis JL, Bussieres E, Pinsolle J. Outcome of squamous cell carcinoma of the gingiva: a follow-up study of 83 cases. J Craniomaxillofac Surg 2000;28:331–335. [From the Bergonie Institute, Regional Cancer Center, Bordeaux, France]

Squamous cell carcinoma of the gingiva is relatively uncommon. Standard treatments involve surgery and radiation therapy. From 1985 to1996, 83 patients with squamous cell carcinoma of the gingiva were treated at the Department of Surgery, the Bergonie Institute and at the Department of Maxillofacial and Plastic Surgery of the University Hospital, Bordeaux, France. A retrospective review of panoramic radiographs and clinical records was used to evaluate bone involvement from the gingival carcinomas. Outcomes were calculated using the Kaplan-Meier method. Primary local control was achieved in 72 patients (87%). Overall survival and rate of recurrence were comparable to those reported for other squamous cell carcinomas of the oral cavity and oropharynx.

Commentary: *The panoramic radiograph is frequently used in screening oral oncology patients prior to cancer therapy and in subsequent follow-up evaluations. (Oncologic dentistry is overviewed in Chapter 16.)*

Jaw Fractures

Maxillofacial trauma: Panoramic radiographs proved significantly more reliable than mandibular plain film radiographic series for the detection of mandibular jaw fractures.

Nair MK, Nair UP. Imaging of mandibular trauma: ROC analysis. Acad Emerg Med 2001;8:689–695. [From the Department of Oral and Maxillofacial Radiology, University of Pittsburgh, USA]

The objective of this study was to compare the diagnostic efficacy for detection of mandibular fractures of panoramic radiography versus mandibular trauma series presented both as analog and as digitized radiographs. Fractures were induced using blunt trauma to 25 cadaver mandibles. Panoramic radiographs and mandibular series comprising an antero-posterior view, two lateral oblique, and a reverse Towne's projection were made. The mandibular series was viewed both in analog and in digitized forms. Six observers recorded their interpretations using a five-point confidence rating scale. The data was studied using receiver operating characteristic curve analysis. Significant differences based on imaging modalities were found ($p < 0.0015$) in the area under the curves (A_z): mandibular series, 0.75; digitized mandibular series, 0.77, panoramic radiograph, 0.87; and panoramic plus antero-posterior radiographs in combination, 0.89. No observer-based differences were found. Intra- and inter-observer agreements were high ($kappa_w = 0.81$ and 0.76, respectively). It is concluded that panoramic radiographs are adequate for the detection of mandibular fractures. The addition of an antero-posterior view only marginally improved diagnostic accuracy.

Commentary: *The panoramic radiograph equal to a several view mandibular series for detection of fractures of the lower jaw; however, computed tomography is preferable to either when maxillary fractures are possible. (See Chapter 14.)*

Jaw fracture and third molar impaction: This study did provide evidence that patients with retained or impacted third molars are significantly more susceptible to angle fracture than those without third molars.

Meisami T, Sojat A, Sandor GK, Lawrence HP, Clokie CM. Impacted third molars and risk of angle fracture. Int J Oral Maxillofac Surg 2002;31:140–144. [From the Department of Oral and Maxillofacial Surgery, University of Toronto, Ontario, Canada]

This investigation assessed the influence of the presence, position, and severity of impaction of the mandibular third molars on the incidence of mandibular angle fractures. A retrospective cohort study was designed for patients presenting to the Division of Oral and Maxillofacial Surgery, Toronto General Hospital, Canada, for treatment of mandibular fractures from January 1995 through June 2000. The study sample comprised 413 mandibular fractures in 214 patients. Demographic data collected included age, sex, mechanism of injury, and number of mandibular fractures. Independent variables studied were the presence, position, and severity of impaction of third molars; the outcome variable was the incidence of mandibular angle fractures. Panoramic radiographs and hospital records were used to determine and classify these variables. The incidence of angle fractures was found to be significantly higher in the male population and was most commonly seen in the third decade of life. Assault was the most frequent causative factor. This study did provide evidence that patients with retained or impacted third molars are significantly more susceptible to mandibular angle fracture than those without third molars. Patients with third molars had a three times increased risk of angle fractures when compared to patients without ($p < 0.001$), and impaction of third molars significantly increased the incidence of mandibular angle fractures ($p < 0.001$). The severity and angulation of third molar impactions did not prove to be significantly associated with angle fractures.

Commentary: *The panoramic radiograph can be used to detect impacted third mandibular molars. In patients at high risk of traumatic injury to the face, extraction of impacted third molars might be warranted. (See Chapter 14.)*

Dental Impactions

Canine ectopia: Using panoramic radiographs, approximately half the subjects with palatal ectopia of canines also have other dental anomalies. Buccal ectopia of the canine was not associated with such additional dental anomalies.

Becker A, Chaushu S. Dental age in maxillary canine ectopia. Am J Orthod Dentofacial Orthop 2000;117:657–662. [From the Department of Orthodontics, Hebrew University-Hadassah, Jerusalem, Israel]

An etiologic connection between palatally ectopic canines and small and missing teeth is well established in the literature. Additionally, it has been observed that patients with palatally ectopic canines have delayed dental development. This report examined the validity of this latter observation. The authors assessed radiographically the subjects' dental ages using criteria of tooth calcification, rather than tooth eruption pattern. A similar determination was made in relation to subjects in whom buccally ectopic canines were present. The experimental group consisted of panoramic radiographs of 55 consecutively treated patients with palatally displaced maxillary canines and of 47 consecutively treated patients with buccally displaced canines. The panoramic radiographs were compared with those from a control group of 57 consecutively treated patients with normally placed canines. Approximately half the subjects with palatal displacement exhibited a late-developing dentition, whereas the timing of dentition in the remaining subjects appeared to be normal. Buccal displacement was not associated with a retarded dental development, and the ranges of the dental age values were similar to those seen in the control group. The results support the idea that there are different etiologies for the occurrence of buccal versus palatal ectopia of maxillary canines. They also suggest that dentitions with a palatal canine could be of two distinct varieties, with different dental characteristics and, perhaps, different etiologies.

Commentary: *This report suggests an association between canine ectopia and delayed development of the dentition. (See Chapters 6 and 7.)*

Impacted canines: Panoramic radiography combined with a lateral cephalometric image is useful in treatment planning impacted maxillary canines.

Stivaros N, Mandall NA. Radiographic factors affecting the management of impacted upper permanent canines. J Orthod 2000;27:169–173. [From the Orthodontic Department, University Dental Hospital, Manchester, UK]

The investigators used a retrospective, cross-sectional design to evaluate radiographic factors influencing the orthodontists' decision whether to expose or remove an impacted upper permanent canine. Panoramic and lateral cephalometric radiographic records of patients referred between 1994 and 1998 to the Orthodontic Department at Manchester University Dental Hospital having impacted upper permanent canines ($n = 44$) were evaluated. Canine position measurements made from the panoramic radiograph were angulation to the midline, vertical height, antero-posterior position of the root, overlap of the adjacent incisor, and presence of root resorption of adjacent incisor(s). The labio-palatal position of the impacted canine was assessed from the lateral skull radiograph. Whether the impacted canine had been exposed and orthodontically aligned or removed was also recorded. Stepwise logistic regression analysis showed that the labiopalatal position of the crown influenced the treatment decision, with palatally positioned impacted canines more likely to be surgically exposed and those in the line of the arch, or labially situated, removed ($p < 0.05$). Additionally, as the canine angulation to the midline increased, the canine was more likely to be removed ($p < 0.05$). The orthodontists' decision to expose or remove an impacted upper permanent canine, based on radiographic information, seems to be primarily guided by two factors: labio-palatal crown position and angulation to the midline. These can be readily assessed using a combination of panoramic radiography and a lateral cephalometric image.

Commentary: *The panoramic radiograph can be used in combination with other views such as the lateral cephalo-*

metric radiograph to improve assessment of the position of anterior dental impactions. (See Chapter 7 for more details on use of panoramic radiographs for evaluation of dental impactions.)

Impacted canines: **The probability of impaction of a maxillary canine is very high when the canine overlaps the midline of the lateral incisor.**

Warford JH Jr, Grandhi RK, Tira DE. Prediction of maxillary canine impaction using sectors and angular measurement. Am J Orthod Dentofacial Orthop 2003;124:651–655. [From the Department of Orthodontics and Dentofacial Orthopedics, University of Missouri, USA]

Maxillary canine impaction has an incidence of one in a hundred in the general population. Because patients with canine impactions generally have relatively long orthodontic treatment times, early identification of impaction is of importance to the orthodontist. In this investigation, angulation of the unerupted canine was measured from panoramic radiographs and added to sector location to see whether the combination of these factors could predict impaction more accurately than sector alone. Logistic regression analysis determined that once the canine overlaps the midline of the lateral incisor, there is a greater than 0.87 chance of impaction. Sector location was found to be the better predictor of impaction, with angulation providing little supplementary predictive value.

Commentary: *Impacted maxillary canines are a fairly frequent finding. The panoramic radiograph can help in early detection—and early detection potentially facilitates better treatment outcomes. (See Chapter 7 for more details on use of panoramic radiographs for evaluation of dental impactions.)*

Impacted teeth: **Panoramic radiographs revealed impacted teeth in more than 28% of the study population in Hong Kong.**

Chu FC, Li TK, Lui VK, Newsome PR, Chow RL, Cheung LK. Prevalence of impacted teeth and associated pathologies: a radiographic study of the Hong Kong Chinese population. Hong Kong Med J 2003;9:158–163. [From Prince Philip Dental Hospital Faculty of Dentistry, University of Hong Kong]

The records of 7,486 patients were examined and a total of 2,115 (28%) patients were determined to have at least one impacted tooth. The prevalence of impacted teeth was high, with a predilection for impacted third molars in the mandible. As more than 50% of maxillary third molars had erupted in patients having impacted mandibular third molars, this created potential trauma to the pericoronal tissues overlying the impacted mandibular third molars. Roughly one-third of patients with dental impaction reported associated symptoms. Of a total of 3,853 impacted teeth, mandibular third molars were the most frequent (83%), followed by maxillary third molars (16%), and maxillary canines (1%). Some 8% of mandibular second molars associated with impacted third molars had periodontal bone loss of more than 5 mm on their distal surfaces. Caries were also found on the distal surface of 7% of the associated second molars. Caries and periodontal diseases were commonly seen in relation to the impacted third molars, yet cystic pathoses and root resorption were rarely observed.

Commentary: *Dental impactions have a very high frequency of occurrence in many populations. Panoramic radiography is an efficient method for the detection of dental impactions (See Chapter 7 for more details on use of panoramic radiographs for evaluation of dental impactions.)*

Impacted third molars: **An intimate association between the tooth and the inferior alveolar canal often resulted in a darkening of the root of the affected tooth when viewed with panoramic radiography.**

Bell GW. Use of dental panoramic tomographs to predict the relation between mandibular third molar teeth and the inferior alveolar nerve. Radiological and surgical findings, and clinical outcome. Br J Oral Maxillofac Surg 2004;42:21–27. [From the Oral and Maxillofacial Surgery Department, Dumfries and Galloway Royal Infirmary, UK]

Preoperative radiological observations from dental panoramic tomographs were compared with surgical findings at removal of third molars with respect to relationship of the tooth to the inferior alveolar nerve. One surgeon viewed the radiographs of 219 patients and recorded the radiological observations of the mandibular third molar tooth and the inferior alveolar canal. The same surgeon removed the teeth and made detailed records of morphology of the root and its relation to the inferior alveolar nerve. Patients were reviewed postoperatively. A total of 300 teeth were removed and the neurovascular bundle observed during surgery. The roots were grooved or deflected due to their proximity to the neurovascular bundle in 12% of the cases ($n = 35$). There was an intimate relation between the mandibular third molar tooth and the inferior alveolar nerve in 51% of cases when darkening of the root was observed ($n = 12$), but only in 11% of cases ($n = 11$) when there appeared to be interruption of the radio-opaque outline of the inferior alveolar canal radiographically.

Commentary: *Panoramic radiography is an efficient method for the detection of dental impactions. Some au-*

thors believe that it is possible to assess the relationship of the inferior dental/mandibular canal to the third molar when these two are superimposed on the panoramic radiographic image. They use morphologic signs rather than measurements. Nevertheless, imaging to disclose the third dimension is still advised in the opinion of the editor of this book. (See Chapter 7 for more details on use of panoramic radiographs for evaluation of dental impactions.)

Impacted third molars: Radiographic changes in the position of impacted third molar teeth can be considerable even after the usual age for eruption of such teeth.

Venta I, Turtola L, Ylipaavalniemi P. Radiographic follow-up of impacted third molars from age 20 to 32 years. Int J Oral Maxillofacial Surg 2001;30:54–57. [From the Department of Oral Medicine, University of Helsinki, Finland]

Nineteen patients (13 male, six female) with 34 impacted third molars (21 in the mandible and 13 in the maxilla) were followed using panoramic radiographs from age 20 to 32 years. All were examined clinically and panoramic radiographs were made at baseline and at the end of the study. Radiographic criteria included tooth resorption, follicular enlargement, root development, change in inclination of the third molar, state of impaction, and the relative depth of the third molar in bone and its relation both to the ramus of the mandible and to the second molar tooth. In the mandible, the mean change in inclination was 19° with 76% of teeth changing in angulation. In the maxilla, only 23% of the teeth changed in inclination. The state of impaction (soft tissue, partially in bone, completely in bone) had changed for 44% of the teeth. According to a questionnaire, no pain or other symptoms in the region of the third molars were reported by 74% of the subjects during the 12-year study period. The authors conclude that considerable radiographic changes, without notable symptoms, can occur in terms of tooth inclination and the state of impaction of third molars after the usual age for their eruption.

Commentary: *While panoramic radiographs provide a general screening assessment of the impacted mandibular third molar, additional imaging is justified to provide a view of the third dimension where there is apparent overlap of the tooth and the mandibular canal. (The use of panoramic radiographs to assess dental impactions is discussed in Chapter 7.)*

Third molars that appear impacted at age 18 years can often erupt into normal occlusion by age 26 years.

Kruger E, Thomson WM, Konthasinghe P. Third molar outcomes from age 18 to 26: findings from a population based New Zealand longitudinal study. Oral Surg Oral Med Oral Pathol Oral Radiol Endod 2001;92:150–155. [From the Department of Oral Health, University of Otago, Dunedin, New Zealand]

This study evaluated the presence and impaction status of third molars in persons at age 18 years, as well as the observed changes in their clinical status between ages 18 and 26 years. This prospective cohort study was performed on 821 individuals for whom panoramic radiographs were taken at age 18 years. For each tooth, its radiographic impaction status at age 18 years was compared with the clinical status by age 26 years. Of the 2,857 third molars assessed at age 18 years, 93% were followed clinically to age 26 years. Approximately 55% of the teeth that were not impacted by age 18 had erupted by 26 years. Of the teeth that were impacted by age 18, 34% had fully erupted by age 26, 3% had been extracted, and 13% remained unerupted. Of the maxillary teeth that were categorized as impacted at age 18 years, 36% had fully erupted by age 26, whereas 26% of the mandibular teeth had done so ($p < .01$). Fewer mandibular teeth than maxillary teeth remained unerupted by the time the patient was 26 years old (27% and 41%, respectively; $p < .01$), but there was no significant difference between the jaws in the proportion of impacted teeth at age 18 years that had been extracted by age 26 years (both 30%). For mesioangularly impacted third molars, 39% of maxillary teeth and 20% of mandibular teeth had fully erupted by age 26, whereas almost one-third of each had been extracted. Of the distoangularly impacted third molars, 20% of the maxillary teeth and one-third of the mandibular teeth erupted by age 26, with 23% of the maxillary teeth and 32% of the mandibular teeth having been extracted. It was concluded that other than horizontally impacted third molars, a substantial proportion of other impaction types do erupt fully, and radiographically apparent impaction in late adolescence should not be sufficient grounds for their prophylactic removal in the absence of other clinical indications.

Commentary: *Sequential panoramic radiographs can provide a useful method for assessing the development of mandibular third molars. Extraction of these teeth is not an invariable need. (The use of panoramic radiographs to assess dental impactions is discussed in Chapter 7.)*

Second molar eruption patterns: Panoramic radiographs can be used to assess the eruption patterns and space availability for second permanent molars.

Tsai LLLI. Eruption process of the second molar. ASDC J Dent Child 2000;67:275–281. [From the Department of Pedodontics, School of Dentistry, China Medical College, Taichung, Taiwan, Republic of China]

This study observed the eruption process of maxillary and mandibular second molars by evaluating 238 panoramic radiographs. The developmental of the second molars was divided into four stages: completion of crown calcified = stage 1; initial root formation = stage 2; initial formation of the radicular bifurcation = stage 3; and root length equal to crown height = stage 4. The mesiodistal crown width of the first and second molars, axial inclination and eruption rate of these teeth, and the space available for their emergence was measured at each stage. Statistical analysis was performed to assess changes in development. Mandibular second molars began to erupt at stage 3 and maxillary second molars at stage 2. The axial inclination of the mandibular second molars was essentially unchanged from stages 1 to 4 but maxillary second molars uprighted gradually from stage 1 to 4. The available space increased significantly from stages 1 to 2 in both jaws. It is suggested that the space available for emergence of the second molar is prepared before stage 2, and the tooth begins to erupt. For the maxillary second molars, there was a further increase in the available space after stage 3. A negative correlation was determined between the mesiodistal crown width of the mandibular second molar and the available jaw space at stage 2. A positive correlation was seen between the mesiodistal crown width of maxillary second molars and the available jaw space at stage 3.

Commentary: *Panoramic radiographs can provide a rough guide to space needs and availability during orthodontic assessment. (The use of panoramic radiographs to assess dental impactions is discussed in Chapter 7.)*

Dental Anomalies

Developmental abnormalities: **Abnormalities affecting dental treatment planning were found in panoramic radiographs from >20% of adolescents aged 10–15 years.**

Cholitgul W, Drummond BK. Jaw and tooth radiographs in New Zealand children aged 10–15 years. N Z Dent J 2000;96:10–13. [From the Department of Radiology, Faculty of Dentistry, Chulalongkorn University, Bangkok, Thailand]

Panoramic radiographs of 1,608 children and adolescents aged 10 to 15 years (797 males and 811 females) were reviewed to determine the prevalence of tooth and jaw abnormalities. Abnormalities were detected on 21% of the radiographs (23% for females and 17% for males); 879 teeth were diagnosed with abnormalities in 331 panoramic radiographs. The more common abnormalities were malpositioned teeth, missing teeth, morphologic anomalies of teeth, and teeth with structural defects such as hypoplasia. Bony abnormalities and growth problems were detected on occasion. These findings demonstrates the value of panoramic radiography in detecting or confirming dental abnormalities, and supports recommendations on the use of panoramic radiography to aid in the assessment of dental development.

Commentary: *The panoramic radiograph provides a useful overview for assessment of developmental anomalies of the dentition, particularly when such anomalies involve the tooth roots. (See Chapter 6.)*

Hypodontia: **Panoramic radiographs showed that hypodontia is more frequent in patients having hemifacial microsomia than in matched individuals without this condition.**

Maruko E, Hayes C, Evans CA, Padwa B, Mulliken JB. Hypodontia in hemifacial microsomia. Cleft Palate Craniofac J 2001;38:15–19. (From the Department of Oral Health Policy and Epidemiology, Harvard School of Dental Medicine, Boston, USA)

This study described the patterns of missing teeth in patients having hemifacial microsomia and compared the prevalence of missing teeth in subjects with hemifacial microsomia with a group of unaffected subjects. Missing teeth were determined by evaluation of panoramic radiographs. Records of 125 patients with hemifacial microsomia were available from the Craniofacial Center at Boston's Children's Hospital. Seventy-six met inclusion criteria for radiographic analysis of hypodontia. Fifty-two patients met inclusion criteria for comparing the prevalence of hypodontia with a group of patients from the Department of Orthodontics at Harvard School of Dental Medicine. A Fisher's exact test was conducted to test the hypothesis that hemifacial microsomia patients have a greater prevalence of missing teeth than individuals without the anomaly. A Chi^2 test for trend was conducted to determine whether hypodontia was more prevalent with increasing severity of the mandibular deformity in hemifacial microsomia. Hypodontia was more prevalent among hemifacial microsomia patients (26.9%) versus the comparison group ($p < .0001$). Additionally, the degree of hypodontia was correlated with the grade of mandibular hypoplasia ($p = .024$). Hypodontia was found to be more prevalent in patients with hemifacial microsomia than in comparison subjects.

Commentary: *The panoramic radiograph provides a useful overview for assessment of developmental anomalies of the dentition, including hypodontia. (See Chapter 6.)*

Supernumerary teeth: Sequential panoramic radiographs evidenced the late development of a post-dentition supplemental supernumerary tooth.

Gibson N. A late developing mandibular premolar supernumerary tooth. Aust Dent J 2001;46:51–52. [From the Torbay Hospital, Torquay, UK]

Supplemental supernumerary premolar teeth can become radiographically apparent at a stage much later than that for the regular dentition. The case of a patient who developed a mandibular premolar supernumerary tooth between the age of 11 and 20 years is reported. Evidence for the late development of the supernumerary tooth came from consecutive panoramic radiographs.

Commentary: *The panoramic radiograph can reveal unanticipated findings such as late developing supernumerary teeth. (See Chapter 6 for more details concerning developmental anomalies of the dentition.)*

Amelogenesis imperfecta: Molecular biology makes inroads into explaining the causation of varieties of this group of phenotypes.

Kida M, Ariga T, Shirakawa T, Oguchi H, Sakiyama Y. Autosomal-dominant hypoplastic form of amelogenesis imperfecta caused by an enamelin gene mutation at the exon-intron boundary. J Dent Res 2002;81:738–742. [From the Research Group of Human Gene Therapy, Hokkaido University Graduate School of Medicine, Sapporo, Japan]

Amelogenesis imperfecta is currently classified into 14 distinct subtypes based on various phenotypic criteria; however, the gene responsible for each phenotype has not been defined. Previous studies have mapped an autosomal-dominant human amelogenesis imperfecta locus to chromosome 4q11-q21, where two candidate genes, ameloblastin and enamelin, are located. The authors performed molecular genetic studies on a Japanese family with a possible autosomal-dominant form of amelogenesis imperfecta. They studied amelogenesis imperfecta patients in this family, focusing on the ameloblastin and enamelin genes, and found a mutation in the enamelin gene. The mutation detected was a heterozygous, single-G deletion within a series of 7 G residues at the exon 9-intron 9 boundary of the enamelin gene. The mutation was detected only in the amelogenesis imperfecta patients and was not detected in unaffected family members or control individuals. The male proband and his brother showed hypoplastic enamel in both primary and permanent dentitions, and their father showed local hypoplastic defects in the enamel of his permanent teeth. The findings are consistent with heterogeneous mutations in the enamelin gene being responsible for an autosomal dominant hypoplastic amelogenesis imperfecta.

Commentary: *The panoramic radiograph provides a good overview of the dentition that can help differentiate between local and more generalized conditions. (See Chapter 6 for more details concerning developmental anomalies of the dentition.)*

Osteogenesis imperfecta: Panoramic radiography revealed a high prevalence of dentinogenesis imperfecta.

Malmgren B, Norgren S. Dental aberrations in children and adolescents with osteogenesis imperfecta. Acta Odontol Scand 2002;60:65–71. [From the Department of Pediatrics, Huddinge University Hospital, Karolinska Institute, Stockholm, Sweden]

The investigators studied dental aberrations in a large sample of unrelated patients having different types and forms of osteogenesis imperfecta. Sixty-eight nonrelated patients aged 0.3 to 20 years (mean 10 years) were examined clinically and panoramic radiographs from 49 patients were analyzed. Dentinogenesis imperfecta Type I was found in 27 of 65 patients and was significantly more common in osteogenesis imperfecta Type III than in Types I and IV. The presence of dentinogenesis imperfecta was almost completely in accordance with affected parents, siblings and children. The percentage of patients with no apparent dental aberrations was approximately the same in patients with osteogenesis imperfecta Types I and III and in patients with mild and more severe forms of osteogenesis imperfecta. The high prevalence of dental aberrations in osteogenesis imperfecta shows the importance of clinical and radiographic dental examinations in the osteogenesis imperfecta population. In patients with mild forms of the disease in whom the medical diagnosis is uncertain, demonstration of disturbances in dental development can be crucial for establishing the osteogenesis imperfecta diagnosis.

Commentary: *The panoramic radiograph provides a good overview of the dentition that can help differentiate between local and more generalized conditions. Occasionally dental anomalies can be associated with systemic disease. (See Chapter 6 for more details concerning developmental anomalies of the dentition.)*

Osteogenesis imperfecta: Mortality rates depend on the type of osteogenesis imperfecta involved.

Singer RB, Ogston SA, Paterson CR. Mortality in various types of osteogenesis imperfecta. J Insur Med 2001;33:216–220. [From the Department of Epidemiology and Public Health, Ninewells Hospital and Medical School, University of Dundee, UK]

Osteogenesis imperfecta comprises a group of closely related inherited diseases characterized by abnormal bone fragility. Six clinical types are recognized, one of which (Type II) is so severe that intrauterine or perinatal mortality is 100%. Types are differentiated by clinical groups, severity, and by the presence or absence of features such as blue sclerae and dentinogenesis imperfecta. From a registry created in association with the Brittle Bone Society, 743 patients with osteogenesis imperfecta in England and Wales were observed from 1980 through 1993. Patients were classified into 3 groups (Type IA, Type III, and Types IB, IVA, and IVB combined). Average osteogenesis imperfecta annual mortality rates were determined and compared with 1981 rates in the general population of England and Wales matched by sex and age. In Type IA (52% of the osteogenesis imperfecta cases), there was no significant excess mortality (mortality ratio 108%, based on 15 deaths). In Type III, on the other hand, excess mortality was very high in children, adolescents and young adults. In the combined group of Types IB, IVA, and IVB, the mortality ratio was 157% in patients aged 45 and up (not significant at the 95% confidence level); however, higher ratios at younger ages were statistically significant, even though based on a total of only five deaths.

Commentary: *The panoramic radiograph provides a good overview of the dentition that can help differentiate between local and more generalized conditions. Occasionally dental anomalies can be associated with systemic disease. Evidence is often based upon small numbers of cases where the disease subclassification is particularly rare in occurrence. (See Chapter 6 for more details concerning developmental anomalies of the dentition.)*

Jaw Pathoses

Jaw cysts: Panoramic images were used to compare the radiographic features of the mandibular keratocystic odontogenic tumors and the dentigerous cysts associated with third molars.

Tsukamoto G, Sasaki A, Akiyama T, Ishikawa T, Kishimoto K, Nishiyama A, Matsumura T. A radiologic analysis of dentigerous cysts and odontogenic keratocysts associated with a mandibular third molar. Oral Surg Oral Med Oral Pathol Oral Radiol Endod 2001;91:743–747. [From the Department of Oral and Maxillofacial Surgery II, Okayama University Dental School, Japan]

The objective was to discriminate radiographically between dentigerous cysts and keratocystic odontogenic tumors associated with a mandibular third molar. Panoramic radiographs were studied for cases of dentigerous cysts (44 patients, 45 cysts) and keratocystic odontogenic tumors (15 patients, 16 cysts). All cysts were associated with a mandibular third molar. The panoramic images were analyzed with reference to patient age and symptoms. The mean age of patients in whom keratocystic odontogenic tumors were detected was less than that of patients having dentigerous cysts. The mean size of keratocystic odontogenic tumors was larger than that of dentigerous cysts. The mean distance from the second to the third molar for dentigerous cysts was greater than that for keratocystic odontogenic tumors. While there was a significant correlation between the lesion size and the distance between the second and third molars in the dentigerous cyst versus the keratocystic odontogenic tumor, patient age did not significantly correlate with these features. Keratocystic odontogenic tumors tended to grow more rapidly than dentigerous cysts, but did not cause as much tooth displacement. No evidence was found for either cyst type to develop gradually from the time of initiation of the dental follicle or the dental lamina. They rather arose randomly at various stages.

Commentary: *Panoramic radiographs can be used to outline jaw pathoses in two dimensions and provide a wider area of coverage that doe intraoral radiographs. (Chapter 10 describes the effects of jaw pathoses on the mandibular canal. Chapter 11 describes the effects of jaw pathoses on the outline of the maxillary sinus.)*

Minor oral surgery: Complications could have been prevented if a panoramic radiograph had been appropriately evaluated. Ordering and reading appropriate radiographs prior to surgery should be considered the normal standard of care.

Mozaffari E, Mupparapu M, Otis L. Undiagnosed multiple myeloma causing extensive dental bleeding: report of a case and review. Oral Surg Oral Med Oral Pathol Oral Radiol Endod 2002;94:448–453. (From the Department of Oral Medicine, University of Pennsylvania, Philadelphia, USA)

Radiology plays an important role in the detection of bone changes associated with undiagnosed myeloma. Extensive bleeding that occurred during a minor dental surgical procedure could have been prevented if the panoramic radiograph had been evaluated carefully before initiation of the treatment. Etiologic factors responsible for the formation of such abnormalities in multiple myeloma are reviewed and the value of panoramic radiology used in diagnostic assessment of the disease is presented.

Commentary: *Appropriate radiographic evaluation prior to surgery can help the clinician avoid complications. Sometimes the panoramic radiograph provides an adequate overview of the field of operation; however ad-*

ditional imaging procedures are not infrequently advisable.

Pre-treatment orthodontic radiographs should be carefully scrutinized to rule out pathoses.

Bondemark L, Jeppsson M, Lindh-Ingildsen L, Rangne K. Incidental findings of pathology and abnormality in pretreatment orthodontic panoramic radiographs. Angle Orthod 2006;76:98–102. (From the Department of Orthodontics, Malmo University, Sweden)

The investigators evaluated the prevalence and location of incidental findings of pathology and abnormalities orthodontic panoramic radiographs made pre-treatment. A total of 496 subjects (232 girls and 264 boys; mean age 11.2 years) were randomly selected from the Orthodontic Clinic, University of Malmo, Sweden. Two observers independently examined the panoramic radiographs for abnormalities, excluding dental caries, eruption disturbances and missing or supernumerary teeth. All panoramic radiographs with positive findings were re-examined by a third examiner, an oral radiologist. A total of 56 findings in 43 patients (8.7%) were recorded, and significantly more findings were detected in girls than in boys ($p = .007$). The most common findings were radio-opacities (idiopathic osteosclerosis) in alveolar bone ($n = 22$), thickening of mucosal lining of the maxillary sinuses ($n = 15$), and periapical inflammatory lesions ($n = 10$). The majority of the periapical lesions and radio-opacities were found in the mandible. As issues related to orthodontic assessment such as eruption disturbances and supernumerary teeth were excluded it is perhaps not surprising that most findings had no consequence for the orthodontic treatment plan. Nevertheless, the authors conclude that the clinician should be aware of the potential to detect pathologic abnormalities in pre-treatment orthodontic panoramic radiographs.

Commentary: *Non-dental pathoses of clinical significance are uncommon; hence, in the absence of signs and symptoms of disease they do not constitute a reason for making screening radiographs. However, when a panoramic radiograph has been prescribed the image must be reviewed for all signs of pathosis.*

Mucocele: A lesion close to sensitive structures in the skull was an important incidental finding from panoramic radiography.

Patinen P, Hietanen J, Peltola J. Sphenoid sinus mucocele: case report of an appearance on a panoramic radiograph. Oral Surg Oral Med Oral Pathol Oral Radiol Endod 2002;93:747–750. [From the Institute of Dentistry, University of Helsinki, Finland]

Mucoceles of the sphenoid bone are significant as they are located deep in the skull close to such sensitive structures as the optic chiasm and the upper six cranial nerves. A case of an incidental finding of a sphenoid sinus mucocele on a dental panoramic radiograph is described in a totally symptom-free, 22-year-old woman. Thorough knowledge of the manifestations of oral and paranasal disease plays a vital role in early diagnosis of a variety of diseases of the head and neck region. This requires systematic evaluation of the whole panoramic radiograph.

Commentary: *Detection of pathoses of the sphenoid sinus using panoramic radiography can be considered unusual in view of the midline location of this sinus. Lesions affecting this sinus are more likely to be found on lateral cephalograms.*

Systemic Diseases

Osteoporosis: Panoramic radiographic evidence of thinning of the mandibular cortex corresponds to a history of osteoporotic fractures in patients older than 60 years.

Bollen AM, Taguchi A, Hujoel PP, Hollender LG. Case-control study on self-reported osteoporotic fractures and mandibular cortical bone. Oral Surg Oral Med Oral Pathol Oral Radiol Endod 2000;90:518–524. [From the Department of Orthodontics, University of Washington, Seattle, USA]

The purpose of this case-control study was to determine whether the radiographic appearance of the mandibular cortical bone in elderly, noninstitutionalized patients correlated with the history of osteoporotic fractures. Patients older than 60 years, and who had a panoramic radiograph were invited to be interviewed regarding their fracture history and risk factors for osteoporosis. The study population comprised 93 individuals reporting osteoporotic fractures (fractures occurring after minor impact). Controls ($n = 394$) were individuals reporting traumatic fractures ($n = 105$) or no fractures ($n = 289$). Blinded to case control status, the investigators evaluated the mandibular cortex on a panoramic radiograph and classified them as normal (even and sharp endosteal margin), moderately eroded (evidence of lacunar resorption or endosteal cortical residues), or severely eroded (unequivocal porosity). In addition, cortical thickness was measured below the mental foramen. After adjustment for potentially confounding factors, the odds ratio for an osteoporotic fracture associated with moderately eroded and severely eroded mandibular cortices was 2.0 (95% Cortical Index 1.2 to 3.3) and 8.0 (95% Cortical Index 2.0 to 28.9), respectively. After adjusting for all potentially confounding factors, it was determined that the cortex was 0.54 mm (or 12%) thinner in subjects with an osteoporotic fracture compared with controls (95% CI, 0.25 to 0.84 mm). Patients with a history of osteoporotic fractures tend to have increased resorption and thinning of the mandibular lower cortex that can be measured from panoramic radiographs.

Commentary: *Details concerning the controversy of using panoramic dental radiographs for detection of osteoporosis are given in Chapter 15.*

Osteoporosis: **Mandibular cortical shape was significantly associated with biochemical mark so dentists may be able to identify postmenopausal women with low BMD by using dental panoramic radiographs.**

Taguchi A, Sanada M, Krall E, Nakamoto T, Ohtsuka M, Suei Y, Tanimoto K, Kodama I, Tsuda M, Ohama K. Relationship between dental panoramic radiographic findings and biochemical markers of bone turnover. J Bone Miner Res 2003;18:1689–1694. [From the Department of Oral and Maxillofacial Radiology, Hiroshima University, Japan]

Recent studies suggest that mandibular inferior cortical shape and width on dental panoramic radiographs may be useful screening tools for low skeletal bone mineral density or increased risk of osteoporotic fracture. Of 609 women who visited the authors' clinic for bone mineral density assessment between 1996 and 2002, 82 Japanese postmenopausal women (age range 46–68 years; mean age 54 ± 5 years), were recruited for a study to further examine this relationship. Biochemical markers of bone turnover and lumbar spine bone mineral density measurements were compared with panoramic radiographic findings. Mandibular inferior cortical shape (normal, mild/moderate erosion, severe erosion) and width were evaluated on dental panoramic radiographs. Bone mineral density at the lumbar spine (L2–L4) was measured by dual energy X-ray absorptiometry and categorized as normal (T-score above −1.0), osteopenia (T-score, −1.0 to −2.5), or osteoporosis (T-score less than −2.5). Bone turnover was estimated by serum total alkaline phosphatase and urinary N-telopeptide cross-links of type I collagen, corrected for creatinine. The odds of low spine bone mineral density in subjects with mandibular cortical erosion were 3.8 (95% CI, 1.2–12.5). Mandibular cortical erosion was significantly associated with increased N-telopeptide cross-links of type I collagen ($p < 0.001$) and serum total alkaline phosphatase ($p < 0.05$) levels. Mandibular cortical width was significantly associated with spine bone mineral density but not with N-telopeptide cross-links of type I collagen and serum total alkaline phosphatase levels. In conclusion, the results suggest that mandibular inferior cortical shape on dental panoramic radiographs might be an indicator of bone turnover and spine bone mineral density in postmenopausal women. Dentists might be able to identify postmenopausal women with increased risk of osteopenia and osteoporosis on dental panoramic radiographs.

Commentary: *Details concerning the controversy of using panoramic dental radiographs for detection of osteoporosis are given in Chapter 15.*

Patients having calcifications detected on panoramic radiography in the region of the carotid arteries should be referred to their physician with a recommendation of formal evaluation for potentially life-threatening atheroma.

Almog DM, Illig KA, Khin M, Green RM. Unrecognized carotid artery stenosis discovered by calcifications on a panoramic radiograph. J Am Dent Assoc 2000;131:1593–1597. [From the Eastman Department of Dentistry, University of Rochester, New York, USA]

Approximately 730,000 strokes occur each year in the United States, costing an estimated $40 billion annually. One-half of all strokes are the result of atherosclerotic plaques found in the carotid artery. Such plaques frequently are heavily calcified and can be identified on a panoramic radiograph by the incidental finding of calcifications overlying the carotid bifurcation. The authors found that a 67-year-old asymptomatic woman had calcium deposits overlying both carotid bifurcation regions on a panoramic radiograph. Subsequent duplex ultrasonic examination indicated bilateral, high-grade carotid arterial stenoses. The patient had critical carotid arterial stenoses associated with significant risk of stroke that had not been identified otherwise. The findings on the panoramic radiograph led to appropriate and potentially life-saving treatment. The patient underwent uneventful bilateral carotid endarterectomy.

Commentary: *Discussion concerning the use of panoramic dental radiographs for detection of carotid calcified atheroma is to be found in Chapter 15. Given the demonstrated high incidence of atherosclerosis in the US population, perhaps it is best to advocate mass screening using periodic ultrasonography of the carotids for individuals of middle age and older.*

TEST: Selected abstracts

1. Third molars that appear impacted on panoramic radiographs at age 18 years should invariably be extracted as they are very unlikely to erupt normally.

   True ☐ **False** ☐

2. Stylohyoid ossification shows age-related differences in incidence, length and topography.

   True ☐ **False** ☐

3. Cholitgul and Drummond did not support the use of panoramic radiography to aid in the assessment of dental development.

   True ☐ **False** ☐

4. Significant reciprocal associations have been found between aplasia of second premolars, small size of maxillary lateral incisors, infraocclusion of primary molars, ectopic eruption of first molars, and palatal displacement of maxillary canines.

   True ☐ **False** ☐

5. At the stage of initial root formation, a positive correlation has been determined between the mesiodistal crown width of the mandibular second molar and available jaw space.

   True ☐ **False** ☐

6. Hemifacial microsomia is associated with hypodontia and mandibular prognathism.

   True ☐ **False** ☐

7. In the use of panoramic radiology for the assessment of patient age, there is a need to develop population specific dental development standards.

   True ☐ **False** ☐

8. Ionizing radiation is a likely cause of intracranial meningioma.

   True ☐ **False** ☐

9. Premolar extraction has no impact on the frequency of third molar impaction.

   True ☐ **False** ☐

10. Panoramic radiography is an efficient method for the detection of dental impactions.

    True ☐ **False** ☐

Frequently Asked Questions About Panoramic Radiography

19

Panoramic Radiology Corporation staff led by Steve T. Yaggy in association with Allan G. Farman

Learning Objectives
A question and answer approach is used to cover information requests most commonly submitted to a leading manufacturer and distributor of panoramic equipment by their customers. While some of the issues are independent of the detector, many are peculiar to use of X-ray film and screens.

Q: What are these clear artifacts on our panoramic images?

A: Clear artifacts fall into four general categories:

1. Clear artifacts caused by metal or radio-opaque objects on or in the patient. Jewelry, eyeglasses, and radio-opaque dental prostheses should be removed before the radiograph is made (see Chapter 2).
2. Clear triangular shape in the lower anterior caused by improper position of the patient lead shield. Make sure the shield is placed low enough on the patient's shoulder and neck so as not interfere with the X-ray beam (see Chapter 2).
3. Tube Side decal is visible on the developed image. With some systems a decal will appear when using film if the intensifying screens are inverted (inside out) or the film was not between the screens. For the Panoramic Corporation PC 1000, orient the screens so that the Tube Side decal is on the outside and the left and right markers (L and R) are inside. Make sure the Tube Side decal side of the screens is aligned with the "This Side Toward Tube" side of the cassette sleeve. Insert the film between the intensifying screens. They can also be caused on occasion by reverse placement of a solid cassette containing a spring latch mechanism (Fig. 19.1).
4. Distinct clear lines, scratches, or cracks, visible on the developed radiograph. These odd artifacts are usually caused by cracks or splits in the intensifying screens when analog film is used. Examine the screens for damage. If the screens are damaged it is permanent. Make sure the screens are not handled roughly, folded, or stored in an unsafe location.

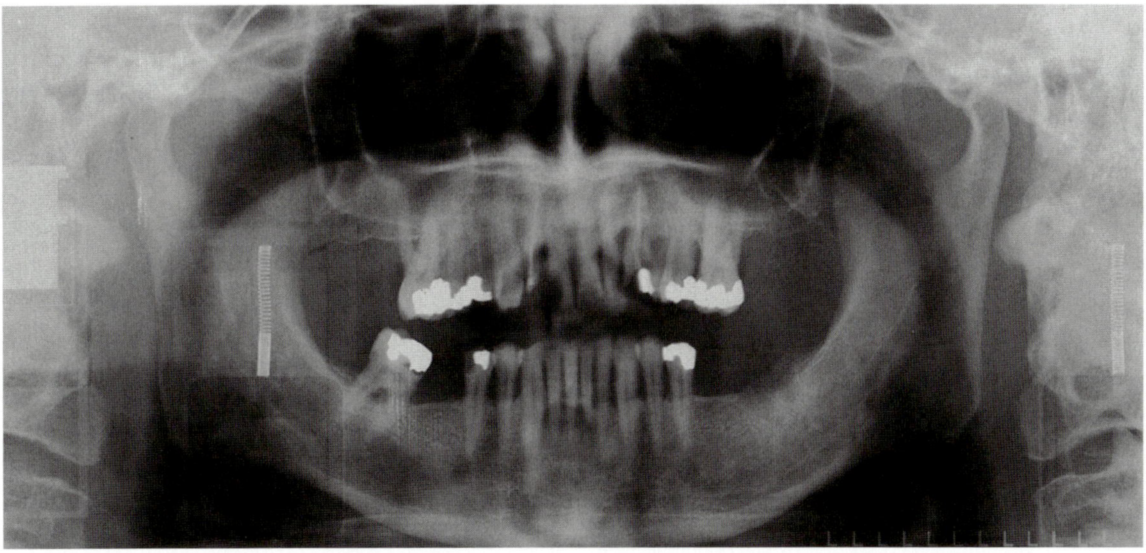

Fig. 19.1 Especial care needs to be taken with reversed cassettes such as that indicated by the spring shown in this image. It also indicates that the side indicators may be reversed in position so structures may be on the opposite side to that labeled

Q: What are these black marks on our panoramic images?

A: Black artifacts on films fall into four general categories:

1. Black ends or corners can be caused by exposure of X-ray film to white light. For film radiography either a torn cassette or an exposed box of film is usually the culprit. Physically check the cassette sleeve for tears and replace sleeve if necessary. To check a box of film for exposure take one sheet of film out of the box, under safelight conditions, and process it at normal time and temperature settings. The film should develop clear/translucent. If the film develops with artifacts similar to the problem film, the box of film needs to be replaced.
2. Black spots or smudges can be caused by a foreign substance contaminating X-ray film. Glove powder residue is usually the source of this artifact. Any substance on the film before it is developed will affect the chemical reaction between the film and the developing solution. Keep your hands and the area where you handle the film, cassettes, and screens clean.
3. Black "starburst," "tree branch," or "lightning bolt" artifacts are caused by static electric discharges. The intensifying screens need to be treated with antistatic screen cleaner solution or mild soapy water. Apply solution to intensifying screens only, not the cassette sleeve. Remove screens from the cassette and place them on a clean countertop. Apply solution to inside and outside of the screens. Partially dry the screens and allow the remaining solution to air dry. Make sure the screens are completely dry before reloading into the cassette.
4. Black "crescent" or "half moon" artifacts are caused by dented film or intensifying screens. Any stress to the film, thumbnail dent, a sharp crease, a heavy object dropped onto the film, will develop black. If no dents are visible on the film surface examine the screens. Damage to the screens is permanent. Make sure the area where you handle films is accessible and uncluttered. Store cassettes in a location where they will not be damaged.

Q: Why are we getting light film radiographs?

A: Light film radiographs can be the result of any one or combination of the following:

1. The intensifying screens could be reversed or turned inside out.
2. The chemicals in the film processor could be weak.
3. The temperature in the film processor could be low.
4. Developing time could be short for analog film radiography.
5. Intensifying screens could be worn out.

For all forms of detector, a light image can result from under exposure due to too low a kVp or mA setting. Tubehead could be out of alignment for any detector type.

Q: What causes dark film radiographs?

A: Dark film radiographs can be a result of any one or combination of the following:

1. Light exposure from light leaks in darkroom or daylight loader (Fig. 19.2).
2. Light exposure from too great of safelight bulb wattage.
3. Safelight being mounted closer than 4 feet from work surface.
4. Exposure from equipment with operational lights in the darkroom.
5. Processing temperature is set too high.
6. Processing time is set too long.
7. Incorrect type of film for the intensifying screens being used.

For all forms of detector, a dark image can result from over exposure due to too high a kVp or mA setting.

Q: How can we eliminate the whiteout in the anterior region of a panoramic image?

A: The whiteout in the anterior region is a result of patient positioning:

For panoramic systems employing a standing position for the patient, first you want the patient to stand as straight as possible, position the patient's feet under the chinrest, this will make sure the neck is straight, next lower the machine so the Frankfort Plane (imaginary line from the middle of the ear opening to the bottom of the eye orbit) is parallel to the ground. This will help stretch the patient's neck enough to allow X-rays to pass between the vertebrae in the neck, allowing radiation to reach the anterior region of the detector. With systems using a seated patient, the patient needs to sit up as straight as possible.

Q: What infection control precautions or practices should be applied to the use of a panoramic X-ray machine?

A: Universal precautions as recommended by the CDC, OSHA, ADA, and OSAP should be applied.

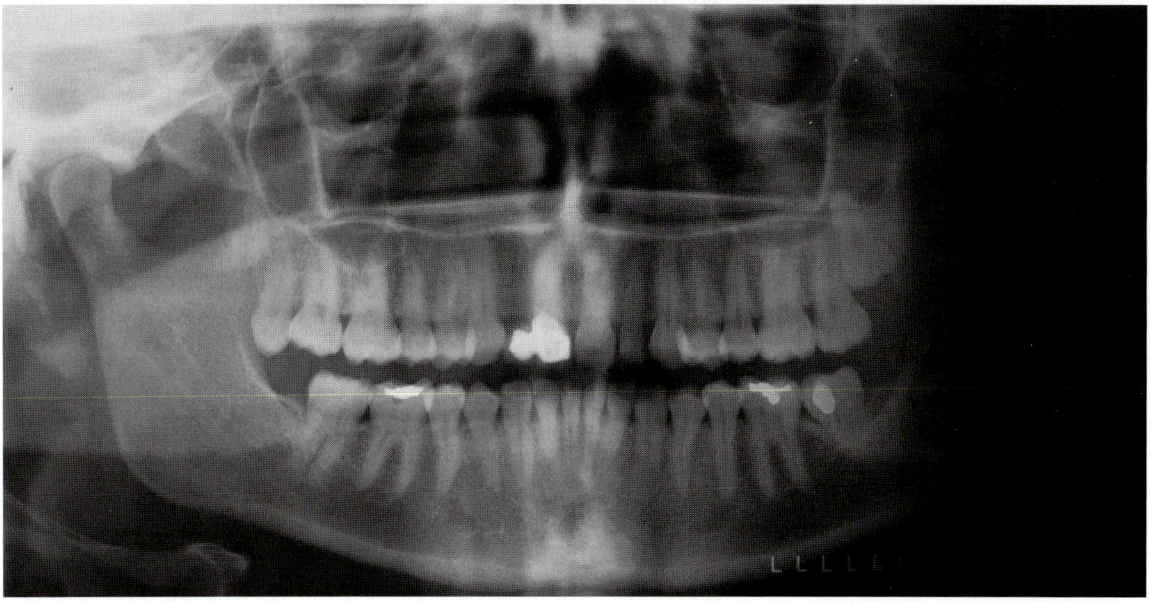

Fig. 19.2. The dark shadow over the right hand side of the film (patient's left) is caused by light leakage into the film drawer, cassette, or during loading into the processor

Wearing of exam gloves is recommended. The hand grips, chin rest, forehead support, temple supports, and any surface that may potentially come in contact with the patient, either directly or secondary from the operator, should be disinfected with a hard surface disinfectant or should be draped. Disposable bite-guides used to position the patient should be disposed of between patients unless autoclavable. Discard and replace disposable biteblocks and covers after each use. When using a cephalometric attachment, disposable rubber covers should be placed over the ear rods. Surface disinfectants should be used on any direct or secondary contact surfaces.

Q: Is there a method for reading panoramic radiograms to assure a thorough review of everything being shown in the panoramic radiograph?

A: One approach is suggested in Chapter 1 of this book:

One can start with the bony landmarks from the midline of the upper jaw and nasal cavity, then working back in the maxilla and zygomatic complex on each side. The soft tissue shadows of the tongue and soft palate are incorporated at this stage. This is followed by evaluation of the cervical spine and associated structure. Then evaluate the contents of the mandible starting from the midline and progressing posteriorly on each side. Any examination would be incomplete without a thorough evaluation of the soft tissues anterior to the spine and inferior to the mandible. The last part of the evaluation should be the area of chief complaint and the dental arches. You can sequence your evaluation in many ways; however, it is very important to develop a consistent approach that ensures that all diagnostic information in the radiograph is indeed read.

Q: Can a panoramic radiograph replace the full mouth radiographic series?

A: The panoramic radiograph supplemented by bitewings and an occasional periapical is frequently all that is needed.

All radiographs should be selected according to the professional judgment of the licensed practitioner. This follows the taking of a health history and careful clinical inspection of the oral and para-oral structures. The panoramic radiograph has the advantage of providing a wide overview of the dental arches in which the structures can be clearly related. It provides a greater area of coverage than the full mouth periapical image series, while using a lower average dosage of radiation. The time taken to make a panoramic image is a small fraction of that required to make and mount a full mouth intraoral survey. It is much more comfortable for the patient than the cutting edge of films inserted into the mouth, and it simplifies issues of infection control in the operatory and in the darkroom. The panoramic radiograph is ideal for assessment of growth and development of the dentition at ages 6, 12, and 18 years and as a baseline in the assessment of the jaws of the edentulous adult. It is also recognized as being the method of choice for evaluation of possible mandibular fractures following trauma to the jaws.

One might ask why so many practitioners continue using full mouth intraoral series as the principal baseline imaging regimen for their patients. The probable answer is "force of habit" following indoctrination during dental school training and the perception that panoramic radiographs are of poorer quality. For the practitioner that feels that panoramic radiographs are inadequate in quality, it is time to check out the new machines that are available. There have been many improvements over the past decades in beam geometry. Film and patient positioning for reliable results are much easier for panoramic radiography than for periapical imaging.

The panoramic radiograph also permits a clear identification of the patient, procedure date and laterality of structures. It is difficult to replace periapical radiographs lost from film mounts individual intraoral radiographs cannot be labeled.

Admittedly, radiographs made using intraoral direct emulsion film have a somewhat higher spatial resolution than those made using extraoral film-screen combinations. The question to be asked is where such fine resolution is needed? It is possible to supplement the baseline panoramic radiograph with bitewings to assist in detection of early proximal dental caries. Where endodontics is to be performed, the periapical radiograph is needed to assess the numbers and positions of a fine root canals as these are not adequately displayed on the panoramic image. For all other radiographic assessments of the teeth and jaws the panoramic radiograph is generally adequate alone.

Perhaps it is time to rethink imaging strategies and try something new if you are still bound to the use of full mouth intraoral surveys. There is certainly no need for a panoramic radiograph plus a full mouth intraoral survey. The panoramic radiograph, supplemented by bitewings and an occasional periapical is all that is needed. This provides savings in time and reduces patient discomfort. As the radiation scatter from a panoramic radiographic machine is very small, the substitution of a panoramic radiograph for a full mouth intraoral radiograph series has the potential to reduce the radiation dose that might inadvertently affect the dental office personnel.

Subject Index

A

abscess 55, 56, 120, 133, 139, 142
acute sinusitis 120, 128, 130
adenomatoid odontogenic tumor 78, 82, 96, 123, 146, 148, 151
adrenogenital syndrome 97
age and maturity 91
airspace 4
ALARA principle 25, 27, 31
ameloblastic fibro-odontoma 96, 145, 147, 149
ameloblastic fibroma 78, 79, 96, 147, 149
ameloblastoma 78, 79, 81, 82, 96, 109, 110, 112, 115, 118, 121, 122, 124, 130, 145–147, 151, 153
amelogenesis imperfecta 41, 56, 58–61, 66, 67, 71, 72, 219
analog film 15–17, 19, 23, 24, 62, 207, 208, 225, 226
anterior nasal spine 4
Apert syndrome 97
apical periodontal cyst 136, 163
artifact 7, 10, 14, 107, 131, 192, 225, 226
aspergillosis 139, 141
augnathus 107, 109

B

benign neoplasm 110, 120, 121, 123, 124, 128, 130, 147
bifid mandibular canal 115, 117
bisphosphonate 190, 193
bit-depth 15
biteblocks 227
black marks 226
blow-out fracture 164

C

calcifying epithelial odontogenic tumor 110
calcifying odontogenic cyst 147, 153
caries 33, 35–37, 41, 42, 67, 73, 75, 80, 83, 104, 135, 138, 175, 186–188, 190, 193, 205, 216, 221, 228
cementifying-ossifying fibroma 96, 109, 123, 124, 140
cementoblastoma 110, 112, 116, 118
cephalogram 29, 39, 96, 98, 100, 101, 105, 195–197, 207, 211, 213, 221
cephalostat 4, 7, 14, 49, 195–197, 199, 210
cervical vertebrae 7, 98, 104, 167, 213
charge-coupled device (CCD) 15, 19, 28
cherubism 96, 113, 114, 145, 148, 150, 153, 196
chondrosarcoma 79, 113, 117
clear artifact 225
cleft 44, 66, 69
cleidocranial dysplasia 47–49, 66, 69, 70, 73, 74, 80, 82, 97, 103
complementary metal oxide semiconductor (CMOS) 15, 19
computed tomography (CT) 160
concrescence 41, 49, 53, 71
condensing osteitis 133, 137
cone beam volumetric computed tomography (CBVCT) 75, 161, 209
connation 41, 49, 53, 55
coronoid process 4, 48, 164
cushing syndrome 97
cyst 34, 41, 47–49, 56, 74, 78, 79, 81, 91, 96, 109–112, 117, 119–121, 128, 129, 133, 134, 136, 138–140, 142, 151–153, 155, 163, 175, 197, 201, 220

D

dark image 226
delayed eruption 47, 73, 74, 97
dens evaginatus 41, 56, 57, 67, 71
dens invaginatus 41, 56, 57, 67
dental eruption 73, 91, 96, 97, 101, 103
dental impaction 42, 73, 74, 79, 83, 87, 155, 157, 215–218, 223
dental implant 45, 46, 62, 66, 190, 193, 194, 209, 210
dental maturation 92, 96–98, 101, 103, 104
dentigerous cyst 34, 41, 48, 74, 78, 79, 81, 96, 109–112, 117, 121, 143–146, 148, 151–153, 197, 220
dentin dysplasia 41, 62–65, 67, 68, 71
dentinogenesis imperfecta 41, 60–63, 67, 68, 72, 219, 220
diabetes 169, 170, 174, 180–182
DICOM 23, 24
digital cameras 15, 16
digital imaging 17, 24, 32, 40, 208
dilaceration 41, 47, 52, 53, 66, 71
Down syndrome 44, 45, 66, 69, 97

E

ectodermal dysplasias 45, 46, 69, 70

ectopic eruption 51, 78, 81, 223
Ellis-van Crevald syndrome 97
enamel hypoplasia 41, 56, 58, 67, 71
enamel pearl 41, 53, 55, 67, 71
endarteritis obliterans 186, 190
endo-antral syndrome 138, 139, 141, 142
endodontics 39, 133, 141, 206, 228
epidermolysis bullosa 103
epiglottis 4, 167
eruption cyst 143
ethmoid 4, 165, 198

F
FDA/CDRH 15
fibrous dysplasia 96, 114, 115, 124, 125, 130
film 1–3, 7, 15–17, 19, 20, 22–24, 29, 34, 62, 75, 84, 85, 88, 98, 159, 160, 164, 167, 181, 195, 197, 198, 206–210, 214, 225–228
film scanner 15–17
Fishman classification 98–100
fistula 38, 124
florid osseous dysplasia 114, 115
focal dermal hypoplasia 97
focal trough 20, 84, 177, 210, 214
follicular cyst 47, 96, 143
fractured tooth 121
fractures 78, 155, 157–166, 178, 195, 197, 198, 200, 214, 215, 221, 222, 228
full mouth radiographic series 227
fusion 41, 49, 53, 67, 98–101

G
Gardner syndrome 47–50, 70, 97
gemination 41, 49, 53, 55
ghost images 7, 9, 10, 14, 124, 167
Goltz syndrome 97
granuloma 56, 133, 134, 139, 142, 175
gunshot injury 164

H
hand-wrist radiograph 97, 98, 100, 101, 105, 213
hemangioma 97, 113
Hertwig Root Sheath 53, 133
Hutchinson-Gilfords syndrome 97
Hutchinson incisor 58
hyoid 4, 167, 168
hypergonadism 97
hyperparathyroidism 140, 174–176, 181, 182
hypodontia 41–46, 48, 66, 69, 70, 96, 191, 218, 223
hypopituitarism 97, 103
hypothyroidism 97

I
image layer 1, 3, 5, 7, 10, 23, 76, 83–85, 87, 88, 119, 120, 124, 128, 131, 210, 214
infraorbital canal 4, 164
interoperability 16, 22–24

J
jaw fractures 155, 164, 214

K
keratitis 187
keratocystic odontogenic tumor 78, 79, 81, 82, 121, 122, 130, 140, 142, 145, 146, 151, 153, 220

L
latent image 3, 17, 24
lateral-oblique 84, 89, 147, 163, 200–202
lateral skull projection 195, 196
lead apron artifacts 14
Le Fort fracture 165
leiomyosarcoma 110, 111, 116
leukemia 66, 145, 148, 149, 191
lingula 4, 107
luxation 155, 156

M
macrodontia 41, 49, 50, 66, 69, 70
malignant neoplasia 124
mandibular canal 4, 74, 75, 107–118, 140, 142, 185, 217, 220
mandibular foramen 4, 107, 110
mandibular ramus 7, 107, 147, 162, 164, 167, 196
mastoid 4, 198
maxillary sinus 4, 7, 10, 14, 119–124, 126, 128–131, 138–142, 164, 165, 197–199, 202, 220, 221
mental foramen 4, 107, 109, 140, 221
mesenchymal chondrosarcoma 79
mesiodens 46, 47, 55, 66, 70, 94
metacarpal 99
microdontia 41, 51, 70, 191
mucocele 120, 129, 221
mucositis 186, 187, 193, 194
mucous retention phenomenon 119, 120
myeloma 109, 113, 117, 118, 220

N
nasal septum 4, 198
nasolacrimal canal 4, 164
NCRP 25, 26, 31
neural tumors 97, 110
neurilemmoma 109, 110, 115
neurofibromas 110
nevoid basal cell carcinoma syndrome 122, 145
non-Hodgkin lymphoma 110
nose 4, 119, 120, 128, 177, 195, 197–199, 202

O
occipitomental projection 120, 197
occupational safety 28
odontodysplasia 41, 63, 65, 68, 72, 96, 145, 148, 150, 152, 153
odontogenic myxoma 96, 113, 117, 147
oncologic dentistry 183, 194, 214

orbit 4, 165, 226
orthodontics 76, 83–85, 87–89, 91, 209–212, 215, 216, 218, 221
OSHA 226
ossifying fibroma 96, 109, 123, 124, 140, 142
osteogenesis imperfecta 60, 61, 67, 71, 72, 219, 220
osteogenic sarcoma 97, 109, 113, 114, 117, 118
osteomyelitis 109, 111, 117, 136, 137, 176–178, 190
osteonecrosis 186, 190, 193, 194
osteoporosis 171–175, 181, 182, 190, 221, 222
osteoradionecrosis 180, 183, 186, 188–190, 193
osteosclerosis 175, 221

P
Paget disease of bone 124, 125
palate 3, 4, 44, 66, 80, 104, 126, 165, 178–180, 218, 227
paradental cyst 143, 145
paragnathus 107, 109
paranasal sinus 83, 119, 128
pedodontics 212, 217
periapical disease 38
periapical periodontitis 133, 138, 142
pericoronitis 75, 109
periodontal disease 35–39, 43, 44, 53, 55, 83, 173–175, 181, 186, 205, 216
phalanx 99, 100
pharynx 214
phosphor plate 15–20, 23, 24, 28, 195
photostimulable phosphor 2, 16–20, 23, 24, 88, 195
pituitary giantism 49, 97
pixel 15, 19
polyps 49, 119, 120
posterior-anterior (PA) projection 195, 197
premature eruption 73, 97, 149
proliferative periostitis 137
prostheses 10, 14, 46, 192–194, 225
prosthodontics 183, 210
pterygoid plates 4, 165
pterygomaxillary fissure 4
pulp necrosis 156
pyknodysostosis 97

Q
quality assurance 1, 39, 212

R
radiation dose 25, 28, 29, 31, 32, 40, 83, 207, 208, 228
radiation exposure 25, 26, 28, 31, 37, 39, 88, 207
radiation protection 25, 26, 31, 39, 207
radiation therapy 37, 43, 58, 97, 170, 183, 186, 188–194, 214
radicular cyst 109–111, 139
radiographic use guidelines 33, 40
radiograph selection 25, 33–35, 155, 205
regional odontodysplasia 63, 65, 68, 96, 145, 148, 150, 152
residual cyst 121, 201
rests of Malassez 133
retrofit 16, 19, 20, 24
risk 25, 27, 28, 31–32, 35–37, 40, 44, 45, 77, 146, 157–159, 165, 167, 169–172, 174, 180, 181, 186, 189, 190, 207–209, 214, 215, 221, 222
root parallelism 83–87, 89

S
scanner 15–20, 29
screening 33–35, 38, 39, 172, 173, 179, 182, 183, 214, 217, 221–223
secondary capture 15, 16, 24
selection criteria 25, 26, 33–35, 39, 206
sinus 4, 7, 10, 14, 38, 119–131, 138–142, 164, 165, 173, 176, 197–199, 220, 221
squamous cell carcinoma 109, 111, 113, 117, 119, 124, 126–128, 152, 184, 192, 198, 214
Stafne bone cavity 140, 142
storage phosphor 7, 15, 17, 18, 20, 23, 28, 29
stylohyoid ligament 213, 214
subluxation 155
sunburst appearance 113, 114
supernumerary root 41, 56, 57, 67
supernumerary teeth 41, 43, 46–49, 51, 70, 74, 77, 82, 83, 97, 219, 221
syphilis 58, 67, 72, 176–178, 182

T
talon cusp 41, 56, 57, 67, 71
taurodontism 41, 53, 54, 60, 66, 67, 70–72
temporomandibular joint (TMJ) 38, 155, 162–164, 176, 179, 214
tomography 61, 75, 107, 108, 111, 113, 116, 119, 120, 123, 127–129, 140, 155, 160–162, 165, 166, 172, 173, 180, 192, 198, 209, 214
tongue 1, 3, 4, 10, 11, 192, 227
traumatic injuries 155, 156
turbinate 4
Turner syndrome 97, 103, 104
Turner tooth 58

V
vertebral index 102

W
Waters projection 119, 120, 128

X
X-ray film 1, 15, 17, 19, 24, 29, 75, 195

Z
zygomaticomaxillary fractures 164
zygomatic process 4